Illustrated Toxicology

Illustrated Toxicology
With Study Questions

PK Gupta

*Director of Toxicology Consultant Group, Patron and Founder
President of the Society of Toxicology of India*

*President of the Academy of Sciences for Animal Welfare,
and Former adviser of World Health Organization (Geneva),
Rajendra Nagar, Bareilly (UP), India*

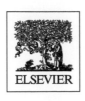

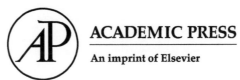

ACADEMIC PRESS

An imprint of Elsevier

Academic Press is an imprint of Elsevier
125 London Wall, London EC2Y 5AS, United Kingdom
525 B Street, Suite 1800, San Diego, CA 92101-4495, United States
50 Hampshire Street, 5th Floor, Cambridge, MA 02139, United States
The Boulevard, Langford Lane, Kidlington, Oxford OX5 1GB, United Kingdom

Notices
Knowledge and best practice in this field are constantly changing. As new research and experience broaden our
understanding, changes in research methods, professional practices, or medical treatment may become necessary.

Practitioners and researchers must always rely on their own experience and knowledge in evaluating and using any
information, methods, compounds, or experiments described herein. In using such information or methods they
should be mindful of their own safety and the safety of others, including parties for whom they have a professional
responsibility.

To the fullest extent of the law, neither the Publisher nor the authors, contributors, or editors, assume any liability
for any injury and/or damage to persons or property as a matter of products liability, negligence or otherwise, or
from any use or operation of any methods, products, instructions, or ideas contained in the material herein.

Library of Congress Cataloging-in-Publication Data
A catalog record for this book is available from the Library of Congress

British Library Cataloguing-in-Publication Data
A catalogue record for this book is available from the British Library

ISBN: 978-0-12-813213-5

For Information on all Academic Press publications
visit our website at https://www.elsevier.com/books-and-journals

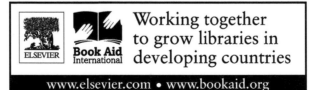

ELSEVIER • Book Aid International

Working together
to grow libraries in
developing countries

www.elsevier.com • www.bookaid.org

Publisher: John Fedor
Acquisition Editor: Rafael Teixeira
Editorial Project Manager: Kathy Pallida
Production Project Manager: Anusha Sambamoorthy
Cover Designer: Mark Rogers

Typeset by MPS Limited, Chennai, India

Contents

Disclaimer

The information including illustrations and questions in the book is based on standard textbooks in the area of specialization. However, it is well-known that with the advancement of science the standard of care in the practice of medicine changes rapidly. Many drugs that were indicated for the treatment of a certain ailment in the beginning get superseded by others. With long-term use their effects and effectiveness become apparent or else the use was advocated for some other problem. Though all the efforts have been made to ensure the accuracy of the information, the possibility of human error still remains. Therefore, neither the author nor the publisher guarantees that the information contained in the book is absolute. Anyone using the clinical information contained in this book has to be, therefore, duly cautious. It is particularly important to check drug dosages, indications, interactions, and contraindications with the manufacturer's most recent product information. Neither the author nor the publisher should be responsible for any damage that results from the use of the information contained in any part of this book.

Preface

The book *Illustrative Toxicology, With Study Questions* is aimed to make the study of toxicology simple and understandable through illustrations, images, custom-made drawings, self-explanatory tables, and questions and answers collated from standard and authoritative textbooks which are widely scanned. Author's own experience in different branches of toxicology including environmental and veterinary toxicology is also abstracted in this book. The book is written in a manner to stimulate interest on various facets of the subject and make it more exciting. It is a general experience that theoretical descriptions do not attract as much attention and interest as illustrations and images do. At the same time the information learnt through questions and their satisfactory answers makes the topics easier to grasp.

This book serves as a comprehensive and quick reference for various examinations. However, it should be noted that this book serves only as a supplement and not as a replacement for any textbook and classroom learning.

The book has 17 chapters that cover several topics such as general toxicology, principles of toxicology, risk assessment, disposition, mechanism of toxicity, toxic effects of various xenobiotics, poisonings of poisonous and venomous organisms, plant toxins, poisonous and food poisonings, radiation hazards, and abuse of drugs. It also deals with the adverse effects on environment and ecosystem exposed to various toxicants and poisonings as relevant to domestic and other animals. One chapter is exclusively devoted to clinical toxicology, principles of diagnosis, followed by general management of poisoning of the patients including methods of removal of poisons from the body and treatment of poisoning. Finally, a chapter deals with brainstorming questions that will be helpful as a review for students so that they understand the concepts delivered.

Each chapter is in the format of questions and answers, data interpretation, multiple choice questions, true/false or correct/incorrect statements, fill in the blanks, and matching the statements. It is a unique book in toxicology having more than 31 self-explanatory tables, 237 custom-made illustrations and images, and about 3400 questions and answers. It is equally useful for students and teachers practicing in medical sciences, toxicology, pharmacology, medicine, pharmacy, environmental toxicology, and veterinary sciences. Therefore, I believe that this book would serve the students, academic institutions and industry as follows:

- It is a good alternative to be used for various courses and an excellent contribution for the students who need a study aid for toxicology but want more than a textbook as they need a self-testing regime.
- It will be a useful tool for the teachers of toxicology who need inspiration when composing questions for their students.

- It will also help the established toxicologists to test their own knowledge of understanding the subject matter.
- It will be useful at universities and colleges and in industry for in-house training courses in toxicology, which I know exist in some pharmaceutical and chemical companies.
- It is required for those studying for the toxicology boards and other examinations.

Thus, the main strength of this book is that it reflects the breadth and multi-disciplinary nature of toxicology with illustrative approach to the subject needed to improve the engagement with and understanding of the subject having a very wide audience.

Toxicology is a rapidly evolving field. Suggestions and comments are welcome to help the author improve the contents of the book. Please also suggest the deficiencies need to be covered at drpkg_brly@yahoo.co.in or drpkg1943@gmail.com if you have any topics you feel should be better covered in any future editions.

PK Gupta

General toxicology

CHAPTER OUTLINE

Illustrated Toxicology. DOI: http://dx.doi.org/10.1016/B978-0-12-813213-5.00001-8
© 2018 Elsevier Inc. All rights reserved.

1.1 DEFINITIONS AND SUBDISCIPLINES OF TOXICOLOGY

Q. Definition

The traditional definition of toxicology is "the science of poisons." As our understanding of how various agents can cause harm to humans and other organisms, a more descriptive definition of toxicology is "the study of the adverse effects of chemicals or physical agents on living organisms."

Explanation: The word "toxicology" is derived from the Greek word "toxicon" which means "poison" and logos means to study. It also includes study of special effects of toxicants developmental toxicity, teratogenicity, carcinogenicity, mutagenesis, immune-toxicity, neurotoxicity, endocrine disruption, etc. Adverse effects may occur in many forms, ranging from immediate death to subtle changes not realized until months or years later. They may occur at various levels within the body, such as an organ, a type of cell, or a specific biochemical. Knowledge of how toxic agents damage the body has progressed along with medical knowledge. It is now known that various observable changes in anatomy or body functions actually result from previously unrecognized changes in specific biochemicals in the body.

Q. Define xenobiotics.

Xenobiotic: Xenobiotics (xeno is a Greek word which means "strange or alien") are the substances which are foreign to the body and are biologically active. These cannot be broken down to generate energy or be assimilated into a biosynthetic pathway. It is a very wide class and structurally adverse agents, both natural and synthetic chemicals such as drugs, industrial chemicals, pesticides, alkaloids, secondary plant metabolites and toxins of molds, plants and animals, and environmental pollutants.

Q. What are the subdisciplines of toxicology?

Biochemical toxicology
Reproductive toxicology
Development toxicology
Teratology
Genetic toxicology
Clinical toxicology
Forensic toxicology
Analytical toxicology
Nutritional toxicology
Veterinary toxicology
Environmental toxicology
Occupational (industrial) toxicology
Regulatory toxicology
Mechanistic toxicology
Aquatic toxicology
Ecotoxicology
Food toxicology

Formal toxicology

Descriptive toxicology.

Q. Define occupational (industrial) toxicology.

Occupational (industrial) toxicology is concerned with health effects from exposure to chemicals in the workplace. It deals with the clinical study of workers of industries and environment around them.

Q. Define regulatory toxicology.

It deals with administrative functions concerned with the development and interpretation of mandatory toxicology testing programs and controlling the use, distribution, and availability of chemicals used commercially and therapeutically. For example, Food and Drug Administration (FDA) regulates drugs, cosmetics, and food additives. Regulatory toxicology gathers and evaluates existing toxicological information to establish concentration-based standards of "safe" exposure. The standard is the level of a chemical that a person can be exposed to without any harmful health effects.

Q. Define regulation.

Regulation is the control, by statute, of the manufacture, transportation, sale, or disposal of chemicals deemed to be toxic after testing procedures or according to criteria laid down in applicable laws.

Q. Describe in brief requirements of the following regulations.

Brief requirements of selected regulations (question and answer format) in United States are summarized in Table 1.1.

Table 1.1 Requirements of Selected Regulations in the United States

Regulation Questions	Answers (Brief Requirements)
Under Clean Air Act, EPA requires	the registration of fuels and fuel additives. Part of the registration process includes in vivo fertility assessment/teratology testing (a rat is the preferred species for testing).
Under FIFRA, teratogenicity and reproduction studies require	two generation testing in two mammalian species (e.g., rat, mouse, rabbit, hamster).
Under TSCA (Toxic Substances Control Act), testing requirements for reproduction and fertility effects call for	the use of rats, although other mammalian species are acceptable with justification.
Specific guidelines for evaluation of developmental toxicity under the Federal Food, Drug, and Cosmetic Act (FFDCA) may vary depending on the Center but typically require	testing of rats and/or rabbits.
The Center for Food Safety and Applied Nutrition identifies testing for	reproductive and developmental toxicity under "Toxicological Principles for the Safety Assessment of Direct Food Additives and Color Additives Used in Food."

Q. Define food toxicology.

It deals with natural contaminants, food and feed additives, and toxic and chemoprotective effects of compounds in food.

Explanation: Food toxicology is involved in delivering a safe and edible supply of food to the consumer. During processing, a number of substances may be added to food to make it look, taste, or smell better. Fats, oils, sugars, starches, and other substances may be added to change the texture and taste of food.

All of these additives are studied to determine if and at what amount they may produce adverse effects. A second area of interest includes food allergies. Almost 30% of the American people have some food allergy. For example, many people have trouble digesting milk and are lactose intolerant. In addition, toxic substances such as pesticides may be applied to a food crop in the field, while lead, arsenic, and cadmium are naturally present in soil and water, and may be absorbed by plants. Toxicologists must determine the acceptable daily intake (ADI) level for those substances.

Q. Define formal toxicology.

It deals with the formal toxicological studies which are prerequisite for release of a new drugs/chemical, e.g., calculation of lethal dose-50 (LD_{50}) and minimum toxic dose.

Q. Define descriptive toxicology.

Descriptive toxicology is concerned with gathering toxicological information from animal experimentation. These types of experiments are used to establish how much of a chemical would cause illness or death. The US Environmental Protection Agency (EPA), the Occupational Safety and Health Administration (OSHA), and the Food and Drug Administration (FDA) use information from these studies to set regulatory exposure limits.

Q. Define mechanistic toxicology.

Mechanistic toxicology makes observations on how toxic substances cause their effects. The effects of exposure can depend on a number of factors, including the size of the molecule, the specific tissue type, or cellular components affected, whether the substance is easily dissolved in water or fatty tissues, all of which are important when trying to determine the way a toxic substance causes harm, and whether effects seen in animals can be expected in humans.

Q. Define nutritional toxicology.

Nutritional toxicology is the study of toxicological aspects of food/feed stuffs and nutritional products/habits.

Q. Define toxicodynamics.

It deals with the study of biochemical and physiological effects of toxicants and their mechanism of action.

Q. Define toxicokinetics.

It deals with the study of absorption, distribution, metabolism, and excretion of toxicants in the body.

Q. Define toxicovigilance.

It deals with the process of identification, investigation, and evaluation of various toxic effects in the community with a view of taking measures to reduce or control exposures involving the substances that produce these effects.

Q. Define toxinology.

It deals with assessing the toxicity of substances of plant and animal origin and those produced by pathogenic bacteria/organism.

Q. Define toxicoepidemiology.

It refers to the study of quantitative analysis of the toxicity incidences in organisms, factors affecting toxicity, species involved, and the use of such knowledge in planning of prevention and control strategies.

1.2 TYPES OF TOXICANTS

Q. Define poison.

Poison is derived from Latin "potus," a drink that could harm or kill. It is any substance which when taken inwardly in a very small dose or applied in any kind of manner to a living body depraves the health or entirely destroys life. Although the word toxicant has essentially the same medical meaning, there are psychological and legal implications involved in the use of the word poison that makes manufacturer reluctant to apply it to chemicals, particularly those intended for widespread use in large quantities, unless they are required to do so by law. The term toxicant is more acceptable to both manufacturer and legislators.

Q. Define toxicant.

Toxicant is synonym of poison, produced by living organism in small quantities and is generally classified as biotoxin. These may be phytotoxins (produced by plants), mycotoxins (produced by fungi), zootoxins (produced by lower animals), and bacteriotoxins (produced by bacteria).

Q. Define different types of toxins.

1. Endotoxins are found within bacterial cells.

2. Exotoxins: elaborated from bacterial cells.

Q. Define venom.

Venom is a toxicant synthesized in a specialized gland and ejected by the process of biting or stinging. Venom is also a zootoxin but is transmitted by the process of biting or stinging.

Q. Define pollutant.

It is any undesirable substance to solid, liquid, or gaseous matter resulting from the discharge or admixture of noxious materials that contaminate the environment and contributes to pollution.

Q. Define systemic toxicant.

It is a toxicant that affects the entire body or many organs rather than a specific site. For example, potassium cyanide is a systemic toxicant that affects virtually every cell and organ in the body by interfering with the cell's ability to utilize oxygen.

Q. Define organ toxicant.

It is toxicant that affects only specific organs or tissues (may be called tissue toxicant) while not producing damage to the body as a whole. For example, benzene is a specific organ toxicant in that it is primarily toxic to the blood-forming tissues.

1.3 TOXICITY AND TOXIC EFFECTS

Toxic and toxicity are relative terms commonly used in comparing one chemical with another.

Q. Define toxicity.

It is a state of being poisonous or capacity to cause injury to living organisms.

Q. Define toxicosis.

It is the condition or disease state that results from exposure to a toxicant. The term toxicosis is often used interchangeably with the term poisoning or intoxication.

Q. Define toxic effects.

These are undesirable effects produced by a toxicant/drug which are detrimental to either survival or normal functioning of the individual.

Q. Define side effects.

These are undesirable effects which result from the normal pharmacological actions of drugs. These results may not be detrimental or harmful to the individual.

Q. Define selective toxicity.

It is the toxicity produced by a chemical to one kind of living matter without harming another form of life even though the two exist in intimate contact.

Q. Define plant toxins.

Different portions of a plant may contain different concentrations of chemicals. Some chemicals made by plants can be lethal. For example, taxon, used in chemotherapy to kill cancer cells, is produced by a species of the yew plant.

Q. Define animal toxins.

Animal toxins can result from venomous or poisonous animal releases. Venomous animals are usually defined as those that are capable of producing a poison in a highly developed gland or group of cells, and can deliver that toxin through biting or stinging. Poisonous animals are generally regarded as those whose tissues, either in part or in their whole, are toxic. For example, venomous animals, such as snakes and spiders, and poisonous animals, such as puffer fish, or oysters may be toxic to some individuals when contaminated with *Vibrio vulnificus.*

1.3.1 TOXICITY IN RELATION TO FREQUENCY AND DURATION OF EXPOSURE

The exposure of experimental animals to chemicals can be divided into four categories: acute toxicity and repeated exposure (subacute, subchronic, and chronic).

Q. Define acute toxicity.

Acute toxicity is defined as an exposure to a chemical for less than 24 hours. The exposure usually refers to a single administration; repeated exposures may be given within a 24-hour period for some slightly toxic or practically nontoxic chemicals. Acute exposure by inhalation refers to continuous exposure for less than 24 hours, most frequently for 4 hours.

Q. Define repeated exposure.

Repeated exposure is divided into three categories:

(1) subacute, (2) subchronic, and (3) chronic.

subacute exposure to a chemical is for 1 month or less, subchronic for 1−3 months, and chronic for more than 3 months (usually this refers to studies with at least 1 year of repeated dosing).

Explanation: Acute or repeated exposure can be by any route, but most often they occur by the oral route, with the chemical added directly to the diet. In human exposure situations, the frequency and duration of exposure are usually not as clearly defined as in controlled animal studies. However, almost same terms are used to describe general exposure situations. Thus, workplace or environmental exposures may be described as acute (occurring from a single incident or episode), subchronic (occurring repeatedly over several weeks or months), or chronic (occurring repeatedly for many months or years).

1.3.2 TOXICITY IN RELATION TO TIME OF DEVELOPMENT AND DURATION OF INDUCED EFFECTS

Q. Define transient or reversible or temporary toxicity.

It is the toxicity or harmful effect that remains for short duration of time, e.g., narcosis produced organic solvents.

Q. Define persistent or permanent or irreversible toxicity.

It is the toxicity or harmful effect that persists throughout the life span of the individual and is of permanent nature, e.g., scarring of skin produced by corrosives.

Q. Define immediate toxicity.

It is the toxicity that develops shortly after a single exposure to a toxicant, e.g., cyanide poisoning.

Q. Define delayed toxicity.

It is the toxicity or harmful effect which has delayed onset of action, e.g., peripheral neuropathy produced by some organophosphorus (OP) insecticides and radiation sickness.

Q. Define cumulative toxicity.

It is a progressive toxicity or harmful effect produced by summation of incremental injury resulting from successive exposures, e.g., liver fibrosis produced by ethanol.

Q. Accumulative effects occur in two ways:

1. Accumulation of toxin: exposure to heavy metals (lead, mercury) that have long half-lives result in disease due to metal accumulation.
2. Accumulation of effect: low-level exposure to organophosphate pesticides depresses acetylcholine esterase to a point where symptoms occur.

1.4 OTHER TERMS USED IN TOXICOLOGY

Q. Define cheminformatics.

Cheminformatics (also known as chemoinformatics, chemioinformatics, and chemical informatics) is the use of computer and informational techniques applied to a range of problems in the field of chemistry. These in silico techniques are used in, for example, pharmaceutical companies in the process of drug discovery.

Q. Define end point study record.

End point study record or IUCLID (International Uniform Chemical Information Database) format of the technical dossier is used to report study summaries and robust study summaries of the information derived for the specific end point according to the REACH regulation.

Q. Define end point of study design.

End point: an observable or measurable inherent property/data point of a chemical substance. For example, a physical−chemical property like vapor pressure or degradability or a biological effect that a given substance has on human health or the environment, e.g., carcinogenicity, irritation, and aquatic toxicity.

Q. Define in vitro test.

In vitro test: literally stands for "in glass" or "in tube," refers to the test taking place outside of the body of an organism, usually involving isolated organs, tissues, cells, or biochemical systems.

Q. Define in vivo test.

In vivo test: a test conducted within a living organism.

Q. Define in silico test.

In silico: in silico (a phrase coined as an analogy to the familiar phrases in vivo and in vitro) is an expression used to denote "performed on computer or via computer simulation." It means scientific experiments or research conducted or produced by means of computer modeling or computer simulation.

Q. Define IUCLID flag.

IUCLID flag: an option used in the IUCLID software to indicate submitted data type (e.g., experimental data) or its use for regulatory purposes (e.g., confidentiality).

Q. Define prediction model.

Prediction model is a theoretical formula, algorithm, or program used to convert the experimental results obtained by using a test method into a prediction of the toxic property/effect of the chemical substance.

Q. Define Quantitative structure–activity relationship (QSARs) and Structure–activity relationship (SARs).

QSARs and SARs: theoretical models that can be used to predict in a quantitative or qualitative manner the physical, chemical, biological (e.g., (eco)toxicological), and environmental fate properties of compounds from knowledge of their chemical structure. A SAR is a qualitative relationship that relates a (sub)structure to the presence or absence of a property or activity of interest. A QSAR is a mathematical model relating one or more quantitative parameters, which are derived from the chemical structure, to a quantitative measure of a property or activity.

Q. Define test or assay, validation test, and validation.

Test (or assay): an experimental system set up to obtain information on the intrinsic properties or adverse effects of a chemical substance.

Validation test: a test for which its performance characteristics, advantages, and limitations have been adequately determined for a specific purpose.

Validation: the process by which the reliability and relevance of a test method are evaluated for the purpose of supporting a specific use.

Q. Define vertebrate animal.

Animals that belong to subphylum Vertebrata; chordate with backbones and spinal columns is known as a vertebrate animal.

Q. Define accidental poisoning.

Accidental poisoning may occur when human beings or animals take toxicant accidentally or is added unintentionally in food or through in its feed, fodder, or drinking water. Such toxicants come from either natural or man-made sources. The natural sources include ingestion of toxic plants, biting or stinging by poisonous reptiles, ingestion of food contaminated with toxins, and contaminated water with minerals. Man-made sources include therapeutic agents, household products, and agrochemicals.

Q. Define malicious poisoning.

It is the unlawful or criminal killing of human beings or animals by administering certain toxic/poisonous agents. Incidence of such poisonings is more prevalent in human beings and less in animals.

Q. What is REACH regulation?

REACH regulation is concerned with registration, evaluation, authorization, and restriction of chemicals in European Union (EU). It entered into force on June 1, 2007. It streamlines and improves the former legislative framework on chemicals of the EU.

1.5 CLASSIFICATION OF TOXIC AGENTS

Toxic agents are classified in number of ways depending on the interests and needs of the classifier. There is no single classification applicable for the entire spectrum of toxic agents and hence combinations of classification systems based on several factors may provide the best rating system. Classification of poisons may take into account both the chemical and biological properties of the agent; however, exposure characteristics are also useful in toxicology.

Q. Classify toxic agents.

In toxicology, compounds are classified in various ways, by one or more of the following classes:

1. Use, e.g., pesticides (atrazine), solvents (benzene), food additives (NutraSweet), metals, and war gases
2. Effects, e.g., carcinogen (benzo[a]pyrene), mutagen (methylnitrosamine), and hepatotoxicant ($CHCl_3$).
3. Physical state such as oxidant (ozone), gas (CO_2), dust (Fe_2O_3), and liquid (H_2O).
4. Chemistry such as aromatic amine (aniline) and halogenated hydrocarbon (methylene chloride).
5. Sources of toxicants, e.g., plant or animal or natural.
6. Mechanism of action: cholinesterase inhibitor (malathion), methemoglobin producer (nitrite), etc.

Q. Classification based on sources of toxicants
1. Plant toxins
2. Animal toxicants
3. Mineral toxicants
4. Synthetic toxicants
5. Physical or mechanical agents.

Q. Classification based on physical state of toxicants
1. Gaseous toxicants
2. Liquid toxicants
3. Solid toxicants
4. Dust toxicants.

Q. Classification based on target organ or system
  1. Neurotoxicants
  2. Hepatotoxicants
  3. Nephrotoxicants
  4. Pulmotoxicants
  5. Hematotoxicants
  6. Dermatotoxicants
  7. Development and reproductive toxicants.

Q. Classification based on chemical nature/structure of toxicants
  1. Metals
  2. Nonmetals
  3. Acids and alkalis
  4. Organic toxicants (carbon compounds other than oxides of carbon, the carbonates, and metallic carbides and cyanides).

Q. Classification based on analytical behavior of toxicants
  1. Volatile toxicants
  2. Extractive toxicants
  3. Metals and metalloids.

Q. Classification based on type of toxicity
  1. Acute
  2. Subacute
  3. Chronic.

Q. Classification based on toxic effects
  1. Carcinogens
  2. Mutagens
  3. Teratogens
  4. Clastogens.

Q. Classification based on their uses
  1. Insecticides
  2. Fungicides
  3. Herbicides
  4. Rodenticides
  5. Food additives, etc.

Q. Classification based on symptoms produced
  1. Corrosive poisons
  2. Irritant poisons
  3. Systemic poisons
  4. Miscellaneous poisons.
  In addition, there are other types of classifications that are based on the environmental and public health considerations and so on.

Q. Summarize examples of some poisons (caustics) based on symptoms produced.
  Examples: corrosive poisons (Table 1.2), irritant poisons (Table 1.3), systemic poisons (Table 1.4), and miscellaneous poisons (Table 1.5).

Table 1.2 Corrosive Poisons

Strong Acids		Strong Alkalis	
Inorganic or mineral acids	**Organic acids**	**Hydrates of**	**Carbonates of**
Sulfuric acid Nitric acid	Carbolic acid Oxalic acid Hydrochloric acid	Sodium Sodium	Potassium Potassium

Table 1.3 Irritant Poisons

Inorganic	Organic	Mechanical
Nonmetallic: phosphorus, halogens Metallic: arsenic, mercury, lead, copper, etc.	Vegetable: *Abrus*, castor, croton, calatropia, ergot, etc. Animal: snake or insect bites and stings	Diamond dust, glass powder, hair, nails, pins, etc.

Table 1.4 Systemic Poisons

CNS (Neurotoxins)	Cardiovascular	Lungs (Asphyxiants)
Central somniferous — Opium — Pethidine Inebriants — Alcohols, anesthetics — Sedative hypnotics — Insecticides (hydrocarbons) — Benzodiazepines, etc. Delirients — Datura — Cannabis — Cocaine, etc. Spinal Strychnine, gelsemium, etc. Peripheral Curare, conium, etc.	Oleanders, aconite, nicotine	Carbon monoxide, carbon dioxide, irrespirable gas, cyanogens gas, cyanides

Table 1.5 Miscellaneous Poisons

Domestic poisons	Insecticides (aluminum phosphide, rat kill), kerosene, diesel, petrol, cleaning agents, soaps, detergents, disinfectants, cosmetics, etc.
Therapeutic substance	Salicylates, paracetamol, antidepressants, sedatives, antipsychotics, insulin, etc.
Food poisons	Bacterial, viral, mushrooms, chemicals, etc.
Drugs of dependence	Alcohol, tobacco, hypnotics, hallucinogens, stimulants, organic solvents, etc.

1.6 TOXICITY RATING

Q. Describe briefly the term "toxicity rating."

A system of "toxicity rating" has been evolved for common poisons. The higher the toxicity rating for a particular substance (over a range of 1−6), the greater is the potency. The toxicity rating based on toxic potential of substances (super toxic, extremely toxic, very toxic, moderately toxic, slightly toxic, and practically nontoxic) is summarized in Table 1.6.

Table 1.6 Toxicity Rating

Toxicity Rating or Class	Probable LD (Human)	
	mg/kg	**For 70 kg man**
6 (Super toxic)	Less than 5 mg/kg	A few drops
5 (Extremely toxic)	5−50 mg/kg	"A pinch" to one teaspoonful
4 (Very toxic)	51−500 mg/kg	One tea spoonful to two table spoonful
3 (Moderately toxic)	501 mg/kg to 5 g/kg	One once to 1 pint (1 pound)
2 (Slightly toxic)	5.1 g/kg to 15 g/kg	1 pint to 1 quart (2 pounds)
1 (Practically nontoxic)	More than 15 g/kg	More than 2 pounds

1.7 HISTORICAL STALWARTS

Q. Who is regarded as father of rational medicine?

Hippocrates (460−375 BC) is regarded as the "father of rational medicine" (Fig. 1.1). He created the Hippocratic Oath. He believed that disease came naturally and not from superstitions and god. He advocated hot oil as an antidote in poisoning and induced vomiting to prevent absorption of the poisons.

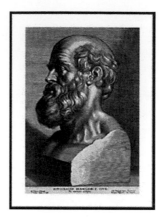

FIGURE 1.1

Hippocrates (460–375 BC).

http://render.fineartamerica.com/images/rendered/search/framed-print/images-medium/1-hippocrates-460-
375-bc-engraving-everett.jpg

Q. Who was Paracelsus?

Theophrastus Paracelsus Bombastus Von Hohenheim (1493–1541), a 1st century Roman physician (Fig. 1.2), promoted a focus on the toxicon, the toxic agent, as a chemical entity. He recognized the dose—response concept and in one of his writings stated, "All substances are poisons, there is none which is not a poison. The right dose differentiates a poison and a remedy."

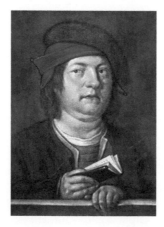

FIGURE 1.2

Theophrastus Paracelsus Bombastus Von Hohenheim (1493–1541).

http://homeoint.org/photo/pq/paracl06.jpg

Q. What is the contribution of Friedrich Serturner?

Friedrich Serturner (1783–1841) was a German pharmacist who isolated the specific narcotic substance from opium and named as morphine after Morpheus (Fig. 1.3), the Roman God of sleep.

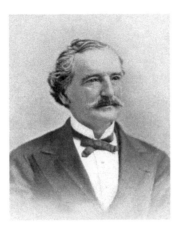

FIGURE 1.3

Friedrich Serturner (1783–1841).

https://upload.wikimedia.org/wikipedia/commons/c/ca/Colton_Gardner_Q.jpg

Q. Who is the father of toxicology?

M.J.B. (Mathieu Joseph Bonaventure) Orfila (1787–1853), a Spanish physician, is considered as a "father of toxicology" (Fig. 1.4).

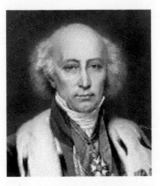

FIGURE 1.4

Father of toxicology—Mathieu Joseph Bonaventure Orfila (1787–1853).

https://encrypted-tbn0.gstatic.com/images?q = tbn:
ANd9GcSsrNZMTcRLMNs2nIvZnnHE19szBbR6Fpd_bHfArIhroJEqTKSIkA

Q. Describe in brief the contributions of M.J.B. Orfila (1787—1853).

He established toxicology as a discipline distinct from others and defined toxicology as the study of poisons. He advocated the practice of autopsy followed by chemical analysis of viscera to prove that poisoning has taken place. His "treatise" Traite des Poisons published in 1814 laid the foundations of forensic toxicology.

Q. Who is the father of experimental pharmacology? Describe in brief his contributions.

Francois Magendie (1783—1855) is known as the "father of experimental pharmacology," a pioneer French physiologist and toxicologist studied the mechanism of action of emetine, morphine, quinine, strychnine, and other alkaloids (Fig. 1.5).

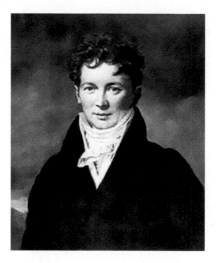

FIGURE 1.5

Francois Magendie.

http://www.culture.gouv.fr/culture/actualites/celebrations2005/images/099.jpg

Q. Who was Claude Bernard?

Claude Bernard (1813—78) was a French physiologist who is considered the "father of modern experimental physiology" (Fig. 1.6). Claude Bernard's first important works were carried out on the physiology of digestion, particularly the role of the pancreas exocrine gland, the gastric juices, and of the intestines. In addition to this, Bernard also made other important contributions to the neurosciences.

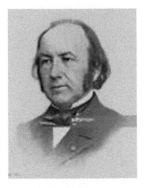

FIGURE 1.6

Claude Bernard (1813–78).

Q. Who was Louis Lewin (1854–1929)?

Louis Lewin (1854–1929) was a German scientist who took up the task of classifying drugs and plants in accordance with their psychological effects (Fig. 1.7). He also published many articles and books dealing with toxicology of methyl alcohol, ethyl alcohol, chloroform, opium, and some other chemicals. His important publications are *Toxicologist's View of World History* and *A Textbook of Toxicology*.

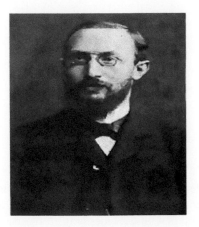

FIGURE 1.7

Louis Lewin (1854–1929).

Q. Who discovered the insecticidal properties of dichlorodiphenyltrichloroethane (DDT)?

Paul Hermann Muller in 1939 (Fig. 1.8) discovered the insecticidal properties of DDT. He was awarded Nobel Prize in 1948 "for his discovery of the high efficiency of DDT as a contact poison against several arthropods." (Fig. 1.9).

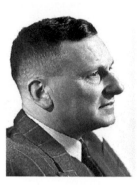

FIGURE 1.8

Paul Hermann Muller (1899–1969)—synthesized DDT.

http://www.nobelprize.org/nobel_prizes/medicine/laureates/1948/muller_postcard.jpg

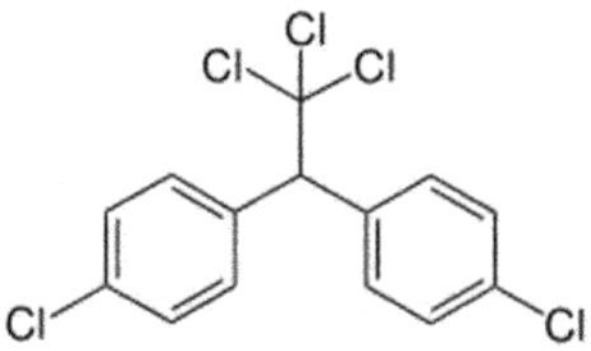

FIGURE 1.9

Dichlorodiphenyltrichloroethane.

https://upload.wikimedia.org/wikipedia/commons/thumb/0/0b/P%2Cp%27-dichlorodiphenyltrichloroethane. svg/300px-P%2Cp%27-dichlorodiphenyltrichloroethane.svg.png

Q. Who is the "father of nerve agents"?

Gerhard Schrader (1903–90) was a German chemist who accidentally developed the toxic nerve agents serin, tabun, soman, and cyclosarin while attempting to develop new insecticides (Fig. 1.10). Schrader and his team, thus, introduced a new class of synthetic insecticides, the OP insecticides, and defined the structural requirements for insecticidal activity of anticholinesterase compounds. He is known as the "father of nerve agents."

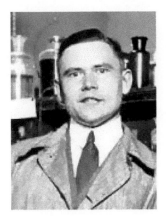

FIGURE 1.10

Gerhard Schrader (1903–90)—"father of nerve agents."

https://encrypted-tbn1.gstatic.com/images?q = tbn:ANd9GcR2tolt3mmeWAkhrqnAMMVPcl2qLvm3-
BcHD5kR-kmEVFI1WwOy

Q. Who is Rachel Carson (1907–64)?

In 1962 Rachel Carson started crusade against the use of DDT and published the great book *Silent Spring* (Fig. 1.11).

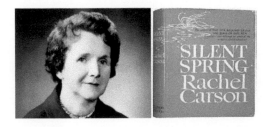

FIGURE 1.11

Rachel Carson (1907–64)—author of *Silent Spring*—campaign against DDT.

http://userscontent1.emaze.com/images/9e391614-3f7f-4447-9c71-2b388ccc79c9/1ddf5e93-4330-4fe8-
9ded-92c2d7047383image1.jpg

Q. What is phocomelia in children?

A rare congenital deformity in which the hands or feet are attached close to the trunk (Fig. 1.12). The limbs are grossly underdeveloped or absent. This condition was a side effect of the drug thalidomide taken during early pregnancy.

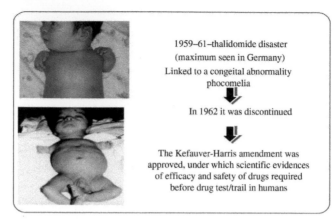

1959–61–thalidomide disaster
(maximum seen in Germany)
Linked to a congeital abnormality
phocomelia

In 1962 it was discontinued

The Kefauver-Harris amendment was
approved, under which scientific evidences
of efficacy and safety of drugs required
before drug test/trail in humans

FIGURE 1.12

Thalidomide tragedy—phocomelia in children.

http://image.slidesharecdn.com/ppvfinal-150403124653-conversion-gate01/95/pharmacovigilance-at-trauma-center-aiims-11-638.jpg?cb = 1428083286, http://farm7.static.flickr.com/6059/6250
205367_686cc54595.jpg

Q. Summarize some important developments in the field of toxicology.

Some important developments in the field of toxicology are summarized in Table 1.7.

Table 1.7 Some Important Developments in the Field of Toxicology

F. Magendie, 1809: study of "arrow poisons," mechanism of action of emetine and strychnine
Marsh, 1836: development of method for arsenic analysis
Reinsh, 1841: combined method for separation and analysis of As and Hg
Fresenius, 1845, and von Babo, 1847: development of screening method for general poisons
Stas-Otto, 1851: detection and identification of phosphorus
C. Bernard, 1850: carbon monoxide combination with hemoglobin, study of mechanism of action of strychnine, site of action of curare
Friedrich Gaedcke, 1855: first isolated cocaine from leaves of *Erthroxylon coca*
Oswald schmiedeberg, 1869: isolated muscarine from *Amanita muscaria*
R. Bohm, c.1890: active anthelmintics from fern, action of croton oil catharsis, poisonous mushrooms
C. Voegtlin, 1923: mechanism of action of As and other metals on the SH groups
K.K. Chen, 1934: demonstrated antagonistic effect of sodium nitrite and sodium thiosulfate in cyanide poisoning
P. Muller, 1944–46: introduction and study of DDT and related insecticide compounds
R.A. Peters, L.A. Stocken, and R.H.S. Thompson, 1945: development of British AntiLewisite (BAL) as a relatively specific antidote for arsenic
Juda Hirsch Quastel, 1946: developed 2,4-D, the first widely used systemic herbicide
G. Schrader, 1952: introduction and study of OP compounds
Rachel Carson, 1962: started crusade against the use of DDT and published the great book *Silent Spring*

1.8 FACTORS AFFECTING TOXICITY

Q. Enumerate at least four group of factors that can affect toxicity.
1. Host factors (factors related to subject)
2. Factors related to toxicant or associated with xenobiotics
3. Environmental factors
4. Individual or nonindividual factors.

1.8.1 HOST FACTORS (FACTORS RELATED TO SUBJECT)

Q. Discuss briefly host-related factors that affect toxicity. Give suitable examples.

Size: Large individuals can tolerate a larger dose than individuals of small size. The metabolism and activity is proportional to the surface area of the body.

Age: Young animals or the human infants are uniquely susceptible to chemicals that are relatively safer at a later period of life. The difference in response during early life is a consequence of the relative inefficiency of various metabolic and excretory pathways, For example, deficiency of glucuronyl transferase activity results in an enhanced toxicity of chemicals which are dependent upon detoxification.

Species, breeds, and strains: Differences in strain of animals also induce a variation in response to chemical agents and such differences have been detected in acute toxicity measurement of various inbred strains of mice. Since man is a remarkably heterogeneous species, the rate of metabolism of any compound may differ greatly from person to person. For example, hemolysis is observed in certain individuals during the administration of drugs like aspirin and sulfonamides because some individuals are deficient in the metabolic enzyme glucose-6-phosphate dehydrogenase (G6PD) (Table 1.8).

Table 1.8 Mechanism of Hemolysis in Individuals Deficient in G6PD

G6PD deficiency causes hemolytic anemia
• Mutations in G6PD results in impairment of NADPH production
• Detoxification of H_2O_2 is inhibited, and cellular damage results—leads to erythrocyte membrane breakdown and hemolytic anemia and jaundice

Similarly, rabbit can survive even after eating *Atropa belladonna* (belladonna leaves) because they contain the enzyme atropinase, which destroys atropine (Fig. 1.13).

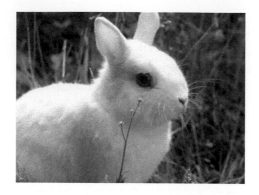

FIGURE 1.13

Rabbit can survive after eating poisonous belladonna leaves.

Reproduced from https://en.wikipedia.org/wiki/File:Kostya2.jpg

Similarly, some breeds of animals are more susceptible to the toxic effects of chemicals. For example, in Koolies, ivermectin easily crosses blood−brain barrier and causes neurological symptom (Fig. 1.14). Mink (species) animal is highly sensitive for polychlorinated biphenyls (PCBs) than other species (Fig. 1.15).

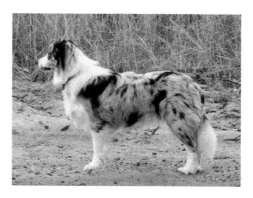

FIGURE 1.14

Koolie breed of dog—more susceptible to ivermectin toxicity.

Reproduced from https://en.wikipedia.org/wiki/Border_Collie#/media/File:Blue_merle_Border_Collie.jpg

Greyhounds (Fig. 1.16) are more susceptible to the toxic effects of barbiturates (used as anesthetics) as they mainly distribute to adipose tissue. Since greyhounds have little body fat resulting in higher circulating concentration of barbiturates causing toxicity.

Sex: The sex of an animal often has an influence on the toxicity of chemical agent. The variation in toxicity due to sex is well known; the chemical agents or drugs must be used with special care during pregnancy

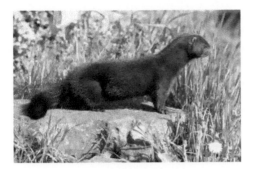

FIGURE 1.15

Mink—most susceptible to PCB poisoning than other animal species.

https://encrypted-tbn2.gstatic.com/images?q = tbn:ANd9GcTkXDdl_DK-RsLIDws6JTDgE6md1AUouVMc33CHtZKfTVLrXiMWVA

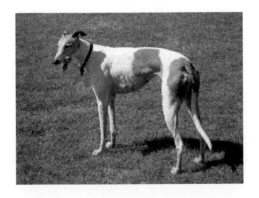

FIGURE 1.16

Greyhound dog breed—more susceptible to barbiturate toxicity.

Reproduced from https://commons.wikimedia.org/wiki/File:GraceTheGreyhound.jpg

because they could lead to teratogenic effects in females, and the differences are shown to be under direct endocrine influence. During lactation, it is important to remember that some chemicals or drugs may be excreted in milk and may even act on the offspring. Thus, it is desirable to measure acute toxicity on both male and female animals of any species.

1.8.2 FACTORS RELATED TO TOXICANTS OR ASSOCIATED WITH XENOBIOTICS

Q. What are the factors associated with toxicants that affect the outcome of response?

1. Physical state and chemical properties of the toxicant
2. Routes and rates of toxicant administration
3. Previous or coincident exposure to other drugs/chemicals (drug–chemical interactions)
4. Tolerance of individuals.

Q. How do physical state and chemical properties of toxicants affect toxicity?

The physical state and chemical properties of the toxicant such as:
(1) solubility in water, (2) solubility in vegetable oils, (3) the suspending medium, (4) the chemical stability of the chemical agent, (5) the particle size, (6) rates of disintegration of formulations of chemicals, (7) the crystal form, and (8) the grittiness of inert substances given in bulk amounts.

For example, fine particles are more readily absorbed than coarse ones (in the case of poisons bearing irritating properties, e.g., α-naphthylthiourea, zinc phosphide). Solvents and other substances included in commercial preparations may also affect the overall toxicity of the active principle(s). Nonpolar solvents may considerably increase the absorption rate of lipophilic poisons, especially when considering the exposure by the dermal route.

Q. How do routes and rate of administration of chemicals affect the toxicity?

Generally, toxicity is the highest by the route that carries the compound to the bloodstream most rapidly. For most xenobiotics, parenteral routes of exposure entail a more prompt and complete bioavailability than the oral one and therefore often result in a lower LD_{50}.

Q. How does previous or coincident exposure to other chemicals (drug–drug interactions) affect the toxicity?

A variety of chemicals (drugs, plant toxins, pesticides, environmental pollutants) are capable of increasing (enzyme inducers) or decreasing (enzyme inhibitors) the expression and the activity of hepatic and extrahepatic phase I and phase II enzyme systems participating in the biotransformation reactions hence modulating the toxicity of several xenobiotics. Thus administration of two or more chemicals of different structures when administered simultaneously may lead to additive effect, "summation," or negative summation, or "antagonism" or "potentiation."

Q. How does repeated administration of drug affect the response of a drug?

It is well known that the toxic reaction of an animal to a given dose of a drug may decrease, remain unchanged, or increase on subsequent administration of that dose. A decrease in toxic response is usually called "tolerance," and an increase in toxic response, "hypersusceptibility." The enzyme induction or the increased activity of enzymes concerned with detoxification and elimination of drug is a common mechanism for the development of tolerance to a drug on repeated administration.

For example, repeated administration of chlorpromazine depresses the central nervous system (CNS) of normal albino rats and lessens their loco motor activity.

Q. How do feed and feeding affect the results of toxicity?

The composition of the feed or food can affect the results of toxicity tests. For example, high-fat diets can sensitize animals to, while high carbohydrate and high protein diets provide protection from, the hepatotoxic effects of chloroform.

1.8.3 ENVIRONMENTAL FACTORS

Q. Discuss in brief environmental conditions that effect toxicity.

The environment can affect the toxic response to chemicals given to animals or human beings. There are three basic factors in the environment of laboratory animals used in toxicity testing, namely:
1. The presence of other species of animals, usually human being
2. The presence of other animals of the same species
3. Physical environment.

Several physical factors such as light, temperature, and relative humidity can influence the LD_{50} of several chemicals.

For example, high ambient temperatures are reported to enhance the toxicity of chlorophenols and nitrophenols that cause an increased production of heat by uncoupling mitochondrial oxidative phosphorylation. Conversely, cold temperatures are predisposing factors for α-chloralose, a rodenticide/avicide formerly used as an anesthetic agent, which may induce a life-threatening hypothermia especially in poisoned cats by acting on hypothalamic thermoreceptors.

Q. How do changes in the internal environment affect toxicity?

Several physiological factors, such as physical activity, stress conditions, hormonal state of animals, and degenerative changes in internal organs, are known to influence the toxicity of any compound. For example, some compounds may induce increased synthesis of liver microsomal enzymes and influence the metabolism of another. The inhibition of drug or chemical agent metabolism, displacement of protein binding of a chemical, or inhibition of its renal clearance can also be accomplished by chemical agents.

1.8.4 INDIVIDUAL OR NONINDIVIDUAL FACTORS

Q. How do habitually used drugs affect the sensitivity of man to toxic doses of chemicals?

The habitual use of certain psychoactive drugs, and particularly excessive use, of these chemicals could affect the sensitivity of human to toxic doses of drugs and other chemicals.

Q. What is idiosyncratic reaction?

Occasionally toxicity peculiar to an individual or which appears in a few persons but not in general population has been observed. Patients with a deficiency of G6PD, for example, develop hemolysis after ingesting certain drugs or foods. Drugs that are known to cause this type of idiosyncratic reaction include troglitazone, valproate, amiodarone, ketoconazole, disulfiram and isoniazid. However, some involvement of allergic mechanism cannot be ruled out.

1.9 NATURAL LAWS CONCERNING TOXICOLOGY

1.9.1 TIME—EFFECT RELATIONSHIP

Q. Describe time—effect relationship of a toxicant.

The relationship between dose and response is usually established when the chemical/drug effect at a particular dose has reached a maximum or a steady level (Fig. 1.17). The chemical effects do not develop instantaneously or continue indefinitely; they change with time. Thus, the magnitude of a chemical effect at any given moment is a function not only of the dose but also of the amount of time elapsed since the chemical made contact with the reactive tissues. This curve represents several important features (there are three distinct phases and a fourth phase that may be present or pronounced with some chemicals while absent with others), which include:

- Time of onset of action (Ta)
- Time to peak effect (Tb)
- Duration of action (Tc)
- Residual effects (Td).

Phase I: Time of onset of action (Ta): Following the administration of a chemical agent to a system, there is a delay in time before the first signs of

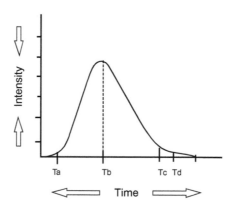

FIGURE 1.17

Hypothetical curve showing time—effect relationship of a toxicant. *Ta*, latency time; *Tb*, peak time; *Tc*, persistence time; *Td*, residual effect.

chemical effects are manifested. The lag in onset is of finite time, but for some chemicals the delay may be so short that it gives the appearance of an instantaneous action. There are various reasons responsible for the chemical effect to reach an observable level.

Phase II: Time to peak effect (Tb): The maximum response will occur when the most resistant cell has been affected to its maximum or when the chemical has reached the most inaccessible cells of the responsive tissue.

Phase III: Duration of action (Tc): The duration of action extends from the moment of onset of perceptible effects to the time when an action can no longer be measured. It will depend upon the rate at which it is metabolized, altered, or otherwise inactivated or removed from the body.

Phase IV: Residual effects (Td): Even after its primary actions are terminated many chemicals are known to exert a residual action. It is not always possible to determine whether the residual effect is caused by a persistence of minute quantities of the chemical or by persistence of subliminal effects.

1.9.2 DOSE–RESPONSE RELATIONSHIP

Q. What is dose relationship?

The dose–response relationship, or exposure–response relationship, describes the change in effect on an organism caused by differing levels of exposure (or doses) to a stressor (usually a chemical) after a certain exposure time. This may apply to individuals (e.g., a small amount has no significant effect, a large amount is fatal) or to populations (e.g., how many people or organisms are affected at different levels of exposure).

Q. What are different types of dose–response relationships?

Dose–response relationship is of two types:

1. Graded or gradual

2. Quantal (all-or-none) such as death.

Q. What is a graded or gradual dose–response relationship?

The individual dose–response relationship, which describes the response of an individual organism to varying doses of a chemical, is often referred to as a "graded" response because the measured effect is continuous over a range of doses (Fig. 1.18).

Explanation: This type of relationship is useful in measuring the incremental responses of a compound and can be seen in an individual organism. e.g., contraction of small intestine produced by carbachol, convulsions produced by strychnine. and inhibition of cholinesterase produced by OP insecticides. This type of relationship is useful in studying the efficiency of therapeutic drugs or toxic symptoms produced by a toxicant(s). A typical dose–response curve in which the percentage of organisms or systems responding to a chemical is plotted against the dose.

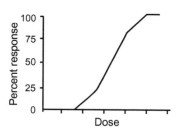

FIGURE 1.18

A typical dose—response curve in which the percentage of organisms or systems responding to a chemical is plotted against the dose.

Q. What are the assumptions of graded dose—response relationship?

The graded dose—response relationship is based on following presumptions:

1. The pharmacological/toxicological effect is a result of the known drug/toxicant.
2. There is a molecular or receptor site(s) with which the drug/toxicant interacts to produce the response.
3. The production of a response and the degree of response are related to the concentration of the drug/toxicant at the molecular or receptor site.
4. The concentration of the drug/toxicant at the molecular or receptor site in turn is related to the administered dose of the agent.
5. The effect of drug/toxicant is proportional to the fractions of molecular or receptor site occupied by the agent; therefore, by increasing or decreasing the dose, the response also increases or decreases, respectively. The maximal effect occurs when the drug/toxicant occupies all molecular or receptor sites.

The logarithmic transformation of dose is often employed for the dose—response relationship because:

1. It permits the display of a wide range of doses on a single graph.
2. It facilitates the visual and mathematical comparisons between dose—response curve for different agents or for different responses to a single agent.
3. Log dose plots usually provide a more linear representation of data.

Q. What is a quantal or all-or-none dose—response relationship?

Quantal dose—response relationship is one involving an all-or-none response, i.e., on increasing the dose of a compound, the response is either produced or not. This relationship is seen with certain responses that follow all-or-none phenomenon and cannot be graded, e.g., death (Fig. 1.19).

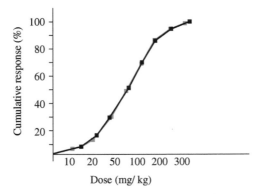

FIGURE 1.19

Typical sigmoid S-shaped curve showing quantal dose–response relationship. The response may be effective dose or morality.

Explanation: In toxicology, quantal dose–response relationship is extensively used for the calculation of lethal dose (LD) because in it we observe only mortality. The quantal dose–response relationship is always seen in a population because the assumption is made that individual responds to maximal possible or not at all. Both are graphs from the same set of experimental data. The log dose scale results in a more linear representation of the data and is more desirable since we will use the linear portion of the curve (from approximately 16% to 84%) to calculate toxic potency (Fig. 1.20).

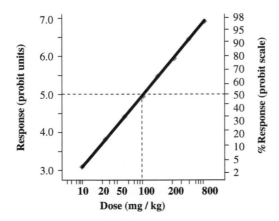

FIGURE 1.20

Quantal dose–response relationship showing linear transformation of dose–response data (typical S-shaped curve shown changed to a straight line by log probit plot). Percentage response may be effective dose or morality.

Explanation: The graph of a quantal dose–response relationship does not show the intensity of effect, but rather the frequency with which any dose produces the all-or-none phenomenon. A widely used statistical approach for estimating the response of a population to a toxic exposure is the "effective dose" (ED) or "lethal dose" (LD). Generally, the midpoint, or 50%, response level is used, giving rise to the "ED_{50}" or LD_{50} value. However, any response level, such as an ED_{01}, ED_{10}, or ED_{30} or LD_{01}, LD_{10}, or LD_{30} could be chosen. A graphical representation of an approximate ED_{50} is shown in Fig. 1.20. Note that these responses may be mortality (LD) or effective dose (ED).

Q. What is the shape of quantal dose–response curve?

In quantal dose–response, the log dose–response curve is sigmoid in character. The sigmoid curve has a relatively linear portion between 16% and 84% (Fig. 1.19), which is used to determine the slope of the curve. A small portion of population at left and right sides of the curve responds to low and high doses and constitutes hyperreactive (hypersensitive) and hyporeactive (hyposensitive) groups, respectively. If a compound produces its effect at very low dosage, the individual is said to be hyperreactive or hypersensitive; if the same effect is produced by the compound at unusually large doses, the individual is said to be hyporeactive or hyposensitive.

Q. What is hormesis dose–response phenomenon?

In toxicology, hormesis is a dose–response phenomenon characterized by a low-dose stimulation and a high-dose inhibition, resulting in either a J-shaped or an inverted U-shaped dose–response (Fig. 1.21).

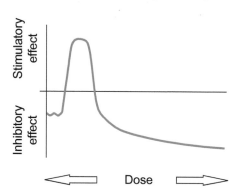

FIGURE 1.21

A low dose of a chemical agent may trigger from an organism the opposite response to a very high dose.

Q. What is U-shaped dose–response curve?

Sometime dose–response curves do not follow typical sigmoidal dose–response curve and *U-shaped dose–response curves* are observed. For example, essential metals and vitamins show U-shaped curves (Fig. 1.22).

At low dose, adverse effects are observed since there is a deficiency of these nutrients to maintain homeostasis. As dose increases, homeostasis is achieved, and the bottom of the U-shaped dose–response curve is reached. As dose increases to surpass the amount required to maintain homeostasis, overdose toxicity can ensue. Thus, adverse effects are seen at both low and high doses.

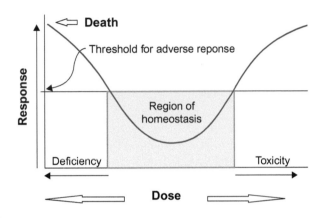

"U"-shaped dose–response curve

FIGURE 1.22

U-shaped dose–response curve for essential metals and vitamins. Vitamins and essential metals are essential for life and their lack can cause adverse responses (plotted on the vertical axis), as can their excess, giving rise to a U-shaped dose-dependent curve.

Q. What do you mean by lethal dose-50 (LD_{50}) and median lethal dose (MLD)?

LD_{50}, also called MLD, is the dose that is lethal for 50% of animals exposed to a given toxicant under defined conditions.

Explanation: The LD_{50} value is the common way of expressing the acute toxicity and may not pertain to the severity of clinical signs observed of the characteristic changes caused by the toxicant but depend only on the lethality produced by the toxicant. Though recently some toxicological organization and government regulatory agencies have greatly reduced the reliance on the LD_{50} (in order to reduce the number of animals needed for study), yet it is still considered an important index to assess the toxicity of chemicals.

The LD_{50} value is obtained by plotting the percentage of individuals succumbing to a given dose of lethal chemical as ordinate against the dose of the compound used as abscissa. In this way one obtains an S-shaped curve as shown in Fig. 1.19. The shape of the curve indicates the degree of variation. The LD_{50} is obtained from the curve by drawing a horizontal line from the 50% mortality point on the ordinate where it intersects the curve. At the point of intersection, vertical line is drawn and this line intersects at the LD_{50} point. This dose is designated as LD_{50}. The same data from the sigmoid curve or a bell-shaped curve will form a straight line when transformed into probit units (Fig. 1.20). These values are statistically obtained and represent the best estimation of the dose required to kill 50% of the animals. The information with respect to the LD for 95% or for 5% of the animals can also be derived by a similar procedure.

1.9.3 VARIABLES OF DOSE—RESPONSE CURVES

Q. Describe different variables of dose—response curve.

The dose—response curve has four characteristic variables:
1. Efficacy
2. Potency
3. Slope
4. Biological variation.

Q. What is efficacy?

The maximal effect or response produced by an agent is called its maximal efficacy or efficacy (Fig. 1.23).

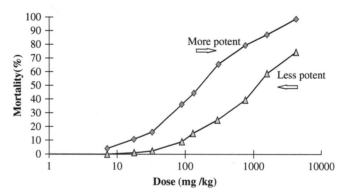

FIGURE 1.23

Comparison of potency of drug/toxicant.

Q. What is potency?

Potency is the dose of drug/toxicant required to produce a specific effect of given intensity as compared to a standard reference. It is a comparative rather than an absolute expression of drug activity. Drug potency depends on both affinity and efficacy. The more potent compound is on the left because less compound is needed to produce an equivalent response compared to the compound depicted on the right (Figs. 1.23 and 1.24).

Q. What is the difference between potency vs efficacy?

From their relative positions along the x-axis, compound "A" is more potent than compound "B." Both "A" and "B" also reach maximum efficacy since their effects both reach the limit of response (Fig. 1.24).

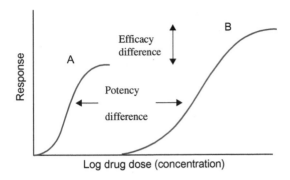

FIGURE 1.24

Typical sigmoid log dose–response curves for two drugs/toxicants, Drug A is more potent than drug B; drug B is more efficacious than drug A.

Q. What is slope?

The slope of a dose–response curve gives the relationship between the receptor/target site and the agent (Figs. 1.23 and 1.24).

Q. What is biological variation?

Biological variation or variance can be defined as the appearance of differences in the magnitude of response among individuals in the same population given the same dose of a compound.

Q. What is a margin of safety?

The *margin of safety* of a drug is the ratio of LD_1/ED_{99} (Fig. 1.25). The farther apart these curves are, the wider the margin of safety.

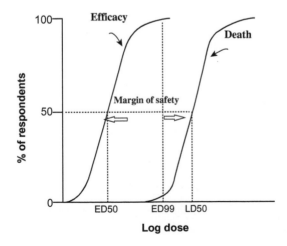

FIGURE 1.25

The margin of safety of a drug may be determined by comparing the 99% dose–response curve for the efficacy with the curve for a toxic or lethal effect.

For example,

$$\text{Safety margin} = LD_1/ED_{99}$$

where LD_1 = dose that is lethal for 1% of the population; ED_{99} = dose that is effective for 99% of the population.

Safety margin is a more conservative estimate than therapeutic index as values are derived from extremes of the respective dose–response curves.

Q. What is the difference between therapeutic index and margin of safety?

The therapeutic index is the ratio of the TD_{50} (or LD_{50}) and the ED_{50}; the margin of safety (a more conservative estimate) is the ratio of the LD_1 and the ED_{99}.

$$\text{Therapeutic index (TI)} = LD_{50}/ED_{50}$$

where LD_{50} = dose that is lethal for 50% of the population; ED_{50} = dose that is effective for 50% of the population.

Therapeutic index measure is commonly used for evaluating the safety and usefulness of therapeutic agents. The higher the index, the safer is the drug.

Q. What is a therapeutic ratio?

Therapeutic ratio may be defined as the ratio of the lethal dose-25 (LD_{25}) and the effective dose-75 (ED_{75}).

$$\text{Therapeutic ratio (TR)} = LD_{25}/ED_{75}$$

where LD_{25} = dose that is lethal for 25% of the population; ED_{75} = dose that is effective for 75% of the population.

Therapeutic ratio is considered a better index of safety of a compound as it includes steepness of curve also. In toxicity cases, a flatter curve is considered more toxic or hyperreactive groups are at a much more risk than hyporeactive or normal group. Shallower curves usually have low therapeutic ratios.

Q. What is a chronicity factor?

Chronicity factor is the ratio of the acute LD_{50} (one dose) to chronic LD_{50} doses.

$$\text{Chronicity factor} = \text{acute } LD_{50}/\text{chronic } LD_{50}$$

Chronicity factor is used to assess the cumulative action of a toxicant. Compounds with cumulative effects have a higher chronicity factor.

Q. What is a risk ratio?

The ratio between the inherent toxicity and the exposure level gives the risk ratio. Risk ratio indicates the risk of a compound. Substances of higher inherent toxicity may pose little risk as access of exposure of individuals to such agents is limited. Compounds of low toxicity may be dangerous if used extensively.

1.9.4 INTERACTION WITH RECEPTORS

Q. What do you understand by interaction with receptors?

Many toxicants/xenobiotics exert their effects by interacting with specific receptors in the body. This xenobiotic—receptor interaction leads to a change in the macromolecule, which in turn triggers a sequence of events resulting in a response of the tissue or organ. The intensity of response produced by a toxicant/xenobiotic depends on its intrinsic activity, which in turn depends on the chemical structure of the compound.

Q. What is a drug affinity?

Affinity is the ability of a xenobiotic to combine with its receptors. A ligand of low affinity requires a higher concentration to produce the same effect than ligand of high affinity. Agonists, partial agonist, antagonist, and inverse agonist have same or similar affinity for the receptor.

Q. What do you mean by intrinsic activity?

Intrinsic activity is defined as a proportionately constant ability of the agonist to activate the receptor as compared to the maximally active compound in the series being studied. It is maximum of unity for full agonist and minimum or zero for antagonist.

Q. What is an agonist?

Agonist (full agonist) is an agent that interacts with a specific cellular constituent (i.e., receptor) and elicits an observable positive response.

Q. What is a partial agonist?

Partial agonist is an agent that acts on the same receptor as other agonists in a group of endogenous ligands or xenobiotics, but regard less of its dose, it cannot produce the same maximal biological response as a full agonist.

Q. What is an antagonism/antagonistic effect?

When the combined effect of two compounds given together is lesser in magnitude to sum of the effects of each compound given alone, or when one compound having no effect of its own decreases or inhibits the effect of other compound, the interaction is called antagonism and the effect produced is called antagonistic effect. The toxic effect of a chemical, A, agonist, can be reduced when given with another chemical, B, the antagonist. Antagonists are often used as antidotes (Fig. 1.26).

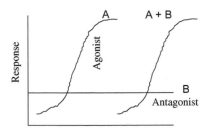

FIGURE 1.26

The toxic effect of a chemical, A, agonist, can be reduced when given with another chemical, B, the antagonist.

Q. What are the possible mechanisms of antagonism?

There are several mechanisms of antagonism:

1. Functional antagonism: It is simple counterbalancing of the toxic effect (caffeine and phenobarbital)
2. Chemical antagonism: Chemical antagonist reacts with the toxin to reduce toxicity (dimercaprol chelates toxic heavy metals such as lead)
3. Receptor antagonism: Receptor antagonist binds to receptor (atropine with organophosphate insecticides)
4. Dispositional antagonism: In disposition antagonism fate of the toxin is altered (cholestyramine can prevent the absorption of organic chemicals by binding with them).

Q. What is an inverse agonist?

Inverse agonist is a compound that interacts with the same receptor as the agonist, but it produces a response just opposite to that of the agonist.

Q. What will be the response if two drugs/xenobiotics are used simultaneously?

When two or more xenobiotics are used together, the pharmacological/ toxicological response is not necessarily the same of two agents used individually. This is because one agent may interfere with the action of another agent called xenobiotic/drug interaction.

Q. What is an addition/additive effect?

When the combined effect of two compounds given together is equal in magnitude to sum of the effects of each compound given alone, the interaction is called an addition and the effect produced is called an additive effect. In this case no specific interactions occur (Fig. 1.27).

$$1 + 1 = 2$$

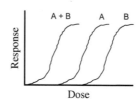

FIGURE 1.27

Additive effect.

Q. What is potentiation/potentiative effect?

When one compound having no effect of its own increases the effect of another compound, the interaction is called potentiation and the effect produced is called potentiative effect.

Explanation: A dose of a compound A is toxic to animals in vivo. Another chemical B is not toxic when given at doses several orders of magnitude higher but when the two are given together the toxic response is greater than that of the given dose of A alone. This means the compound B has a potentiative effect on compound A. This is known as potentiation.

Q. What is synergism/synergistic effect?

The combined effect of the administration of two compounds may be greater than the sum of the two effects; this is called synergism (Fig. 1.28). The synergist piperonyl butoxide is added to some insecticides to greatly increase their toxicity to insects.

For example, $1 + 1 =$ more than two.

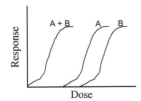

FIGURE 1.28

Synergistic effect.

Q. What is the difference between synergism and potentiation?

The difference between the two concepts is that synergism is the interaction of two or more substances, while potentiation is about a singular substance and how it may act when in a synergy relationship.

Q. Why are toxins often selective to tissues, give suitable examples?

Toxins are often selective to certain tissues because of the following reasons:

1. Preferential accumulation: Toxicant may accumulate in only certain tissues and cause toxicity to that particular tissue, e.g., Cd in kidney, paraquat in lung.

2. Selective metabolic activation: Enzymes needed to convert a compound to the active form may be present in highest quantities in a particular organ, e.g., CCl_4, nitrosamines in liver.

3. Characteristics of tissue repair: Some tissues may be protected from toxicity by actively repairing toxic damage; some tissues may be susceptible because they lack sufficient repair capabilities, e.g., nitrosamines in liver.

4. Specific receptors and/or functions: Toxicant may interact with receptors in a given tissue, e.g., curare—a receptor-specific neuromuscular blocker.

5. Physiological sensitivity: The nervous system is extremely sensitive to agents that block utilization of oxygen, e.g., nitrite, oxidizes hemoglobin (methemoglobinemia), cyanide, inhibits cytochrome oxidase (cells not able to utilize oxygen), and barbiturates, interfere with sensors for oxygen and carbon dioxide content in blood.

Q. What are the main target organs most frequently affected by toxicants?
1. Central nervous system
2. Circulatory system (blood, blood-forming system)
3. Visceral organs (liver, kidneys, lung)
4. Muscle and bone.

Q. Why effect or response is observed after administration of any chemical? Give primary assumptions.

Primary assumptions include:
1. There is a molecular site (or receptor) with which the chemical interacts to produce a response.
2. Production of response is related to the concentration of the compound at the active site.
3. The concentration of the compound at the active site is related to the dose administered.

1.10 RISK ASSESSMENT

1.10.1 DEFINITIONS

Q. Define risk.

Risk is defined as the probability of an adverse outcome based upon the exposure and potency of the hazardous agent(s).

Q. Define safety.

Means practical certainty that injury will not result from the use of a substance under specified condition of quantity and manner of use.

Q. Define benefit-to-risk ratio.

This implies that even a toxic agent may warrant use if its benefits for a significant number of people are much greater than the dangers.

Q. Describe briefly risk assessment.

Risk assessment is a quantitative assessment of the probability of deleterious effects under given exposure conditions. It requires an integration of both qualitative and quantitative scientific information. For example, qualitative information about the overall evidence and nature of the end points, and hazards are integrated with quantitative assessment of the exposures, host susceptibility factors, and the magnitude of the hazard. A description of the uncertainties and variability in the estimates is a significant part of risk characterization and an essential component of risk assessment.

Q. Define hazard.

It is the qualitative description of the adverse effect arising from a particular chemical or physical agent with no regard to dose or exposure. The term hazard is related to the risk, but it mainly expresses likelihood or probability of danger, irrespective of dose or exposure.

Or

A property or set of properties of the chemical substance that may cause an adverse health or ecological effect provided if there is an exposure at a sufficient level.

Q. Define acceptable risk.

It is the probability of suffering a disease or injury during exposure to a substance, which is considered to be small but acceptable to the individual.

Q. Define acceptable exposure.

It is the unintentional contact with a chemical or physical agent that results in the harmful effect.

Q. Define margin of exposure.

Margin of exposure is defined as the ratio of the no-observed adverse-effect level (NOAEL) for the critical effect to the theoretical, predicted, or estimated exposure dose or concentration.

Q. Define threshold limit values (TLVs).

The TLVs refer to the airborne concentration of a substance to which it is believed a worker can be exposed day after day for a working lifetime without adverse effects. These values are expressed as time weight concentration for 7- to 8-hour workday and for 40 weeks.

Q. Define no-observed effect level/concentration (NOEL/NOEC).

NOEL/NOEC is the highest dose level/concentration of a substance that under defined conditions of exposure causes no effect (alteration) on morphology, functional capacity, growth, development, or life span of the test animals.

Q. Define no-observed adverse-effect level/concentration (NOAEL/NOAEC).

NOAEL/NOAEC is the highest dose level/concentration of a substance that under defined conditions of exposure causes no observable/detectable adverse effect (alteration) on morphology, functional capacity, growth, development, or life span of the test animals. NOAEL/NOAEC is a variant of NOEL/NOEC that specifies only that the effect in question is adverse (Fig. 1.29).

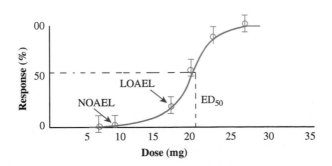

FIGURE 1.29

NOAEL and LOAEL.

Q. Define lowest observed adverse-effect level/concentration (LOAEL/LOAEC).

LOAEL/LOAEC is the highest exposure level/dose level/concentration of a substance under defined conditions of exposure, an observable/ detectable effect (alteration) on morphology, functional capacity, growth, development, or life span of the test animals is observed.

Q. Define reference dose/concentration (RfD/RfC).

For noncancerous effects oral intake (RfD) or an inhalation RfC for airborne materials is calculated using the NOAEL or LOAEL as a starting point. These values are developed from experimentally determined NOAEL or LOAEL.

1.10.2 PRELIMINARY EVALUATION OF RISK ASSESSMENT

Q. Describe briefly the requirement of data for preliminary evaluation of risk assessment in human health.

The type of data required for preliminary evaluation is summarized in Table 1.9.

Table 1.9 Data Required for Preliminary Evaluation of Risk Assessment in Human Health

Data Required	Quality Data
Physiochemical processes	Observed effects on humans
Toxicity	Derived from animal studies
Release/transport/uptake	Applicable to expected dosage
Chemical physical interaction	Most current to support specific conclusions

1.10.3 BASIC ELEMENTS OF RISK ASSESSMENT

Q. What are the basic elements involved in the process of risk assessment?

Four steps used in risk analysis are shown in Fig. 1.30. These steps include:

1. Hazard identification
2. Dose−response evaluation
3. Exposure assessment
4. Risk characterization.

Explanation: The initial step is hazard identification, which identifies the chemical that presents a risk to human health. This is a qualitative step, which involves a thorough evaluation of current scientific evidence, including animal studies, human studies, epidemiological studies, and cellular studies. If a chemical is identified as a potential hazard to human health, the process continues.

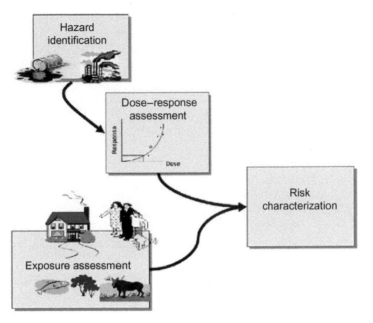

FIGURE 1.30

The four major elements of risk assessment. The information developed in the risk assessment process is utilized in risk management, whereby decisions are made based on the need for and degree of the steps that should be taken to control exposures of chemicals of concern.

NRC, 2007. Models in Environmental Regulatory Decision Making. The National Academies Press, Wasington, DC. Available from: <http://www.nap.edu/read/11972/chapter/4>

    The second step of risk analysis is the dose–response evaluation, which is a quantitative step. This step measures the magnitude of the response at different doses. If available, human studies showing the potency of the agent, or its ability to produce negative health effects in humans, are also assessed.

    The next step is the exposure assessment. This step seeks to estimate people's level of exposure. Exposure refers to the amount of a substance in the environment, and such an estimation includes the length of exposure, duration of exposure, and route of exposure, among other considerations. The difference between the actual dose, or level of a substance taken in, and the amount of the substance measured (exposure) is included in this assessment. This assessment must also quantify various properties of a substance, e.g., volatility, as well as the group exposed and whether the exposure is continuous, intermittent, short term, long term, or chronic.

    The final step is risk characterization. This step uses all of the previously gathered information through the first three steps and creates a picture of risk that describes its likelihood, severity, and consequences. This characterization includes an estimate of the negative effects, e.g., deaths or cancer cases per 100,000 people. The final step also takes into account any limitations and/or uncertainties that were involved in creating the estimate.

1.10.3.1 Hazard identification

Q. Name four steps involved in hazard identification used for risk assessment process.

Hazard identification involves the following four steps:
1. Epidemiology
2. Animal studies
3. Short-term assays
4. Structure—activity relationship.

1.10.3.2 Dose—response assessment

Q. Name three steps involved in dose—response assessment used for risk assessment process.

Dose—response assessment involves the following three steps:
1. Quantitative toxicity information collected
2. Dose—response relationship established
3. Extrapolation of animal data to human.

1.10.3.3 Exposure assessment

Q. Name three steps involved in exposure assessment used for risk assessment process.

Exposure assessment involves the following three steps:
1. Identification of exposed populations
2. Identification of routes of exposure
3. Identification of degree of exposure.

1.10.3.4 Risk characterization

Q. Name three steps involved in risk characterization used for risk assessment process.

Risk characterization involves the following three steps:
1. Estimation of the potential for adverse health effects to occur
2. Evaluation of uncertainty
3. Risk information summarized.

Q. Discuss at least three limitations inherent in risk analysis.

Limitations to risk analysis include:
1. Uncertainty of effect
2. Variability of exposure
3. Possibility of multiple exposures.

Explanation: Often, too little is known about any substance to provide any real assurance. Despite laboratory testing and careful risk analysis, uncertainty will remain. Interpersonal variability may also strongly affect a specific individual's risks, as a general overview may not identify people who may be more sensitive to exposures than others, and thus may have a higher "safe" dose. Multiple exposures are difficult to study, although they certainly exist in the real world. In addition, any additive effects are ignored, which may heighten the risk and which are sure to occur outside of the laboratory. However, despite its limitations, risk analysis is still an important tool to explore and understand risks in the modern world.

1.10.4 ESTABLISHMENT OF AN ACCEPTABLE RFD

Q. How an acceptable RfD is established for risk assessment?

Acceptable RfD is established by the following relationship.

$$RfD = NOAEL/(UF \times MF)$$
$$ADI = NOAEL/(UF \times MF)$$

where the uncertainty factor (UF) is typically equal to 100 and modifying factor (MF).

For cancer end points, the only strictly safe exposure level is at zero dose, although for very small doses the risk is extremely low and is not considered significant.

Explanation: Approaches for characterizing dose—response relationships include identification of effect levels such as LD_{50} (dose producing 50% lethality), LC_{50} (concentration producing 50% lethality), ED_{10} (dose producing 10% response), as well as NOAELs. NOAELs have traditionally served as the basis for risk assessment calculations, such as RfDs or ADI values. RfDs or RfCs are estimates of a daily exposure to an agent that is assumed to be without adverse health impact in humans. The ADIs are used by WHO for pesticides and food additives to define "the daily intake of chemical, which during an entire lifetime appears to be without appreciable risk on the basis of all known facts at that time." RfDs and ADI values typically are calculated from NOAEL values by dividing uncertainty (UF) and/or modifying factors (MF). Tolerable daily intakes can be used to describe intakes for chemicals that are not "acceptable" but are "tolerable" as they are below the levels thought to cause adverse health effects. These are calculated in a manner similar to ADI. In principle, dividing by the uncertainty factors allows for interspecies (animal-to-human) and intraspecies (human-to-human) variability with default values of 10 each. An additional uncertainty factor is used to account for experimental inadequacies—e.g., to extrapolate from short exposure—duration studies to a situation more relevant for chronic study or to account for inadequate numbers of animals or other experimental limitations. If only a LOAEL value is available, then an additional 10-fold factor commonly is used to arrive at a value more comparable to a NOAEL. Traditionally, a safety factor of 100 is used for RfD calculations to extrapolate from a well-conducted animal bioassay (10-fold *factor animal-to-human variability) and to account for human variability in response (10-fold factor human-to-human variability).*

Assumption is made that exposure below a certain level, the NOAEL, will have no adverse health consequences. An acceptable RfD is then established.

1.11 QUESTION AND ANSWER EXERCISES

1.11.1 SHORT QUESTIONS AND ANSWERS

Exercise 1

Q.1 What is toxicology
   The study of adverse effects of agents on living organisms (their identification, chemical properties, biological effects, intervention/prevention).

Q.2 What is the duration of exposure for acute toxicosis/toxicity?
   Less than 24 hours (single or multiple).

Q.3 What is the duration of exposure for subacute toxicosis/toxicity?
   Multiple/continuous: less than 1 month.

Q.4 What is the duration of exposure for subchronic toxicosis/toxicity?
   Multiple/continuous: more than 1 month and less than 3 months.

Q.5 What is the duration of exposure for chronic toxicosis/toxicity?
   Multiple/continuous: more than 3 months.

Q.6 What will be the toxicity rating of a toxic compound having LD_{50} values more than 1000 mg/kg?
   Practically nontoxic.

Q.7 What will be the toxicity rating of a toxic compound having LD_{50} values less than 1000 mg/kg?
   Mild/slightly toxic.

Q.8 What will be the toxicity rating of a toxic compound having LD_{50} values less than 500 mg/kg?
   Moderately toxic.

Q.9 What will be the toxicity rating of a toxic compound having LD_{50} values less than 50 mg/kg?
   Highly toxic.

Q.10 What will be the toxicity rating of a toxic compound having LD_{50} values less than 1 mg/kg?
   Severe/extremely toxic.

Exercise 2

Q.1 What are the assumptions for the dose–response relationship?
   1. Exposure effects—casualty
   2. The target site is affected
   3. The exposure dose gets concentrated at the target site.

Q.2 What do you mean by dose–response characteristics?
1. The severity increases with increase in dose.
2. But variation between individuals is not apparent.

Q.3 What do you interpret from population single dose–response?
1. Spectrum of responses
2. Normal distribution across population
3. Median response.

Q.4 What are end point responses after population dose curve?
1. Lethality
2. Increase in range of doses
3. Minimum dose
4. Maximal dose
5. 50% response dose (LD_{50})
6. Therapeutic index
7. Margin of safety.

Q.5 What is therapeutic index?

LD_{50}/ED_{50}

Q.6 What is margin of safety?

LD_1/ED_{99}

Q.7 What do you mean by the terms, LD_1, ED_{99}, threshold, and threshold dose?

LD_1 = lethal dose for 1% of the population.
ED_{99} = effective dose for 99% of the population.

Threshold = point at which the detoxification pathways and/or the repair mechanisms become saturated/overwhelmed: once threshold is crossed, adverse toxic response is observed.

Threshold dose = theoretical dose where the dose–response curve approaches the x-axis (0% response).

Q.8 Which term(s) is (are) used to determine the population dose–response relationship?
1. LD_{50}
2. Minimum toxic dose
3. Median population response to a single dose plus outliers.

Q.9 What three factors that determine toxicity?
1. Chemical factors
2. Biological factors
3. Exposure factors.

Q.10 What are chemical additive factors?

$1 + 1 = 2$

Exercise 3

Q.1 What are chemical antagonism factors?

$1 + 1 = <2$

Q.2 What are chemical synergism factors?

$1 + 1 = >2$

Q.3 What are biological factors that affect toxicity?

Host: species, age, nutrition, health status

Individual

Environment: housing, ventilation, temperature, soil pH, precipitation.

Q.4 What are species-related factors that affect toxicity?

1. Sex
2. Breed
3. Excretion pathways
4. Anatomy/physiology of gastrointestinal (GI) tract
5. Respiratory tract
6. Target receptor density/subtypes.

Q.5 What are host factors for toxicity, things associated for age?

1. Sex
2. Species/strains
3. Enzyme expression
4. Organ function
5. Presence of protective barriers.

Q.6 Why would a newborn be more sensitive to malathion toxicity than an adult?

Newborn does not have liver enzymes to break it down, and adults do, so more toxic to malathion.

Q.7 Why would a newborn be less toxic to DDT, and adults more toxic?

In newborn, liver enzymes that activate DDT are not present, so not as toxic as in adults.

Q.8 What is the difference between "poison," "toxicant," and "toxin"?

1. Poison is a broader term which includes any/every substance causing harmful effects to living beings.
2. Toxicant is any toxic substance introduced into the environment, e.g., a pesticide, metals, solvents, and gases.
3. Toxin is a poison of plant or animal origin, especially one produced by or derived from microorganisms. This could be of plant (plant toxin), fungal (mycotoxin), animal (zootoxin), or bacteria (bacteriotoxins—endo- and exotoxins) origin.

Q.9 How "toxicosis" differs from "toxicity"?

Toxicosis is the disease or condition (effect) which results due to the exposure to a poison, whereas "toxicity" is the degree of the disease or condition. However, the term toxicity is also used to mean the adverse effects of a poison.

Q.10 How you will categorize toxicity occurring due to repeated exposures?
Within 24 hours: acute toxicity
Within 30 days or less: subacute toxicity
Within 1−3 months: subchronic toxicity
More than 3 months: chronic

Exercise 4

Q.1 What are harmful or adverse effects?
Harmful or adverse effects are those that are damaging to either the survival or normal function(s) of the individual.

Q.2 What is toxicity?
The word "toxicity" describes the degree to which a substance is poisonous or can cause injury. The toxicity depends on a variety of factors: dose, duration and route of exposure, shape and structure of the chemical itself, and individual human factors.

Q.3 What is toxic?
This term relates to poisonous or deadly effects on the body by inhalation (breathing), ingestion (eating), or absorption, or by direct contact with a chemical.

Q.4 What is a toxic symptom?
This term includes any feeling or sign indicating the presence of a poison or foreign substance in the system/body.

Q.5 What are toxic effects?
This term refers to the health effects that occur due to exposure to a toxic substance; also known as a poisonous effect on the body.

Q.6 What is selective toxicity?
Selective toxicity means that a chemical will produce injury to one kind of living matter without harming another form of life, even though the two may exist close together.

Q.7 How does toxicity develop?
Before toxicity can develop, a substance must come into contact with a body surface such as skin, eye, or mucosa of the digestive or respiratory tract. The dose of the chemical, or the amount one comes into contact with, is important when discussing how "toxic" a substance can be.

Q.8 Repeated oral toxicity of a compound is tested in rats for a period of 28 days. What kind of toxicity is being studied here?
It is termed as subacute toxicity.

Q.9 What is the difference between lethal dose (LD_{50} or L_{99}) and lethal concentration (LC)?
Both LD and LC cause death in exposed population. LD refers to the "lethal dose" of the toxicant administered to the animal in any route. LC refers to the "lethal concentration" of toxicant present in feed, water, or air.

Q.10 What is the meaning of the subscripts in the terms LD_{50} or L_{99} and LC_{50}?

The subscripts indicate the percent of mortality (deaths) in exposed population.

Exercise 5

Q.1 For a given compound, between maximum tolerated dose (MTD) and NOAEL, which one will be higher?

NOAEL is the highest dose which will not cause any adverse effect but MTD refers to the highest dose which will cause adverse effects. Hence, MTD is higher than NOAEL (MTD is also referred to as LD).

Q.2 What is the relationship between various toxicity doses with respect to given compound?

LD > MTD > NOAEL > NOEL > ADI > MRL

Q.3 What is a dose?

The dose is the actual amount of a chemical that enters the body. The dose received may be due to either acute, subacute, or chronic (long-term) exposure.

Q.4 What is dose—response?

Dose—response is a relationship between exposure/dose and response/effect that can be established by measuring the response relative to an increasing dose. This relationship is important in determining the toxicity of a particular substance. It relies on the concept that a dose, or a time of exposure (to a chemical, drug, or toxic substance), will cause an effect (response) on the exposed organism. Usually, larger the dose, the greater is response, or the effect. This is the meaning behind the statement "the dose makes the poison."

Q.5 What is the threshold dose?

The threshold dose is the exposure level below which the harmful or adverse effects of a substance are not seen in a population. This dose is also referred to as the NOAEL, or the NOEL. These terms are often used by toxicologists when discussing the relationship between exposure and dose. However, for substances causing cancer (carcinogens), no safe level of exposure exists, since any exposure could result in cancer.

Q.6 What do you mean by "individual susceptibility?"

This term describes the differences in types of responses to hazardous substances, between people. Each person is unique, and because of that, there may be great differences in the response to exposure. Exposure in one person may have no effect, while a second person may become seriously ill, and a third may develop cancer.

Q.7 What is a "sensitive subpopulation?"

A sensitive subpopulation describes those persons who are more at risk from illness due to exposure to hazardous substances than the average, healthy person. These persons usually include the very young, the chronically ill, and the very old. It may also include pregnant women and women of childbearing age. Depending on the type of contaminant, other factors (e.g., age, weight, lifestyle, sex) could be used to describe the population.

Q.8 Define the action of poisons.

Poisons act usually by three ways: locally, remotely, and both locally and remotely.

Locally acting: The chemicals act only at the site of application such as skin/mucosa, e.g., corrosive poisons.

Remotely acting: These act only after being absorbed into the circulatory system, e.g., narcotic poisons and cardiac poisons.

Both locally and remotely acting: These act by local and remote actions, e.g., carbolic acid.

Q.9 Why hemolysis is observed in certain individuals during the administration of drugs like aspirin and sulfonamides?

Some individuals are deficient in the metabolic enzyme G6PD. Drugs like aspirin and sulfonamides cause hemolysis in these individuals.

Q.10 Why rabbit can survive even after eating belladonna leaves?

Rabbit can survive the consumption of *Atropa belladonna* (Belladonna) because they contain the enzyme atropinase, which destroys atropine.

Exercise 6

Q.1 Which breed of dog is more susceptible to the toxic effects of ivermectin?

In Koolies (a breed of dog), ivermectin easily crosses blood—brain barrier and causes neurological symptoms.

Q.2 Why greyhounds are more susceptible to the toxic effects of barbiturates (used as anesthetics)?

Barbiturates mainly distribute to adipose tissue. Greyhounds, have little body fat, resulting in higher circulating concentration of barbiturates causing toxicity.

Q.3 Define lethal dose (LD).

LD is the lowest dose that causes death in any animal during the period of observation. Various percentages can be attached to the LD value to indicate doses required to kill 1% (LD_1), 50% (LD_{50}), or 99% (LD_{99}) of the test animals in the population.

Q.4 Define lethal dose-50 (LD_{50}).

LD_{50} is also known as MLD. It is the dose of the toxicant that causes death of the 50% animals under defined conditions like species, route of exposure, and duration of exposure. It is a commonly used measure of toxicity.

Q.5 Define lethal concentration (LC).

LC is the lowest concentration of the compound in feed (or water in case of fish) that causes death during the period of observation. It is expressed as milligrams of compound per kilogram of feed (or water).

Q.6 Define lethal concentration-50 (LC_{50}).

LC_{50} is the concentration of the compound in feed (or water in case of fish) that is lethal for 50% of exposed population. It mainly expresses acute lethal toxicity.

Q.7 Define maximum allowable or admissible/acceptable concentration (MAC).

MAC is the regulatory value defining the upper limit of concentration of certain atmospheric contaminants allowed in the ambient air of the workplace.

Q.8 Define maximum residue limit/maximum residue level (MRL).

MRL is the maximum amount of a pesticide or grog (mainly veterinary pharmaceutical) residue that is legally permitted or recognized as acceptable in or on food commodities and animal feeds. Although both the terms have the same meaning, in practice the term maximum residue limit is used for the pesticide residue, while the term maximum residue level is applicable for the drug residue.

Q.9 Define maximum tolerated dose (MTD).

MTD is the highest dose/amount of a substance that causes the toxic effects but no morality in the test organism. In chronic toxicity study, the MLD can cause limited toxic effects in the test organism, but it should not decrease the body weight more than 10% compared with control group or produce the overt toxicity (death of cells or organ dysfunction). The value is often denoted by LD_0.

Q.10 Define maximum tolerated concentration (MTC).

MTC is the highest concentration of a substance in an environment medium that causes the toxic symptoms and no mortality in the test organism.

Exercise 7

Q.1 Define absolute lethal dose (LD_{100}).

LD_{100} is the lowest dose of a substance that under defined conditions is lethal for 100% exposed animals. The value is dependent on the number of organisms used in its assessment.

Q.2 Define absolute lethal concentration (LC_{100}).

LC_{100} is the lowest concentration of a substance in an environment medium that under defined conditions is lethal to 100% exposed organisms or species.

Q.3 Define acceptable daily intake (ADI).

ADI is the estimated amount of a substance in food or drinking water that can be ingested daily over a lifetime by humans without appreciable health risk. ADI is normally used for food additives (the term tolerable daily intake is used for contamination).

Q.4 What do you mean by alternative tests (other than use of animals)?

Alternative test is an alternative technique that can provide the same level of information as current animal tests, but which use fewer animals, cause less suffering, or avoid the use of animals completely. Such methods, as they become available, must be considered wherever possible for hazard characterization and consequent classification and labeling for intrinsic hazards and chemical safety assessment.

Q.5 Name different routes of drug administration.

1. GI tract (ingestion, oral, or diet)
2. Lungs (inhalation)
3. Skin (topical, percutaneous, or dermal)
4. Parenteral routes (IV, IP, IM, SC, intradermal, i.e., other than intestinal canal).

Q.6 Describe briefly different routes of drug administration in descending order of effectiveness.

IV > inhalation > IP > SC > IM > intradermal > oral (per os) > dermal > diet.

Q.7 Discuss the route(s) having highest toxicity.

Generally, toxicity is the highest by the route that carries the compound to the bloodstream most rapidly. However, a compound could be more toxic orally than parenterally if an active product is formed in the GI tract. The GI absorption of a compound varies widely. The difference between oral and parenteral LD_{50}'s gives some indication as to the extent of absorption of a compound. The IV toxic dose is greatly influenced by the rate of injection.

Q.8 Describe in brief tolerance.

The toxic reaction of an animal to a given dose of a drug may decrease, remain unchanged, or increase on subsequent daily administration of that dose. A decrease in toxic response is usually called "tolerance," and an increase in toxic response, "hypersusceptibility."

Q.9 How tolerance is developed?

The enzyme induction or the increased activity of the enzymes concerned with detoxification and elimination of the compound is a common mechanism for the development of tolerance to a drug/toxicant on repeated administration.

A decrease in the sensitivity of the end organs to the toxic effects of the drug is also known to cause tolerance. Chlorpromazine, for example, on repeated administration depresses the CNS of normal albino rats and lessens their locomotor activity. On abrupt withdrawal of the drug, the excitatory feedback is no longer balanced by the depressant action of the drug. This is followed by a marked increase in the activity of the brain with insomnia and an increase in locomotor activity.

Q.10 Define benefit-to-risk ratio.

This implies that even a toxic agent may warrant use if its benefits for a significant number of people are much greater than the dangers.

1.11.2 MULTIPLE CHOICE QUESTIONS (CHOOSE THE BEST STATEMENT, IT CAN BE ONE, TWO OR ALL OR NONE)

Exercise 8

Q.1 A toxic substance produced by biological system is specially referred to as a
a. toxicant
b. toxin
c. xenobiotic
d. poison

Q.2 Allergic contact dermatitis is
a. a nonimmune response caused by a direct action of an agent on the skin
b. an immediate type I hypersensitivity reaction
c. a delayed type IV hypersensitivity reaction
d. characterized by the intensity of reaction being proportional to the elicitation dose
e. not involved in photo-allergic reactions

Q.3 The RfD is generally determined by applying which of the following default procedures?
a. An uncertainty factor of 100 is applied to the NOAEL in chronic animal studies
b. A risk factor of 1000 is applied to the NOAEL in chronic animal studies
c. A risk factor of 10,000 is applied to the NOAEL in subchronic animal studies
d. An uncertainty factor between 10,000 and 1 million is applied to the NOEL from chronic animal studies
e. Multiplying the NOAEL from chronic animal studies by 100

Q.4 Which of the following concerning the use of the "benchmark dose" in risk assessment is NOT correct?
a. Can use the full range of doses and responses studied.
b. Allows the use of data obtained from experiments where a clear "no-NOAEL has been attained.
c. May be defined as the lower confidence limit on the 10% effective dose.
d. Is primarily used for the analyses of carcinogenicity data and has limited utility for analyses of developmental and reproduction studies that generate quantal data.
e. Is not limited to the values of the administered doses.

Q.5 Administration by oral gavage of a test compound that is highly metabolized by the liver vs subcutaneous injection will most likely result in

a. less parent compound present in the systemic circulation

b. more local irritation at the site of administration caused by the compound

c. lower levels of metabolites in the systemic circulation

d. more systemic toxicity

e. less systemic toxicity

Q.6 The phrase that best defines "toxicodynamics" is the

a. linkage between exposure and dose

b. linkage between dose and response

c. dynamic nature of toxic effects among various species

d. dose range between desired biological effects and adverse health effects

e. loss of dynamic hearing range due to a toxic exposure

Q.7 Which of the following was banned under the Delaney clause of the Food Additive Amendment of 1958?

a. Butylated hydroxytoluene

b. Sulfamethazine

c. Cyclamate

d. Phytoestrogens

e. Aflatoxin

Q.8 Which of the following is NOT an initiating event in carcinogenesis?

a. DNA adduct formation

b. DNA strand breakage

c. Mutation of proto-oncogenes

d. Oxidative damage of DNA

e. Mitogenesis

Q.9 Which of the following toxicity can occur due to single exposure?

a. Acute toxicity

b. Subacute toxicity

c. Subchronic toxicity

d. Chronic toxicity

Q.10 Which of the following assumptions is NOT correct regarding risk assessment for male reproductive effects in the absence of mechanistic data?

a. An agent that produces an adverse reproductive effect in experimental animals is assumed to pose a potential reproductive hazard to humans.

b. In general, a nonthreshold is assumed for the dose—response curve for male reproductive toxicity.

c. Effects of xenobiotics on male reproduction are assumed to be similar across species unless demonstrated otherwise.

d. The most sensitive species should be used to estimate human risk.

e. Reproductive processes are similar across mammalian species.

Answers

1. b; 2. c; 3. a; 4. d; 5. a; 6. b; 7. c; 8. e; 9. a; 10. b.

Exercise 9

Q.1 Which of the following is characteristic of a nongenotoxic carcinogen?
  a. Has no influence on the promotional stage of carcinogenesis.
  b. Would be expected to produce positive responses in in vitro assays for mutagenic potential.
  c. Typically exerts other forms of toxicity and/or disrupts cellular homeostasis.
  d. Generally shows little structural diversity.
  e. Typically has little effect on cell turnover.

Q.2 A newly formed hapten protein complex usually stimulates the formation of a significant amount of antibodies in
  a. 1−2 minutes
  b. 1−2 hours
  c. 1−2 days
  d. 1−2 weeks

Q.3 Prolonged muscle relaxation after succinylcholine is an example of a/an
  a. immunoglobulin E (IGE)-mediated allergic reaction
  b. idiosyncratic reaction
  c. immune complex reaction
  d. reaction related to a genetic increase in the activity of a liver enzyme

Q.4 Increased production of methemoglobin is due to decreased activity of
  a. cytochrome P450 2B6
  b. NADH cytochrome b5 reductase
  c. cytochrome oxidase
  d. cytochrome a3

Q.5 The most common target organ of toxicity is the
  a. heart
  b. lung
  c. CNS (brain and spinal cord)
  d. skin

Q.6 The organs least involved in systemic toxicity are
  a. brain and peripheral nerves
  b. muscle and bone
  c. liver and kidney
  d. hematopoietic system and lungs

Q.7 If two organophosphate insecticides are absorbed into an organism, the result will be
  a. additive effect
  b. synergistic effect
  c. potentiation
  d. substraction effect

Q.8 If ethanol and carbon tetrachloride are chemically absorbed into an organism, the effect on the liver would be
  a. additive effect
  b. synergy
  c. potentiation
  d. substraction effect
Q.9 If propyl alcohol and carbon tetrachloride are chronically absorbed into an organism, the effect on the liver would be
  a. additive effect
  b. synergistic
  c. potentiation
  d. substraction effect
Q.10 The treatment of strychnine-induced convulsions by diazepam is an example of
  a. chemical antagonism
  b. dispositional antagonism
  c. receptor antagonism
  d. functional antagonism

Answers
1. c, 2. d, 3. b, 4. b; 5. c; 6. b; 7. a; 8. b; 9. c; 10. D.

Exercise 10
Q.1 The use of antitoxin in the treatment of snakebite is an example of
  a. dispositional antagonism
  b. chemical antagonism
  c. receptor antagonism
  d. functional antagonism
Q.2 The use of charcoal to prevent the absorption of diazepam is an example of
  a. dispositional antagonism
  b. chemical antagonism
  c. receptor antagonism
  d. functional antagonism
Q.3 The use of tamoxifen in certain breast cancer is an example of
  a. dispositional antagonism
  b. chemical antagonism
  c. receptor antagonism
  d. functional antagonism
Q.4 Chemicals known to produce dispositional tolerances are
  a. benzene and xylene
  b. trichloroethylene and methylene chloride
  c. paraquat and diaquat
  d. carbon tetrachloride and cadmium

Q.5 The most rapid exposure to a chemical would occur through which of the following routes?
- **a.** Oral
- **b.** Subcutaneous
- **c.** inhalation
- **d.** intramuscular

Q.6 A chemical that is toxic to the brain but which is detoxified in the liver would be expected to be
- **a.** more toxic orally than intramuscularly
- **b.** more toxic rectally than intravenously
- **c.** more toxic via inhalation than orally
- **d.** more toxic on the skin than intravenously

Q.7 The LD_{50} is calculated from
- **a.** a quantal dose–response curve
- **b.** a hormesis dose–response curve
- **c.** a graded dose–response curve
- **d.** a log–log dose–response curve

Q.8 An U-shaped graded toxicity dose–response curve is seen in humans with
- **a.** pesticides
- **b.** sedatives
- **c.** opiates
- **d.** vitamins

Q.9 The TD_1/ED_{99} is called
- **a.** margin of safety
- **b.** therapeutic index
- **c.** potency ratio
- **d.** efficacy ratio

Q.10 All of the following are reasons for selective toxicity except
- **a.** transport differences between cell
- **b.** biochemical differences between cell
- **c.** cytology of male neurons vs female neurons
- **d.** cytology of plant cells vs animal cells

Answers

1. b; 2. a; 3. c; 4. d; 5. c; 6. c; 7. a; 8. d ;9. a ;10. c.

Exercise 11

Q.1 Regulatory toxicology aims at guarding the public from dangerous chemical exposures and depends primarily on which form of study?
- **a.** Observational human studies
- **b.** Controlled laboratory animal studies
- **c.** Controlled human studies
- **d.** Environmental studies

Q.2 Risk from a public health perspective is best described as which of the following?

    a. Undesirable end point is reached

    b. A possibility of a bad outcome

    c. Likelihood of an unwanted outcome combined with uncertainty of when it will occur

    d. A bad outcome is assured and its mechanism is well understood

Q.3 Which of the following statements is true regarding risk analysis?

    a. It is a field of study that has been around for the last century.

    b. It was developed by the pharmaceutical companies in response to concerns over new medications.

    c. It is a relatively new field of study, spurred by new technologically based risks.

    d. It was largely a private sector venture.

Q.4 Which of the following are tools used in risk analysis?

    a. Toxicology

    b. Epidemiology

    c. Clinical trials

    d. All of the above

Q.5 Which of the following are common end points?

    a. Death

    b. No-observable effect level

    c. No-observable adverse-effect level

    d. Lowest observable adverse-effect level

    e. All of the above

Q.6 The LD_{50} is best described as which of the following?

    a. The dose at which 50% of all test animals die

    b. The dose at which 50% of the animals demonstrate a response to the chemical

    c. The dose at which all of the test animals die

    d. The dose at which at least one of the test animals dies

Q.7 The effective dose is best described as which of the following?

    a. The dose at which 50% of all test animals die

    b. The dose at which some of the animals demonstrate a response to the chemical

    c. The dose at which all of the animals demonstrate a response to the chemical

    d. The dose at which 50% of all test animals demonstrate a response to the chemical

Q.8 Extrapolation is best described as which of the following?

    a. Using known information to reach a conclusion

    b. Using known information to infer something about the unknown

    c. Using speculative information to infer something about the known

    d. A "best guess" approach

Q.9 Which of the following assumptions is NOT correct regarding risk assessment for male reproductive effects in the absence of mechanistic data?
  a. An agent that produces an adverse reproductive effect in experimental animals is assumed to pose a potential reproductive hazard to humans.
  b. In general, a nonthreshold is assumed for the dose−response curve for male reproductive toxicity.
  c. Effects of xenobiotics on male reproduction are assumed to be similar across species unless demonstrated otherwise.
  d. The most sensitive species should be used to estimate human risk.
  e. Reproductive processes are similar across mammalian species.
Q.10 Which of the following statements is true?
  a. Chemical carcinogens in animals are always carcinogens in animals.
  b. A chemical that is carcinogenic in humans is usually carcinogenic in at least one animal species.
  c. From a regulating perspective carcinogens are considered to have a threshold dose−response curve.
  d. Arsenic is an example of a chemical that is carcinogenic to humans and nearly all species treated.

Answers

1. b; 2. c; 3. c; 4. d; 5. e; 6. a;7. d; 8. b; 9. b;10. c.

Exercise 12

Q.1 Examples of significant concentrations of a toxicant in a tissue that is not a target organ include all of the following except
  a. lead in bone
  b. DDT in adipose tissue
  c. paraquat in lung
  d. TCDD in adipose tissue
Q.2 The ability of a chemical to cause acute skin and eye irritation is usually evaluated in a
  a. rabbit
  b. rat
  c. mouse
  d. dog
Q.3 Before a potential pharmaceutical compound can be given to humans
  a. an NDA must be filed with the FDA
  b. an IND must be filled with the FDA
  c. acute toxicity studies on four species must be conducted
  d. a 2-year dog carcinogenicity study must be completed
Q.4 Phase I clinical trials are conducted to determine all of the following except
  a. pharmacokinetics
  b. safety
  c. rare adverse effects
  d. preliminary efficacy

Q.5 MTD stands for
  a. minimum tolerated dose
  b. maximum total dose
  c. maximum tolerated dose
  d. maximum threshold dose

Q.6 The acute toxicity study in animals provides
  a. an appropriate lethal dose
  b. information on target organs
  c. information on dose selection for long-term studies
  d. all of the above

Q.7 A subacute toxicity study in rats usually lasts
  a. 3 days
  b. 14 days
  c. 3 months
  d. 6 months

Q.8 The period of organogenesis in rats is
  a. days 3−10
  b. days 7−17
  c. days 12−25
  d. days 17−56

Q.9 A dose of investigational drug that suppresses body weight gain slightly in a 90-day animal study is defined by some regulatory agencies to be
  a. LOAEL
  b. NOAEL
  c. MTD
  d. RfD

Q.10 A subchronic animal study required by the FDA will usually include
  a. two species (usually one rodent and one nonrodents)
  b. both genders
  c. at least three doses (low, intermediate, and high)
  d. all of the above

Q.11 A dose of a compound A is toxic to animals in vivo. Another chemical B is not toxic when given at doses several orders of magnitude higher but when the two are given together the toxic response is greater than that of the given dose of A alone (select the correct answer).
  a. Antagonism
  b. Synergism
  c. Additivity
  d. Potentiation
  e. None of the above

Q.12 Which information may be gained from an acute toxicity study?
  a. No effect level
  b. LD_{50}
  c. Therapeutic index
  d. Target organ
  e. All of the above

Q.13 The therapeutic index is usually defined as
    a. TD_{50}/LD_{50}
    b. ED_{50}/LD_{50}
    c. LD_{50}/ED_{50}
    d. ED_{50}/TD_{50}
    e. LD_{50}/ED_{50}
Q.14 1000 ppm is equivalent to 1%
    a. True
    b. False

Answers

1. c; 2. a; 3. b; 4. c; 5. c; 6. d; 7. b; 8. b; 9. c; 10. d; 11. d; 12. e; 13. c; 14. b.

1.11.3 FILL IN THE BLANKS

Exercise 13

Q.1 The branch of science which deals with the harmful effects of physical and chemical agents of human and animal life is ----------------------------------.
Q.2 In the term toxicology, the word "toxicon" (Greek) means --------------------.
Q.3 The branch of toxicology which deals with diagnosis, treatment, and management of toxic substances is known as ----------------------------------.
Q.4 The development and interpretation of mandatory toxicology testing programs is addressed by ---.
Q.5 Investigating and controlling the toxic effects of various substances on the community is dealt by ----------------------.
Q.6 The study of toxicity produced by substances of plant, animal, and microbial origin is termed as -------------.
Q.7 A foreign chemical substance which is not normally produced in the body or forms a part of the food is known as --------------------.
Q.8 The source of adverse effect/damage is known as ----------------------.
Q.9 The likelihood/probability of adverse effect upon exposure to a hazard is known as --------------------.
Q.10 The statement "all substances are poisons; the dose differentiates poison from a remedy" is associated with -------------------------.

Answers

1. TOXICOLOGY; 2. POISON; 3. CLINICA L TOXICOLOGY; 4. REGULATORY TOX COLOGY; 5 TOXICOVIGILANCE; 6. TOXINOLOGY; 7. XENOIOTIC; 8 HAZARD (e.g., water containing fluoride; here fluoride is the hazard and fluorosis is the adverse effect. Hazard is independent of dose or exposure, i.e., it is present whether someone drinks the water or not). 9. RISK (e.g., while drinking water containing fluoride, the chances of getting fluorosis is called

risk. Risk can range from 0% to 100% depending on dose and exposure, i.e., one should be exposed to a hazard to calculate the risk); 10. PARACELSUS.

Exercise 14

Q.1 The scientist referred to as "father of toxicology" is -----------------------.

Q.2 DDT which is used to control malaria and typhus was discovered by ----------------------------.

Q.3 The person who is known as "father of nerve agents" is ------------------------------.

Q.4 The author of the book *Silent Spring* in which the detrimental effect of DDT and other pesticides on environment—particularly on birds—was documented is -------------------------.

Q.5 Bhopal gas tragedy, which is considered to be the world's worst industrial disaster, was caused due to the leakage of------------------------------------ from Union Carbide fertilizer company.

Q.6 The use of thalidomide in pregnant women for treating women for treating morning sickness led to ------------------------ condition in the infants.

Q.7 If the action of one substance opposes or neutralizes the effect of another substance, the relationship is referred to as -------------------------.

Q.8 Rodents are preferred for oral toxicity testing as they lack ------------------ reflex.

Q.9 Maximum acceptable/permitted amount of a drug present in feed and foods is known as ---.

Q.10 The highest dose of a compound which produces adverse effects but no mortality is called ---.

Answers

1. M.J.B. ORFILA; 2. PAUL HERMANN MULLER; 3 GERHARD SCHRADER; 4. RACHEL CARSON; 5. METHYL-ISOCYANATE (MIC); 6. PHOCOMELIA; 7. ANTAGONISM (all antidotes have antagonistic relationship with their respective toxicants; have antagonistic relationship with the irrespective toxicants); 8. VOMITION; 9. MAXIMUM RESIDUE LEVEL (MRL) (for pesticides—MAXIMUM RESIDUE LIMIT); 10. MAXIMUM TOLERATED DOSE (MTD) (MTD is also referred to as LD_0 (zero) as it will cause adverse effects but no mortality).

Exercise 15

Q.1 If the period of exposure of a toxicant is more than 3 months, the type of study is termed as ---------------------.

Q.2 The type of toxicity which results due to progressive accumulation of a toxicant in the body is known as ------------------------------.

Q.3 The amount of toxicant in food and water which can be consumed daily over a lifetime without any significant health risk is called as ---.

Q.4 Unlawful or criminal killing of animals through administration of poisons is known as ----------------------.

Q.5 Unintentional addition of toxicants and contaminants in feed and water is known as ---------------------.

Q.6 Man-made sources of toxicants are referred to as ----------------------- sources.

Q.7 Genetically determined abnormal reactivity of an individual to a chemical is known as ---------------------------.

Q.8 Failure to elicit a response to an ordinary dose of a substance due prior usage is known as -------------------------.

Q.9 The beneficial effects of toxic substances at low doses are known as -----------------.

Q.10 In the event of irreparable injury, the cell undergoes a process of programmed cell death known as ---------------------------.

Q.11 A substance is classified as extremely toxic if the LD is LESS THAN ------------- and as practically nontoxic if the LD is ------------.

Q.12 The ability of a substance to induce cancer is known as ------------------.

Answers

1. CHRONIC TOXICITY; 2. CUMULATIVE TOXICITY (several toxicants such as heavy metals, alcohol, and DDT cause cumulative toxicity); 3. ACCEPTABLE DAILY INTAKE (ADI); 4. MALICIOUS POISONING; 5. ACCIDENTAL POISONING; 6. ANTHROPOGENIC; 7. IDIOCYNCARY; 8. TOLERANCE (tolerance is generally caused due to the induction of metabolizing enzymes in liver. However, in case of chronic alcoholism, pseudo-tolerance is observed, due to thickened gastrointestinal tract (GIT) mucosa, which reduces absorption); 9. HORMESIS; 10. APOPTOSIS (apoptosis is also involved in a number of physiological processes such as embryogenesis, aging, and cancer prevention); 11.1 mg/kg, 5−15 g/kg (it should be remembered that more the LD of a compound, less is its toxicity); 12. CARCINOGENESIS.

1.11.4 TRUE OR FALSE STATEMENTS (WRITE T FOR TRUE AND F FOR FALSE STATEMENT)

Exercise 16

Q. Write T for true and F for false statement.

Q.1 Environmental risk is a well-understood entity.

Q.2 Cross-sectional studies look at the exposure and disease at the same time.

Q.3 Bias is a problem primarily of clinical trials.

Q.4 Subchronic studies are shorter than acute studies.

Q.5 The lethal dose refers to the dose at which 50% of test animals die.

Q.6 The MTD is the level of chemical exposure where 10% of the animals die.

Q.7 Case–control studies start with the exposure and follow for the disease.
Q.8 Case–control studies are good for rare diseases.
Q.9 Clinical trials look at dose–response in animals.
Q.10 Dose refers to the amount of a substance in the environment.

Answers

1. F; 2. T; 3. F; 4. F; 5. T; 6. F; 7. F; 8. T; 9. F; 10. F.

1.11.5 MATCH THE STATEMENTS

Exercise 17

Q. Match the following statements in Columns A and B.

Column A	Column B
1. Antagonism	a. Program to prevent birth defects
2. TOCP	b. Programs human risk assessment
3. Probit unit	c. Idiosyncratic-prolonged apnea
4. Synergy	d. Delayed neurotoxicity
5. Succinylcholine	e. Normal equivalent derivation plus 5
6. STEPS	f. $4 + 0 = 1$
7. Superfund Act	g. Toxicology and the law
8. Descriptive toxicology	h. $2 + 3 = 10$
9. Regulatory toxicology	i. Performs toxicology testing
10. Forensic toxicology	j. Studies/treats human disease caused by toxins
11. Clinical toxicology	k. Support to clean toxic-waste sites

Answers

1. Antagonism	f. $4 + 0 = 1$
2. TOCP	d. Delayed neurotoxicity
3. Probit unit	e. Normal equivalent derivation plus 5
4. Synergy	h. $2 + 3 = 10$
5. Succinylcholine	c. Idiosyncratic-prolonged apnea
6. STEPS	a. Program to prevent birth defects
7. Superfund Act	k. Support to clean toxic-waste sites
8. Descriptive toxicology	i. Performs toxicology testing
9. Regulatory toxicology	b. Programs human risk assessment
10. Forensic toxicology	g. Toxicology and the law
11. Clinical toxicology	j. Studies/treats human disease caused by toxins

FURTHER READING

Bert Hakkinen, P.J., Kennedy, G., Stoss, F.W., 2000. Information Resources in Toxicology, third ed. Academic Press, San Diego, CA.

Cope, W.G., Leidy, R.B., Hodgson, E., 2010. Classes of Toxicants: Use Classes, A Textbook of Modern Toxicology, fourth ed. John Wiley & Sons, NJ, pp. 49–73.

Eaton, D.L., Gilbert, S.G., 2013. Principles of toxicology. In: Klaassen, C.D. (Ed.), Casarett and Doull's Toxicology: The Basic Science of Poisons, eighth ed. McGraw-Hill, New York, NY, pp. 13–48.

Faustman, E.M., Omenn, G.S., 2013. Risk assessment. In: Klaassen, C.D. (Ed.), Casarett and Doull's Toxicology: The Basic Science of Poisons, eighth ed. McGraw-Hill, New York, NY, pp. 123–150.

Gallo, M.A., 2013. History and scope of toxicology. In: Klaassen, C.D. (Ed.), Casarett and Doull's Toxicology: The Basic Science of Poisons, eighth ed. McGraw-Hill, New York, NY, pp. 3–12.

Gupta, P.K., 1988. Veterinary Toxicology. Cosmo Publications, New Delhi, India (Chapter 2).

Gupta, P.K., 2010. Natural laws concerning toxicology. In: second reprint Gupta, P.K. (Ed.), Modern Toxicology: Basis of Organ and Reproduction Toxicity, vol. 1. PharmaMed Press, Hyderabad, India, pp. 17–70.

Gupta, P.K., 2010. Introduction and brief history. In: 2nd reprint Gupta, P.K. (Ed.), Modern Toxicology: Basis of Organ and Reproduction Toxicity, vol. 1. PharmaMed Press, Hyderabad, India, pp. 1–26.

Gupta, P.K., 2014. Essential Concepts in Toxicology. BSP Pvt Ltd., Hyderabad, India (Chapter 1).

Gupta, P.K., 2016. Fundamental in Toxicology: Essential Concepts and Applications in Toxicology. Elsevier/BSP, San Diego, USA (Chapters 5 and 6).

Hodgson, E.A., 2010a. Future considerations for environmental and human. In: Hodgson, E.A. (Ed.), A Textbook of Modern Toxicology, fourth ed. John Wiley & Sons, NJ, pp. 521–524.

Hodgson, E.A., 2010b. Introduction to toxicology. In: Hodgson, E.A. (Ed.), A Textbook of Modern Toxicology, fourth ed. John Wiley & Sons, NJ, pp. 3–12.

LeBlanc, G.A., 2010. Acute toxicity. In: Hodgson, E.A. (Ed.), A Textbook of Modern Toxicology, fourth ed. John Wiley & Sons, NJ, pp. 213–224.

Merchant, G.E., 2013. Regulatory toxicology. In: Klaassen, C.D. (Ed.), Casarett and Doull's Toxicology: The Basic Science of Poisons, eighth ed. McGraw-Hill, New York, NY, pp. 1413–1426.

Merwe, van der D., Pickrell, J.A., 2018. Toxicity of nanomaterials. In: Gupta, R.C. (Ed.), Veterinary Toxicology: Basic and Clinical Principles, third ed. Academic Press/Elsevier, San Diego, USA, pp. 319–326.

Rao, G.N., 2010. Textbook of Forensic Medicine & Toxicology. JaypeeBrothes Medical Publishers, New Delhi, India (Chapters 31–33).

Ronald, E.B., 2010. Human health risk assessment. In: Hodgson, E.A. (Ed.), A Textbook of Modern Toxicology, fourth ed. John Wiley & Sons, NJ, pp. 423–437.

Semler, D.E., 1992. The rat toxicology. In: Gad, S.C., Chengelis, C.P. (Eds.), Animal Models in Toxicology. Marcel Dekker Inc, pp. 21–164.

Shea, D., 2010. Environmental risk assessment. In: Hodgson, E.A. (Ed.), A Textbook of Modern Toxicology, fourth ed. John Wiley & Sons, NJ, pp. 501−517.

Thorne, P.S., 2013. Occupational toxicology. In: Klaassen, C.D. (Ed.), Casarett and Doull's Toxicology: The Basic Science of Poisons, eighth ed. McGraw-Hill, New York, NY, pp. 1274−1292.

Timbrell, J.A., 2009. Fundamental of toxicology and dose response relationship, Principles of Biochemical Toxicology, fourth ed. Informa, New York, NY, pp. 7−33.

Disposition

2

CHAPTER OUTLINE

2.1 ABSORPTION

Q. Define absorption.

Absorption is defined as the process of movement of unchanged compound from its sites of administration or exposure to the bloodstream.

Q. Define distribution of xenobiotics.

Distribution may be defined as a process by which xenobiotics move throughout the body and reach their site of action (extracellular fluid and tissues).

Explanation: Once absorbed, a toxicant typically enters the interstitial fluid at the site of absorption and then passes into the tissue cells or enters the blood and/or lymph. Blood is moved rapidly through the body by the cardiovascular

Illustrated Toxicology. DOI: http://dx.doi.org/10.1016/B978-0-12-813213-5.00002-X

circulatory system and this process constitutes the major mechanism whereby absorbed chemicals are distributed to the various organs and tissues of the body. The entrance of xenobiotics to some tissues is restricted by special barriers (e.g., blood—brain barrier, blood—testes barrier, and blood—placenta barrier) that form continuous cellular layers with tight junctions that prevent movement of toxicants into tissues by passive diffusion through intercellular spaces. To gain entry into these protected tissues, toxicants must pass through lipid cell membranes, either by penetrating the lipid membranes directly or by active or facilitated transport through transmembrane transporter proteins.

Q. Define excretion of xenobiotics.

Excretion may be defined as a process by which toxicants and/or their metabolites are irreversibly transferred from body to external environment. Thus excretion is one of the primary mechanisms of protecting the body from the toxic effects of toxicants through the elimination of these compounds from the body. Compounds that are rapidly eliminated are less likely to accumulate in tissues and damage critical cells. Although the terms elimination and excretion are sometimes used synonymously, the former term encompasses all the processes that decrease the amount of parent compound in the body, including biotransformation.

Q. Define ADME.

ADME is an abbreviation in pharmacokinetics and pharmacology for "absorption, distribution, metabolism, and excretion," and describes the disposition of a pharmaceutical compound within an organism.

Q. Discuss briefly translocation of xenobiotics and their mechanism of transport across membranes.

Translocations may take place through different mechanisms such as passive process or active process as given in Table 2.1.

Table 2.1 Transfer of Molecules Across Biological Membranes

Transfer Process	Mechanism	Substrate Specificity
Passive diffusion	Diffusion through lipoidal membrane down a concentration gradient	None, most foreign compounds
Filtration	Diffusion through aqueous pores in the membrane down to concentration gradient	Hydrophilic molecules and ions of the molecular weight, e.g., water, urea
Facilitated diffusion	Carrier transport through membrane down a concentration gradient. Saturated by excess substrate	Narrow, mainly for molecules concerned with process of intermediary metabolism, e.g., sugars and amino-acids
Active transport	Carrier transport through membrane against a concentration gradient requires metabolic energy. Saturated by excess substrate	Narrow, mainly for molecules concerned with process of intermediary metabolism, e.g., sugars and amino-acids
Pinocytosis	Invaginations of the membrane absorbs extracellular material	Uncertain

Q. What are the primary routes of exposure for toxic substances?

Following are the routes of exposure:

1. Oral

2. Respiratory

3. Dermal

4. Parenteral.

Explanation: Oral or gastrointestinal (GI), respiratory, and dermal systems are lined with epithelia that present significant barriers to the entry of foreign substances due to tight junctions between their cells, or continuous lipid layers in the case of skin. The onset, duration, and intensity of a substance's toxic effects are therefore dependent on the toxicant's ability to permeate lipid cell membranes directly and its interactions with transporter proteins. Dermal penetration is unique in the sense that the outer epithelial cellular layers (corneocytes) are nonviable and do not contain transporter proteins. Absorption, in this case, is therefore dependent on the ability of the toxicants to penetrate the intercellular lipid matrix found between corneocytes.

The plasma membranes surrounding all these cells are remarkably similar (such as the stratified epithelium of the skin, the thin cell layers of the lungs or the GI tract, capillary endothelium, and ultimately the cells of the target organ). The plasma membranes surrounding all these cells are remarkably similar.

Q. What is plasma membrane?

The biological cell has a fundamental structure, the cell membrane, or, as it is often called, the plasma membrane. The thickness of the membranes is of the order of 100 Å.

Explanation: The majority of chemicals to which most of the population is exposed are organic acids or bases. An acid with a low pKa is a strong acid and one with a high pKa is a weak acid. Conversely, a base with a low pKa is a weak base and one with a high pKa is a strong base. The weak acids are absorbed readily from the stomach because they all are almost completely nonionized at the gastric pH. Weak bases are not absorbed well; indeed, they would tend to accumulate within the stomach at the expense of the chemical agent in the bloodstream. Naturally, in the more alkaline intestine, bases would be absorbed better, acids more poorly.

The concentration of a chemical that is in ionized or in nonionized form depends on both pKa of the chemical and the pH of the solution in which it is dissolved. The relationship may be derived by mathematical transformation of Henderson—Hasselbalch equation:

For weak acidic compound

$$pKa - pH = \log \frac{\text{conc. of unionized compound}}{\text{conc. of ionized compound}}$$

$$\% \text{ ionized compound} = \frac{100}{1 + \text{antilog (pKa} - \text{pH)}}$$

For weak basic compound

$$pH - pKa = \log \frac{\text{conc. of unionized compound}}{\text{conc. of ionized compound}}$$

$$\% \text{ ionized compound} = \frac{100}{1 + \text{antilog (pH - pKa)}}$$

It is therefore assumed that the gastric mucosal wall acts as a simple lipoid barrier which is permeable only to the lipid soluble, nondissociated form of the acid. Thus, in plasma, the ratio of nonionized to ionized drug is 1:1000; in gastric juice, the ratio is 1:0.001. The total concentration ratio between the plasma and the gastric sides of the barrier is therefore 1000:1. For a weak base with a pKa of 4.4, the ratio is reversed.

Q. Draw a schematic representation of absorption, distribution, and excretion, the possible toxicokinetic fate of a chemical after exposure by inhalation, dermal contact, and ingestion.

Fig. 2.1 shows the schematic representation of absorption, distribution, and excretion, the possible toxicokinetic fate of a chemical after exposure by inhalation, dermal contact, and ingestion.

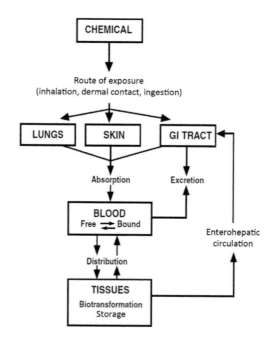

FIGURE 2.1

Schematic representation of absorption, distribution, and excretion, the possible fate of a chemical after exposure by inhalation, dermal contact, and ingestion.

2.2 DISTRIBUTION

Q. Describe the factors that determine a compound's rate and extent of distribution.

Factors that influence distribution include:

1. Molecular size, i.e., physicochemical properties of compound
2. Lipophilicity
3. Plasma protein and tissue binding
4. Blood flow and organ size
5. Special compartmental and barriers, e.g., blood−brain barrier, blood−cerebrospinal barrier, placental barrier, and other barriers
6. Availability of special transport system
7. The ability to interact with transmembrane transporter proteins
8. Disease state, etc.

Explanation: After absorption into the bloodstream, the chemicals penetrate into the various fluid compartments: (1) plasma, (2) interstitial fluid, (3) transcellular fluid, and (4) cellular fluids. The nonionized lipid/soluble fractions penetrate most readily. Some chemicals may accumulate in various areas as a result of binding or due to their affinity for fat.

Q. Describe the important blood−organ barriers for transport of xenobiotics.

For transport of xenobiotics, the effective tight junction occurs at the level of capillary endothelium, e.g., brain, placenta, and thymus barriers. These barriers are called blood−organ barriers. In blood−bile barriers, the blood has direct access to the membranes of the hepatocytes. Tight junctions formed by adjacent hepatocytes constitute the physical barrier immediately interposed between blood and bile. Some of the so-called blood−organ barriers do not directly involve the blood. For example, in blood−urine barrier, tight junction occurs near the luminal surface of bladder epithelial cells and in the blood−testes barriers within the seminiferous tubules. Thus blood−testes barrier resembles the blood−urine barriers more than the blood−brain barriers with which it is often compared. A few important barriers are:

1. Blood−brain barrier
2. Placental barrier
3. Blood−testes barrier.

Q. Describe in brief different factors that affect distribution and tissue retention of drugs.

The following factors affect the distribution and retention of drugs:

1. Blood flow
2. Volume of distribution
3. Enzyme induction
4. Chemical interaction
5. Age and sex differences
6. Genetic factors

7. Binding with proteins
8. Storage in various body tissues including brain and fat.

2.3 EXCRETION

Q. Discuss briefly the routes of excretion of xenobiotics.

The principal organ of excretion is called renal excretion, and excretion by organs other than kidneys is known as extra-renal or nonrenal excretion.

The biliary route of excretion plays a major role in the elimination of anions, cations, and nonionized molecules containing both polar and lipophilic groups. The biliary excretion of foreign compounds varies with species and is generally highest in the dog and rat. The hepatic excretory system is not fully developed in the infants and is an additional reason for some compounds being more toxic in infants than in the adults. More information is required to see if increased toxicity of some compounds in the infants is due to this reason.

In addition to renal excretion, there are nonrenal or extra-renal excretion through GI tract, expired air, sweat, saliva, milk, vaginal secretions, and other routes such as lachrymal fluid, intestinal fluid, and tracheobronchial secretions.

2.4 BIOTRANSFORMATION

Q. What is disposition of a chemical?

The disposition of a chemical or xenobiotic is defined as the composite actions of its absorption, distribution, biotransformation, and elimination.

Explanation: To reach the target site, the toxicant must be absorbed effectively into bloodstream, distributed efficiently to the site of action, and subsequently metabolized and excreted from the body. The processes of absorption and distribution are responsible for the placement or deployment of these toxicants in the body, and metabolism and excretion for elimination of the toxicant from the body. All these processes involve passage across biological membranes.

Q. What are the functions of biotransformation? Give suitable examples.

Biotransformation performs the following functions:

1. It causes conversion of an active compound to less active called inactivation or detoxification. Examples are phenobarbitone to *p*-hydroxyphenobarbitone; dichlorodiphenyltrichloroethane (DDT) to metabolite products dichlorodiphenyldichloroethylene (DDE) and dichlorodiphenyldichloroethane (DDD).

2. It causes conversion of an active compound to more active metabolite(s) called bioactivation. Examples are malathion to malaoxon or parathion to paraoxon and acetonitrile to cyanide.

3. It causes conversion of an inactive compound (i.e., pro-drug or precursor compound) to active metabolite(s) called activation. Examples are phenacetin to paracetamol, thiocyanates to cyanide.

4. It causes conversion of an active compound to equally active metabolite(s) (no change in the activity). Examples are dichrotophos to monochrotophos, digitoxin to digoxin.

5. It causes conversion of an active compound to active metabolite(s) having entirely pharmacological/toxicological activity (change in activity). Examples are iproniazid (antidepressant) to isoniazid (antitubercular), aflatoxin B1 (hepatotoxin) to aflatoxin M1 (carcinogen).

2.4.1 METABOLIZING ENZYMES

Q.1 What are xenobiotic metabolizing enzymes?

These enzymes can be divided into two main groups:

1. Microsomal enzymes
2. Nonmicrosomal enzymes.

Microsomal enzymes: These enzymes are present in the endoplasmic reticulum (ER) (especially smooth) of liver and other tissues.

Nonmicrosomal enzymes: Enzymes occurring in organelles/sites other than microsomes are called nonmicrosomal enzymes. These are usually present in the cytoplasm, plasma, and mitochondria.

Q.2 Describe briefly the fine pathways of biotransformation.

The major transformation reactions for xenobiotics are divided into two phases known as phase I and phase II.

1. Phase I reactions (nonsynthetic or nonconjugative phase)

Phase I reactions modify the compound's structure by adding a functional group. This allows the substance to interact with a reactive group, such as $-OH$, SH, $-NH_2$, or $-COOH$. Most of these reactions involve different types of microsomal enzymes, except a few where reactions involve nonmicrosomal enzymes. Phase I reactions usually yield products with decreased activity. However, some may give rise to products with similar or even greater activity.

Oxidation: It is the most common reaction and may take place in a number of ways such as hydroxylation, deamination, desulfurization, dealkylation, or sulfoxide formation.

In the biotransformation of lipophilic xenobiotics, microsomal oxidation is the most prominent reaction where microsomal enzymes associated with smooth ER of hepatocytes are involved and the enzyme cytochrome P450, a heme protein, which is a part of an enzyme system termed as mixed function oxidase (MFO) system, plays an important role.

The other enzyme systems of phase I biotransformation are involved in metabolism when the appropriate functional groups are available, e.g., alcohol dehydrogenase is involved in the biotransformation of alcohols and aldehydes, monomine oxidase is a flavin adenine dinucleotide (FAD)-containing enzyme that catalyzes the oxidative deamination. Epoxide hydrolases are enzymes that add water across epoxide bonds to form diols. A number of carbroxyl esterases are responsible for biotransformation of certain compounds including organophosphates. The extent to which these metabolic reactions take place appear to vary with the species.

Reduction: Reduction is acceptance of one or more electrons(s) or their equivalent from another substrate. Biotransformation by reduction is also capable of generating polar functional groups such as hydroxyl and amino groups which can undergo further biotransformation or conjugation. Many reductive reactions are exact opposite of oxidative reactions.

Hydrolysis: It is the process of cleaving of a foreign compound by the addition of water. It occurs both in the cytoplasm and in the smooth ER. It is an important metabolic pathway for compounds with an ester linkage (−CO, O−) or an amide (−CO, HN−) bond. The cleavage of esters or amides generates nucleophilic compounds which undergo conjugation.

2. Phase II reactions or conjugation/synthetic reactions

Phase II reactions (conjugation/synthetic reactions) includes reactions that catalyze conjugation of xenobiotics or their phase I metabolites with endogenous substances with a water-soluble molecule. In phase II, most of the reactions involve nonmicrosomal process (except a few that involve microsomal enzyme). Due to biotransformation, the water solubility of a compound is typically increased.

Synthetic reactions may take place when a xenobiotic or a polar metabolite of phase I metabolism containing −OH, −COOH, −NH$_2$, or −SH group that undergoes further transformation to generate nontoxic products of high polarity which are highly water soluble and readily excretable by combining with some hydrophilic endogenous moieties. Conjugating agents are glucuronic acid, acetyl, sulfate, glycine, cysteine, methionine, and glutathione which conjugate with different functional groups of xenobiotics.

Most of the phase II biotransforming enzymes are located in the cytosol with the exception of uridine diphosphate (UDP) glucuronyl transferase (UGT) which is a microsomal enzyme.

Q.3 What do you understand by induction or inhibition of metabolizing enzymes?

1. Induction of enzymes

Several drugs and chemicals have the ability to increase the metabolizing activity of enzymes called enzyme induction. Microsomal enzyme induction by drugs and chemicals usually requires repetitive administration of the inducing agent over a period of several days and the induction, once started, may continue for several days. Metabolizing enzyme induction has great clinical importance because it affects the plasma half-life and duration of action of xenobiotics.

Q.4 Inhibition of enzymes

Contrary to metabolizing enzyme induction, several drugs and chemicals have the ability to decrease the metabolizing activity of certain enzymes called enzyme inhibition. Enzyme inhibition can be either nonspecific of chromosomal enzymes or specific of some nonmicrosomal enzymes (e.g., monoamine oxidase, cholinesterase, and aldehyde dehydrogenase). The inhibition of hepatic microsomal enzymes mainly occurs due to administration of hepatotoxic agents, which cause either rise in the rate of enzyme degradation (e.g., carbon tetrachloride and carbon disulfide) or fall in the rate of enzyme synthesis (e.g., puromycin and dactinomycin). Enzyme inhibition may also produce undesirable xenobiotic interactions.

2.4.2 BIOACTIVATION

Q. Describe briefly bioactivation.

Formation of harmful or highly reactive metabolic from relatively inert/nontoxic chemical compounds is called bioactivation or toxication. The bioactive metabolites often interact with the body tissues to precipitate one or more forms of toxicities such as carcinogenesis, teratogenesis, and tissue necrosis.

The bioactivation reactions are generally catalyzed by cytochrome P450-dependent monooxygenase systems, but some other enzymes like those in intestinal flora are also involved in some cases. The reactive metabolites primarily belong to three main categories—electrophiles, free radicals, and nucleophiles. The formation of electrophiles and free radicals from relatively harmless substances/xenobiotics account for most toxicities.

2.4.3 ELECTROPHILES

Q. Define electrophiles.

Electrophiles are molecules which are deficient in electrons pair with a positive charge that allows them to react by sharing electron pairs with electron-rich atoms in nucleophiles. Important electrophiles are epoxides, hydroxyamines, nitroso and azoxy derivatives, nitrenium ions, and elemental sulfur. These eletrophiles form covalent binding to nucleophilic tissue components such as macromolecules (proteins, nucleic acids, and lipids) or low molecular weight cellular constituents to precipitate toxicity. Covalent binding to DNA is responsible for carcinogenicity and tumor formation.

Q. Define free radicals.

Free radicals are molecules which contain one or more unpaired electrons (odd number of electrons) in their outer orbit.

Q. Define nucleophiles.

Nucleophiles are molecules with electron-rich atoms. Formation of nucleophiles is a relatively uncommon mechanism for toxicants. Examples of toxicity induced through nucleophiles include formation of cyanides from amygdalin, acrylonitrile, and sodium nitroprusside and generation of carbon monoxide from dihalomethane.

2.5 TOXICOKINETICS

Q. What is toxicokinetics?

Toxicokinetics (often abbreviated as "TK") is the description of what rate a chemical will enter the body and what happens to it once it is in the body.

Q. What do you mean by extravascular (EV) administration?

Drug or toxicant administration by any other route than the intravenous (IV) route is called EV administration.

Q. Define minimum effective concentration (MEC)

MEC is the minimum concentration of drug in plasma required to produce the desirable pharmacological/therapeutic response (Fig. 2.2). In case of antimicrobials, the term minimum inhibitory concentration (MIC) is used, which may be defined as the minimum concentration of antimicrobial agent in plasma required to inhibit the growth of microorganisms.

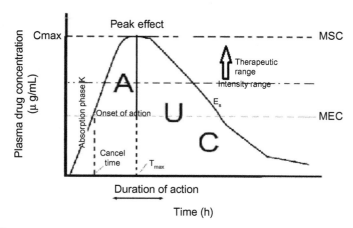

FIGURE 2.2

Plasma concentration—time profile of drug/toxicant after oral administration of a single dose of a toxicant. K_a, absorption rate constants (absorption phase); $E\beta$, elimination rate constant (elimination phase).

Q. Define maximum safe concentration (MSC) or minimum toxic concentration (MTC)

MSC or MTC is the concentration of drug in plasma above which toxic effects are produced. Concentration of drug above MSC is said to be in toxic level. The drug concentration between MEC and MSC represents the therapeutic range (Fig. 2.2).

Q. Define maximum plasma concentration/peak plasma concentration (C_{max} or Cp_{max}).

Maximum plasma concentration/peak plasma concentration is the point of maximum concentration of drug in plasma. The maximum plasma concentration depends on the administered dose and rates of absorption (absorption rate constant, K_a) and elimination (elimination rate constant, β). The peak represents the point of time when absorption equals elimination rate of the drug. It is often expressed as μg/mL.

Q. Define area under curve (AUC).

AUC is the total integrated area under the plasma drug concentration−time curve. It expresses the total amount of drug that comes into systemic circulation after administration of the drug (Fig. 2.2).

Q. Define peak effect.

Peak effect is the maximal or peak pharmacological or toxic effect produced by the drug. It is generally observed at peak plasma concentration (Fig. 2.2).

Q. Define time of maximum concentration/time of peak concentration (t_{max}).

Time of maximum concentration/time of peak concentration is the time required for a drug to reach peak concentration in plasma. The faster the absorption rate, the lower is the t_{max}. It is also useful in assessing the efficacy of the drugs used to treat acute conditions (e.g., pain) which can be treated by a single dose. It is expressed in hours.

Q. Define onset of action.

Onset of action is the beginning of pharmacological or toxicological effect or response produced by the drug. It occurs when the plasma drug concentration just exceeds the MEC (Fig. 2.2).

Q. Define onset time

Onset time is the time required for the drug to start producing pharmacological or toxic response. It usually corresponds to the time for the plasma concentration to reach MEC after administration of the drug (Fig. 2.2).

Q. Define duration of action

Duration of action is the time period for which pharmacological or toxic response is produced by the drug. It usually corresponds to the duration for which the plasma concentration of drug remains above the MEC level (Fig. 2.2).

Q. What is zero-order process or kinetics?

Zero-order process (zero-order kinetics or constant-rate kinetics) is defined as a toxicokinetic process whose rate is independent of the concentration of the xenobiotic/chemical, i.e., the rate of toxicokinetic process remains constant and cannot be increased further by increasing their concentration of xenobiotic.

Q. What is first-order process or kinetics?

First-order process (first-order kinetics or linear kinetics) is defined as a toxicokinetic process whose rate is directly proportional to the concentration of the xenobiotic/chemical, i.e., greater the concentration, faster is the process.

Q. What is mixed-process or mixed-order kinetics?

Mixed-process (mixed-order kinetics, nonlinear kinetics, or dose-dependent kinetics) is defined as a toxicokinetic process whose rate is a mixture of both zero-order and first-order processes. The mixed-order process follows zero-order kinetics at high concentration and the first-order kinetics at lower concentration of the xenobiotic. This type of kinetics is usually observed at increased or multiple doses of some chemicals.

2.5.1 TOXICOKINETIC MODELS

Q. Name three toxicokinetic models that are commonly used.
1. Classic toxicokinetics (traditional)
2. Noncompartment models/noncompartment analysis
3. Physiological models.

Q. What are classic toxicokinetic models?

Classic toxicokinetic modeling (traditional) is simplest mean of gathering information on absorption, distribution, metabolism, and elimination of a compound and examining the time course of blood or plasma toxicant concentration over time. In this approach the body represents a system of one or two compartments (sometimes more than two compartments) even though the compartments do not have exact correspondence to anatomical structures or physiological processes.

Q. What are the advantages of classic models?
1. They do not require information on tissue physiology or anatomic structure.
2. They are useful in predicting the toxicant concentrations in blood at different doses.
3. They are useful in establishing the time course of accumulation of the toxicant, either in its parent form or as biotransformed products during continuous or episodic exposures, in defining concentration−response (vs dose−response) relationships.
4. They provide help/guidance in the choice of effective dose and design of dosing regimen in animal toxicity studies.

Q. Define one-compartment open model.

One-compartment open model is the simplest model which considers the whole body as a single, kinetically homogeneous unit; in this model, the final distribution equilibrium between the chemical in plasma and other body fluids is attained rapidly and maintained at all times (Figs. 2.3 and 2.4).

Q. Define two-compartment open model.

Two-compartment open model assumes that body is composed of two compartments—the central compartment and peripheral compartment. The central compartment (compartment 1) consists of blood and highly perfused organs like liver, kidney, lungs, heart, and brain; the less perfused tissues (compartment 2) like skin, muscles, bone, and cartilage make the peripheral compartment (Fig. 2.5).

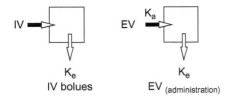

FIGURE 2.3

Schematic representation of one-compartment model. K_a, first absorption rate constant; K_e, first-order elimination rate constant (from central compartment).

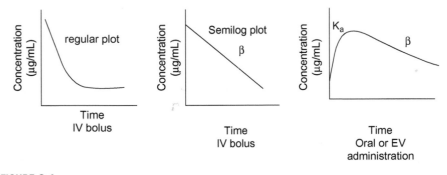

FIGURE 2.4

Graph showing one-compartment open model following IV bolus and oral or EV route of a single dose of toxicant. After IV bolus the curve is a straight line on semilogarithmic paper and shows monophasic decline. In contrast to IV bolus, after oral or EV administration (instead of a straight line), there are two exponents, i.e., absorption and elimination phase.

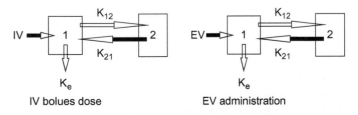

FIGURE 2.5

Schematic representation of two-compartmental model. K_a, first absorption rate constant; K_e, first-order elimination rate constant (from central compartment); K_{12}, first-order rate constant for the toxicant transfer central (1) to peripheral (2) compartments; K_{21}, first-order rate constant for the toxicant transfer peripheral (2) to central (1) compartments.

Q. Describe the shape of time curve in two-compartment model.

In two-compartment open model, after IV bolus or EV administration of a single dose of toxicant the curve is biexponential. As shown in Fig. 2.6 linear terminal portion is elimination phase β (Fig. 2.7).

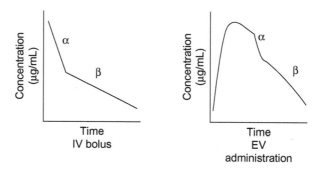

FIGURE 2.6

Graph showing two-compartment open model following IV bolus and EV administration of a single dose of toxicant (curve is biexponential). Linear terminal portion is elimination phase β.

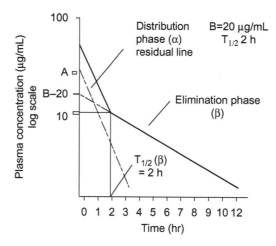

FIGURE 2.7

Time curve in two-compartment model showing half-life and elimination phase.

Q. Describe three-compartment open model.

The toxicokinetic behavior of some chemicals, which have a high affinity for a particular tissue and are under redistribution, is best interpreted according to a three-compartment open model. Body is conceived as consisting of three compartments—one central and two peripheral compartments (Fig. 2.8). The central compartment (compartment 1) comprises

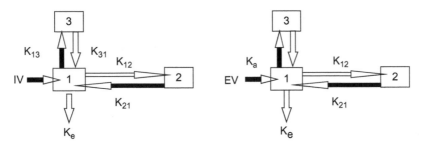

FIGURE 2.8

Schematic representation of various compartmental (one, two, and three) models. K_a, first absorption rate constant; K_e, first-order elimination rate constant (from central compartment); K_{12}, first-order rate constant for the toxicant transfer central (1) to peripheral (2) compartments; K_{21}, first-order rate constant for the toxicant transfer peripheral (2) to central (1) compartments; K_{13}, first-order rate constant for the toxicant transfer central (1) to peripheral (3) compartments; K_{31}, first-order rate constant for the toxicant transfer peripheral (3) to central (1) compartments.

plasma and highly perfused organs, whereas peripheral compartment 2 comprises moderately (e.g., skin and muscles) and compartment 3 poorly perfused tissues (e.g., bone, teeth, ligaments, hair, and fat). If any chemical is administered IV, it is first distributed immediately into the highly perfused tissues (compartment 1), then slowly into the moderately perfused tissues (compartment 2), and thereafter very slowly to the poorly perfused tissues (compartment 3). If plasma level–time profile is plotted on semilogarithmic graph, it gives triexponential appearance.

Q. Define the term half-life.

Half-life ($T_{1/2}$) may be defined as the time taken for the concentration of a compound/toxicant in plasma to decline by ½ or 50% of its initial value (or it may be defined as the time required for the body to eliminate half of the chemical). This value is determined during the elimination phase of a chemical; therefore, it is called elimination half-life (Fig. 2.9).

Q. What is bioavailability?

After oral or EV routes, often only a fraction of the total dose to which an animal or human is exposed gets absorbed systemically. This fraction is referred to as the bioavailability (F). Bioavailability is determined by measuring the area under plasma drug concentration vs time curve (AUC) after oral or EV routes. This is compared with AUC measured after IV bolus administration of the same drug.

If the AUC for both curves are equal, bioavailability is 100% (F = 1). The equation for the same is given as follows:

$$\text{Bioavailability} = \frac{\text{AUC oral } \beta'}{\text{AUC IV } \beta} \times 100 \text{ or } F = \frac{\text{AUC oral } \beta'}{\text{AUC IV } \beta}$$

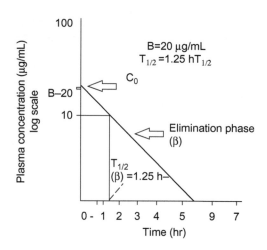

FIGURE 2.9

Semilogarithmic graph exhibiting kinetic behavior conforming to one-compartment model. Plasma concentration profile after IV bolus administration shows half-life ($T_{1/2}$).

where β and β' are the elimination rate constants after IV bolus and EV routes and F is the bioavailability fraction (fraction of the administered dose that enters the systemic circulation).

Bioavailability is a useful parameter which is used to predict the drug efficacy after different routes of administration.

Q. What is the influence of route of administration of drug/toxicant on bioavailability?

It is generally in the following order:

IV > oral route > topical route.

Q. Define volume of distribution (V_d).

The total volume of fluid in which a toxic substance must be dissolved to account for the measured plasma concentrations is known as the apparent volume of distribution (V_d). If a compound is distributed only in the plasma fluid, the V_d is small and plasma concentrations are high. Conversely, if a compound is distributed to all sites in the body, or if it accumulates in a specific tissue such as fat or bone, the V_d becomes large and plasma concentrations are low.

The value of V_d may be determined by area method using the following equation.

$$V_d = \frac{\text{dose (D)}}{C}$$

Q. Define total body clearance, a term used in kinetic studies of toxicants.

In toxicology, the clearance is a pharmacokinetic measurement of the volume of plasma that is completely cleared off of a substance per unit time.

The usual units are mL/min. The total body clearance will be equal to the renal clearance + hepatic clearance + lung clearance.

2.5.2 FLIP-FLOP KINETICS

Q. Define flip-flop kinetics.

Flip-flop kinetics refers to a situation when the rate of absorption of a compound is significantly slower than its rate of elimination from the body. The persistence of the compound in the body therefore becomes dependent on absorption rather than elimination processes (Fig. 2.10). This sometimes occurs when the route of exposure is dermal.

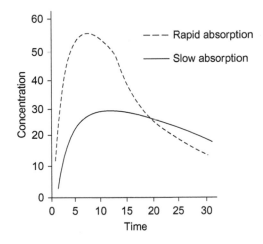

FIGURE 2.10

Concentrations of toxicants comparing a slow rate of absorption to a rapid rate of absorption, demonstrating a "flip-flop" kinetics, where the persistence of the compound is dependent on the rate of absorption, rather than the rate of elimination.

Q. Define PBTK.

It is a physiological-based toxicokinetic (PBTK) model. These models are mathematical simulation of physiological processes that determine the rate and extent of xenobiotics/toxicant ADME. The primary difference between physiological compartmental models and classic compartmental models lies in the basis for assigning the rate constants that describe the transport of chemicals into and out of the compartments. In classic kinetics, the rate constants are defined by the data; thus, these models are often referred to as data-based models. In PBTK models, the rate constants represent known or hypothesized biological processes, and these models are commonly referred to as PBTK models (Fig. 2.11).

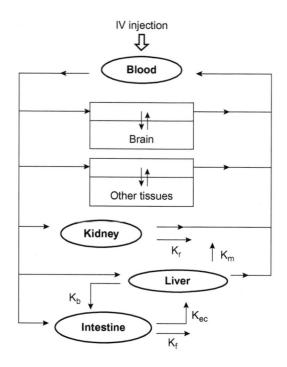

IV injection

FIGURE 2.11

Schematic representation of PBTK for a hypothetical toxicant that is soluble in water. Oval shapes show perfusion-limited compartments (kidney, liver, and intestine) and rectangular shapes show diffusion-limited compartments (brain and other tissues). The toxicant is eliminated through metabolism in the liver (K_m), biliary excretion (K_b), renal excretion (K_r) into the urine, and fecal excretion (K_f). The chemical can also undergo enterohepatic circulation (K_{ec}).

2.6 QUESTION AND ANSWER EXERCISES

2.6.1 SHORT QUESTIONS AND ANSWERS

Exercise 1

Q.1 Define ADME.

ADME is the study of absorption, distribution, metabolism/biotransformation, and excretion of toxicants/xenobiotics in relation to time.

Q.2 What is toxicokinetics?

Toxicokinetics refers to the study of absorption, distribution, metabolism/biotransformation, and excretion (ADME) of toxicants/xenobiotics in relation to time. An important parameter in toxicokinetic is to examine the time course of blood or plasma concentration of the toxicant with time.

Q.3 What is dosage regimen?

Dosage regimen is defined as the manner in which a drug is administered.

Irrespective of the route of administration, a dosage regimen is composed of two important variables:

1. The magnitude of each dose (dose size)
2. The frequency with which the dose is repeated (dosing interval).

Q.4 Define in brief dose size.

Dose or dose size is a quantitative term estimating the amount of drug which must be administered to produce a particular biological response, i.e., to achieve a specified target plasma drug concentration.

Q.5 How the therapeutic dose should be selected?

As the magnitude of both therapeutic and toxic responses depends on plasma drug concentration, size of dose should be so selected that it produces the peak plasma concentration (C_{max}) or steady-state level within the limits of therapeutic range (between MEC and MSC). The therapeutic plasma concentration range is obtained by careful clinical evaluation of the response in a sufficient number of appropriately selected individuals (for microbials, the range is based upon the MIC for susceptible microorganisms).

Q.6 What do you mean by dosing interval?

Dosing interval is the time interval between doses. It ensures maintenance of plasma concentration of a drug within the therapeutic range for entire duration of therapy.

Q.7 What do you mean by EV administration?

Administered of xenobiotic by EV route (e.g., oral, IM, SC, and IP) is called EV administration (other than IV route).

Q.8 Define minimum effective concentration (MEC).

MEC is the minimum concentration of drug in plasma required to produce the desirable pharmacological/therapeutic response. In case of antimicrobials, the term MIC is used, which may be defined as the minimum concentration of antimicrobial agent in plasma required to inhibit the growth of microorganisms.

Q.9 Define maximum safe concentration (MSC) or minimum toxic concentration (MTC).

MSC or MTC is the concentration of drug in plasma above which toxic effects are produced. Concentration of drug above MSC is said to be in toxic level. The drug concentration between MEC and MSC represents the therapeutic range.

Q.10 Define maximum plasma concentration/peak plasma concentration (C_{max} or Cp_{max}).

Maximum plasma concentration/peak plasma concentration is the point of maximum concentration of drug in plasma. The maximum plasma concentration depends on the administered dose and rates of absorption (absorption rate constant, K_a) and elimination (elimination rate constant, β). The peak represents the point of time when absorption equals elimination rate of the drug. It is often expressed as $\mu g/mL$.

Exercise 2

Q.1 Define area under curve (AUC).

AUC is the total integrated area under the plasma drug concentration—time curve. It expresses the total amount of drug that comes into systemic circulation after administration of the drug.

Q.2 Define peak effect.

Peak effect is the maximal or peak pharmacological or toxic effect produced by the drug. It is generally observed at peak plasma concentration.

Q.3 Define time of maximum concentration/time of peak concentration (t_{max}).

Time of maximum concentration/time of peak concentration is the time required for a drug to reach peak concentration in plasma. The faster the absorption rate, the lower is the t_{max}. It is also useful in assessing the efficacy of the drugs used to treat acute conditions (e.g., pain) which can be treated by a single dose. It is expressed in hours.

Q.4 Define onset of action.

Onset of action is the beginning of pharmacological or toxicological effect or response produced by the drug. It occurs when the plasma drug concentration just exceeds the MEC.

Q.5 Define onset time.

Onset time is the time required for the drug to start producing pharmacological or toxic response. It usually corresponds to the time for the plasma concentration to reach MEC after administration of the drug.

Q.6 Define duration of action.

Duration of action is the time period for which pharmacological or toxic response is produced by the drug. It usually corresponds to the duration for which the plasma concentration of drug remains above the MEC level.

Q.7 Define the term half-life.

Half-life ($T_{\frac{1}{2}}$) may be defined as the time taken for the concentration of a compound/toxicant in plasma to decline by ½ or 50% of its initial value (or it may be defined as the time required for the body to eliminate half of the chemical). This value is determined during the elimination phase of a chemical; therefore, it is called elimination half-life.

Q.8 What are the physiochemical properties that affect absorption?

1. Route
2. Duration of exposure
3. Ability to cross cell membrane (passive and active transport, endocytosis).

Q.9 Out of nonionized or ionized forms of chemicals, which form passively diffuse?

Only nonionized.

Q.10 What are the determinants of ionization?
1. pKa = −log[acid dissociation constant]
2. pH of the local environment.

Exercise 3

Q.1 What does it mean when pKa = pH?

It means 50% ionization.

Q.2 What happens to weak acids when they are in an environment where the pH decreases?

More become nonionized and are passively diffusible (e.g., diffuse in the stomach).

Q.3 What happens to weak basic when they are in an environment where the pH decreases?

Becomes more nonionized (e.g., intestine).

Q.4 What is bioavailability?

The proportion of a drug or toxicant which enters the circulation when introduced into the body and so is able to have an active effect.

Q.5 Name six things that affect distribution.
1. Lipid/water soluble
2. Serum protein binding
3. Presence of specialized barriers
4. Degree of organ/tissue perfusion
5. Presence/density of receptors/transporters
6. Tissue storage.

Q.6 What is drug interactions?

Using two drugs at the same time may affect each other's fraction unbound. For example, assume that Drug A and Drug B are both protein-bound drugs. If Drug A is given, it will bind to the plasma proteins in the blood. If Drug B is also given, it can displace Drug A from the protein, thereby increasing Drug A's fraction unbound. This may increase the effects of Drug A, since only the unbound fraction may exhibit activity.

Q.7 Out of bound or unbound toxicant which one is active?

Unbound.

Q.8 Name the proteins to which plasma can bind.

Albumin α-glycoproteins.

Q.9 What is the problem with highly bound toxicants?

Slowly eliminated, so linger longer.

Q.10 What is the meaning of kernicterus?

Kernicterus is a bilirubin-induced brain dysfunction. Bilirubin is a highly neurotoxic substance that may become elevated in the serum, a condition known as hyperbilirubinemia.

Exercise 4

Q.1 In which main tissue/organ biotransformation of toxicants occurs?

Liver.

Q.2 In which tissue/organ excretion of toxicants occurs?

1. Renal
2. Intestinal (bile)—fecal
3. Unabsorbed—fecal.

Q.3 What is elimination $T_{1/2}$?

Time it takes for plasma concentration to drop by 50%.

Q.4 What are the factors that are responsible for renal reabsorption of toxicants?

1. Lipid solubility
2. Weak acids/bases
3. Urine pH.

Q.5 What are the factors that are responsible for biliary excretion?

1. Enterohepatic recirculation
2. Glucuronide conjugates.

Q.6 Name the solute carrier proteins family.

1. OATs (organic anion transporters)
2. OCTs (organic cation transporters)
3. OATPs (organic anion transporter polypeptides).

Q.7 Name main sites for biotransformation.

1. Liver
2. Lung
3. Kidney
4. Skin, intestine, testes, placenta.

Q.8 What is the outcome of biotransformations?

1. Detoxification (inactivation)
2. Bioactivation
3. Facilitate excretion.

Q.9 What are phase I biotransformation reactions?

1. Simple degradation reactions
2. ATP dependent add or expose a functional group such as —hydroxyl, carboxyl, and amino.

Q.10 Write phase I biotransformation reactions.

1. Oxidative reactions
2. Reductive reactions
3. Hydrolytic reactions.

Exercise 5

Q.1 During phase I reactions, which enzymes are used?

Cytochrome P450.

Q.2 During oxidation biotransformation (phase I), cytochrome b contains what?

  Fe-containing heme proteins.

Q.3 Where cytochrome P450 enzymes are located?

  ER membrane (multiple isoforms) (broad range of substrates).

Q.4 What happens (reactions) during biotransformation phase II?

  1. Conjugation reactions that are ATP dependent (alteration of chemicals)

  2. Renders nonpolar compounds to polar

  3. Promotes excretion (larger, charged, water soluble).

Q.5 Name phase II conjugation reactions and their location.

  1. Glucuronidation (ER)

  2. Sulfation (cytosol)

  3. Acetylation (cytosol)

  4. Methylation (cytosol and ER)

  5. Glutathione conjugation (cytosol and ER).

Q.6 What is the influence of route of administration of drug/toxicant on bioavailability?

  It is generally in the following order:

  IV > oral route > topical route.

Q.7 Define volume of distribution (V_d).

  The total volume of fluid in which a toxic substance must be dissolved to account for the measured plasma concentrations is known as the apparent volume of distribution (V_d).

2.6.2 MULTIPLE CHOICE QUESTIONS (CHOOSE THE BEST STATEMENT, IT CAN BE ONE, TWO OR ALL OR NONE)

Exercise 6

Q.1 Toxicants are most likely to be reabsorbed after being filtered at the glomerulus are

  a. organic anions

  b. organic cations

  c. natural polar molecules

  d. highly lipid-soluble molecules

Q.2 A high urinary pH would favor the excretion of

  a. organic acids

  b. organic bases

  c. neutral organic compounds

  d. none of the above

Q.3 Diuretics can enhance the renal elimination of compounds that

  a. are of molecular weight greater than 70 kDa

  b. are ions trapped in the tubular lumen

  c. are highly lipid soluble

  d. are highly protein bound

Q.4 The amount of a volatile liquid excreted by the lungs is
   a. inversely proportional to its lipid−water partition coefficient
   b. directly proportional to its vapor pressure
   c. directly proportional to its molecular weight
   d. inversely proportional to cardiac output

Q.5 Kernicterus results from
   a. enzyme induction leading to decreased glucocorticoid levels
   b. excess ingestion of foods containing tyramine
   c. displacement of bilirubin from plasma proteins
   d. malabsorption of fat-soluble vitamins

Q.6 All of the following could influence the GI absorption of xenobiotics except
   a. pH
   b. intestinal microflora
   c. presence of food
   d. time of day

Q.7 The rate of diffusion of a xenobiotic across the GI tract is proportional to all of the following except
   a. hepatic blood flow
   b. surface area
   c. permeability
   d. residence time

Q.8 Which of the following is not absorbed in the colon?
   a. Water
   b. Sodium ion
   c. Glucose
   d. Hydrogen ion

Q.9 Nanoparticles are considered to have diameter smaller than
   a. 100 μm
   b. 10 μm
   c. 1 μm
   d. 0.1 μm

Q.10 All of the following are true of nanoparticles except
   a. they are capable of exposing the lung to a large number of particles
   b. they are capable of exposing the lung to a large particle surface area
   c. because of turbulence, very few reach the alveoli
   d. they are the focus of recent toxicological research

Answers

1. d; 2. a; 3. b; 4. b; 5. c; 6. d; 7. a; 8. c; 9. d; 10. c.

Exercise 7

Q.1 All of the following are significantly stored in bone matrix except
   a. lead
   b. diquat
   c. strontium
   d. fluoride

Q.2 All of the following can cross the placenta except
   a. heparin
   b. rubella virus
   c. spirochetes
   d. immunoglobulin (IgG) antibody

Q.3 Methylmercury crosses the blood−brain barrier by combining with cysteine and forming a molecular similar to
   a. glycine
   b. glutamine
   c. taurine
   d. methionine

Q.4 Which of the following statements are true?
   a. The blood−brain barrier of a 70-year-old is more permeable than that of a premature infant.
   b. Chemicals/drugs can be excreted into the urine by active secretion.
   c. The kidney lacks cytochrome P450 enzymes.
   d. All mammalian placentas have the same number of tissue layers.

Q.5 All of the following are true of breast milk except
   a. acidic compounds may be more concentrated in milk than that of plasma
   b. toxicants can be passed from mother to offspring
   c. toxicants can be passed from cows to humans
   d. DDT, polychlorinated biphenyls (PCBs), and polybrominated biphenyls (PBBs) can be found in human milk

Q.6 Active transport is characterized by all of the following except
   a. a movement against a concentration gradient
   b. energy requirement
   c. nonsaturability
   d. competitive inhibition

Q.7 All of the following are true of the facilitated diffusion except
   a. does not require energy
   b. movement against a concentration gradient
   c. saturability
   d. involvement of a carrier

Q.8 Which of the following does NOT uncouple oxidative phosphorylation?
   a. Pentachlorophenol
   b. Dinitrophenol
   c. Aconitase
   d. Salicylate
   e. Gramicidin

Q.9 Which of the following is NOT true regarding peroxisome proliferators?
   a. They are a structurally diverse group of chemicals.
   b. They cause marked induction of lipid metabolizing enzymes.
   c. They often are nongenotoxic hepatocarcinogens in rodents.
   d. They induce hepatic CYP1A which is indicative of peroxisome proliferation.
   e. They operate via the peroxisome proliferator activated receptor.
Q.10 For which of the following route of exposure, pre-systemic elimination is possible?
   a. Oral (GI tract)
   b. Inhalation
   c. Intramuscular
   d. Intravenous

Answers
1. b; 2. a; 3. d; 4. b; 5. a; 6. c; 7. b; 8. c; 9. d; 10. a.

Exercise 8

Q.1 Methylation
   a. typically increases the water solubility of xenobiotics
   b. is a major pathway of xenobiotic metabolism
   c. requires *S*-adenosylmethionine (SAM)
   d. requires acetyl coenzyme A
   e. requires taurine
Q.2 Of the more than 40 cytochrome P450 isozymes, which six account for the majority of xenobiotic metabolism in humans?
   a. CYP1E1, CYP2B1, CYP2B19, CYP2F1, CYP3A7, CYP4A6
   b. CYP1A1, CYP2A6, CYP2B6, CYP2D6, CYP2F2, CYP4B2
   c. CYP1B2, CYP2C6, CYP2F2, CYP3A2, CYP3A4, CYP4A2
   d. CYP1A2, CYP2C9, CYP2C19, CYP2D6, CYP2E1, CYP3A4
   e. CYP1A1, CYP2C8, CYP2F2, CYP3A7, CYP4A2, CYP4A6
Q.3 Which of the following is NOT a characteristic of active transport?
   a. Blocked by saxitoxin
   b. Movement against a concentration gradient
   c. Exhibits a transport maximum
   d. Energy dependent
   e. Selectivity
Q.4 Which of the following does NOT inhibit electron transport?
   a. Rotenone
   b. Succinate
   c. Antimycin-A
   d. Formate
   e. Azide

Q.5 Reabsorption of toxicants does NOT occur through

  a. enterohepatic recirculation
  b. glomerular filtration
  c. diffusion
  d. active transport
  e. carriers for physiological oxyanions

Q.6 When all receptors are occupied by a toxicant and there is a maximum amount of receptor–toxicant complexes, the response is labeled

  a. $T_{1/2}$
  b. LC_{max}
  c. E_{max}
  d. C_{max}

Q.7 Which of the following statements is true?

  a. Toxicant receptor interactions are always reversible.
  b. Receptors for toxicants are always enzymes.
  c. The toxic response is related to the toxicant concentration in the plasma more so than the concentration at the site of action.
  d. None of the above.

Q.8 An increase in free drug concentration will

  a. increase the pharmacological effect
  b. decrease the toxic effect
  c. decrease the amount of drug filtered at the glomerulus
  d. none of the above

Q.9 The phrase that best defines "toxicodynamics" is the

  a. linkage between exposure and dose
  b. linkage between dose and response
  c. dynamic nature of toxic effects among various species
  d. dose range between desired biological effects and adverse health effects
  e. loss of dynamic hearing range due to a toxic exposure

Q.10 Which of the following is NOT an initiating event in carcinogenesis?

  a. DNA adduct formation
  b. DNA strand breakage
  c. mutation of proto-oncogenes
  d. oxidative damage of DNA
  e. mitogenesis

Answers

1. c; 2. d; 3. a; 4. b; 5. b; 6. c; 7. d; 8. a; 9. b; 10. e.

Exercise 9

Q.1 A probe drug for human CYP2C19 activity is

  a. mephenytoin
  b. valproic acid
  c. carbamazepine
  d. warfarin

Q.2 All of the following are true of CYP2D6 except
  a. it converts codeine to morphine
  b. it is polymorphic
  c. it is induced by quinidine
  d. poor metabolizers have a lower risk of lung cancer

Q.3 Aryl hydrocarbon receptor agonist includes all of the following except
  a. TCDD
  b. benzopyrene
  c. 3-methylcholanthrene
  d. benzene

Q.4 Enzyme induction in humans has been associated with
  a. osteomalacia
  b. hepatocellular carcinoma
  c. cirrhosis
  d. psoriasis

Q.5 In metabolism-dependent inhibition of cytochrome P450,
  a. the parent compound is a potent inhibitor
  b. the metabolite must be a product of P450 catalysis
  c. the metabolite is a potent inhibitor
  d. the inhibition is always irreversible

Q.6 A compound that induces CYP2D6 is
  a. rifampin
  b. dexamethazone
  c. ethanol
  d. none of the above

Q.7 All of the following are considered phase I biotransformation reactions except
  a. hydrolysis
  b. conjugation
  c. reduction
  d. oxidation

Q.8 All of the following statements are true except
  a. forms of epoxide hydrolase can exist in both microsomes and cytosol
  b. gemfibrozil is conjugated with glucuronic acid before it is oxidized by cytochrome P450
  c. CYP2D6 and CYP2C9 metabolize over half of the drugs in current use
  d. biotransformation can take place in the gut

Q.9 UGT conjugate all of the following endogenous molecules except
  a. thyroid hormone
  b. bilirubin
  c. steroid hormones
  d. parathyroid hormone

Q.10 If codeine were given to a patient who was a 2D6 ultrametabolizer, the most likely result would be
    a. inadequate analgesia
    b. higher-than-normal levels of morphine at 2-hour post-dose
    c. higher-than-normal levels of codeine at 4-hour post-dose
    d. higher-than-normal levels of oxycodone at 4-hour post-dose

Answers

1. a; 2. c; 3. d; 4. a; 5. c; 6. d; 7. b; 8. c; 9. d; 10. b.

Exercise 10

Q.1 Victim drug is
    a. a drug whose clearance is determined mostly by a single route of administration
    b. a drug that induces neutralizing antibodies
    c. a drug that is unstable in plasma
    d. a racemic drug mixture where one isomer inhibits the metabolism of the other isomer

Q.2 Terfenadine and ketoconazole are examples of
    a. enzyme inducers
    b. perpetrator and inhibitor
    c. victim drug and perpetrator
    d. drugs with limited biotransformation

Q.3 All of the following are true except
    a. hyperforin induces CYP3A4
    b. broccoli inhibits 1A2
    c. grapefruit juice inhibits intestinal CYP3A4
    d. drugs that inhibit transporters can help anticancer agents

Q.4 Levels of uridine diphosphoglucuronic acid (UDPGA) and 3-phosphoadenosine-5-phosphosulfate (PAPS) are lowered by
    a. St. John's wort
    b. phenobarbital
    c. rifampin
    d. fasting

Q.5 An example of a pair of enantiomers in which one inhibits CYP2D6 and the other has little inhibiting activity is
    a. R and S methadone
    b. R and S warfarin
    c. R and S mephenytoin
    d. quinidine and quinine

Q.6 Which of the following biotransformation enzyme—subcellular location pairs is correct?
    a. Alkaline phosphatase—cell membrane
    b. Carboxylesterase—blood

c. Sulfotransferase—cytosol

d. All of the above

Q.7 The least likely biotransformation reaction that aniline would undergo is

a. halogenation

b. aromatic hydroxylation

c. *N*-acetylation

d. *N*-glucuronidation

Q.8 The proteins KEAPI and Nrf2

a. suppress CYP expression in response to inflammation

b. induce enzymes in response to oxidative stress

c. promote DNA methylations

d. none of the above

Q.9 All of the following are true to glutathione except

a. germ cells and ovum have high levels

b. conjugation of dibromoethane results in a mutagenic metabolite

c. conjugation of electrophiles is a major means of protecting DNA

d. conjugation always occurs enzymatically

Q.10 Phenobarbital

a. causes liver tumors in human and rodents

b. causes liver tumors in rodents but not humans

c. causes liver tumors in primates but not in rodents

d. causes liver tumors in rodents and nasal tumors in humans

Answers

1. a; 2. c; 3. b; 4. d; 5. d; 6. d; 7. a; 8. b; 9. d; 10. b.

Exercise 11

Q.1 Systemic availability of an orally administered toxicant is dependent on

a. GI absorption

b. intestinal mucosa metabolism

c. first-pass liver metabolism

d. all of the above

Q.2 Which of the following statements are true?

a. Renal clearance is equal to urine formation

b. Hepatic clearance cannot exceed hepatic blood flow

c. A process that increases free drug concentration will decrease hepatic clearance and increase renal clearance

d. Total body clearance equals dose divided by half-life

Q.3 A classic example of a drug inducing its own metabolism is

a. warfarin

b. lovastatin

c. carbamazepine

d. theophylline

Q.4 An example of a thermodynamic parameter used in physiological toxicokinetic models (PBTK) is
   a. tissue partition coefficient
   b. alveolar ventricular rate
   c. cardiac output
   d. liver volume

Q.5 Fick's law of diffusion
   a. is a zero-order process
   b. is a first-order process
   c. applies to active transport
   d. requires energy

Q.6 The method of predicting the toxicokinetic behavior of chemicals and drugs across species is called
   a. Monte Carlo simulation
   b. benchmark kinetics
   c. allometric scaling
   d. linear regression kinetics

Q.7 Which of the following is not theoretically possible?
   a. Volume of distribution greater than volume of human body
   b. Volume of distribution equal to blood volume
   c. Total clearance equal to renal clearance
   d. Bioavailability (F) greater than 1

Q.8 A compartment in which uptake of xenobiotic is dependent on membrane permeability and total membrane area is called
   a. perfusion limited
   b. diffusion limited
   c. blood flow limited
   d. ventilation limited

Q.9 The α-phase of an intravenously administered drug classically represents the
   a. absorption phase
   b. elimination phase
   c. dissolution phase
   d. distribution phase

Q.10 An advantage of a physiological, toxicokinetic model over a classic model is
   a. it may be able to predict tissue concentration
   b. it has only two compartments
   c. the mathematics is less complicated
   d. it can give a better estimation of bioavailability

Answers
1. d; 2. b; 3. c; 4. a; 5. b; 6. c; 7. d; 8. b; 9. d; 10. a.

Exercise 12

Q.1 the hepatic clearance of a drug with a high hepatic extraction ratio is largely dependent on
  a. drug protein binding
  b. hepatic blood flow
  c. drug metabolizing enzyme activity
  d. intestinal blood flow

Q.2 All of the following are true of saturation kinetics with increasing dose except
  a. clearance must decrease
  b. half-life can increase or decrease
  c. volume of distribution will decrease if there is a saturation of serum protein binding
  d. volume of distribution will decrease if there is a saturation of tissue binding

Q.3 All of the following are true of nonlinear kinetics except
  a. ratio of metabolites will remain constant with change in dose
  b. clearance will change with change in dose
  c. AUC will not be dose proportional
  d. decline of xenobiotic is nonexponential

Q.4 All of the following are true of first-order kinetics except
  a. steady-state concentration is proportional to rate of intake
  b. rate of intake will not change time to steady state
  c. half-life is inversely proportional to clearance
  d. a change in half-life will not change time to steady state

Q.5 All of the following are true of first-order kinetics except
  a. the elimination rate constant increases with dose
  b. a semilogarithmic plot of plasma concentration vs time yields a single straight line
  c. the concentration of xenobiotic in plasma decreases by a constant fraction per unit time
  d. the volume of distribution is independent of dose

Q.6 After _____, 93.8% of a dose of drug is eliminated.
  a. three half-lives
  b. four half-lives
  c. five half-lives
  d. six half-lives

Q.7 All of the following are components of the central compartment except
  a. liver
  b. lungs
  c. bone
  d. kidney

Q.8 Which of the following has the largest value of distribution?
   a. Chloroquine
   b. Ethyl alcohol
   c. Albumin
   d. Ethylene glycol
Q.9 The common units used to express total clearance of a toxicant are
   a. mg/mL
   b. mg/min
   c. mL/min
   d. mg/min mL
Q.10 In first-order kinetics
   a. a constant amount of toxicant is removed per unit time
   b. AUC is not proportional to dose
   c. half-life changes with increasing dose
   d. clearance, volume of distribution, and half-life do not change with dose

Answers
1. b; 2. c; 3. a; 4. d; 5. a; 6. b; 7, c; 8. a; 9. c; 10. d.

Exercise 13
   Q.1 All of the following are hydrolytic enzymes except
      a. carboxylesterase
      b. alcohol dehydrogenase
      c. cholinesterase
      d. paraoxonase
   Q.2 All of the following are true of epoxide hydrolyases except
      a. they add oxygen to a double bond and form a three-member ring
      b. they are important in hydrolyzing electrophiles
      c. they play a role in converting benzo[a]pyrene to a carcinogen
      d. some forms are inducible
   Q.3 Nitroreductase plays an important role in
      a. nasal epithelium
      b. lung Clara cells
      c. white blood cells
      d. intestinal flora
   Q.4 A drug that undergoes sulfoxide reduction is
      a. haloperidol
      b. chloramphenicol
      c. thaliomide
      d. sulindac
   Q.5 Quinidine oxidoreductases are thought to play a protective role in
      a. liver toxicity of microcystin
      b. bone marrow toxicity of benzene
      c. renal toxicity of aminoglycosides
      d. neurotoxicity of n-hexane

Q.6 All of the following are mechanisms for removing halogen atoms from aliphatic xenobiotics except
   a. Grignard dehalogenation
   b. reductive dehalogenation
   c. oxidative dehalogenation
   d. double dehalogenation

Q.7 Oxidation of ethanol to acetaldehyde takes place in
   a. cytosol
   b. microsomes
   c. peroxisomes
   d. all of the above

Q.8 Reductive dehalogenation of carbon tetrachloride produces
   a. phosgene
   b. chloroform
   c. trichloromethyl radical
   d. hydrochloric acid

Q.9 Acetaldehyde is converted to acetic acid by ALDH2 in
   a. mitochondria
   b. cytosol
   c. microsomes
   d. all of the above

Q.10 Aldehyde oxidase and xanthene oxidoreductase contain
   a. zinc
   b. molybdenum
   c. selenium
   d. copper

Answers

1. b; 2. a; 3. d; 4. d; 5. b; 6. a; 7. d; 8. c; 9. a; 10. b.

Exercise 14

Q.1 Slow acetylators of *N*-acetyltransferase (NAT) demonstrate all of the following except
   a. peripheral neuropathy from isoniazid
   b. systemic lupus erythematous from procainamide
   c. peripheral neuropathy from dapsone
   d. decreased hypotensive response from hydrazine

Q.2 In contrast to glucuronidation, sulfonation is
   a. a low-affinity, low-capacity pathway
   b. a low-affinity, high-capacity pathway
   c. a high-affinity, high-capacity pathway
   d. a high-affinity, low-capacity pathway

Q.3 Induction of sulfotransferase enzymes by rifampin be clinically relevant for
   a. warfarin
   b. digoxin
   c. ethinyl estradiol
   d. all of the above
Q.4 All of the following statements regarding sulfonation reaction are true except
   a. they can take a molecule less lipid soluble
   b. they always detoxify a molecule
   c. some drugs must be metabolized to a sulfonate conjugate to have pharmacological effect
   d. morphine-6-sulfate is more potent than morphine in the rat
Q.5 All of the following statements are true regarding methylation except
   a. the process generally decreases the water solubility of the parent
   b. the process can mask functional groups that can be metabolized by other conjugation enzymes
   c. inorganic mercury and arsenic can be dimethylated
   d. high methyltransferace activity may lower levels of homocysteine
Q.6 All of the following are methyltransferase enzymes except
   a. S-adenosylmethionine (SAM)
   b. Catechol-O-methyltransferase (COMT)
   c. Nicotinamide-N-methyltransferase (NNMT)
   d. Histamine-N-methyltransferase (HNMT)
Q.7 All of the following are true of glucuronide conjugates of xenobiotics except
   a. they can be excreted into the urine
   b. they are formed from activated xenobiotics
   c. they are substances for β-glucuronidase in the intestinal flora
   d. they can be excreted into the bile
Q.8 All of the following are true of sulfonation reaction except
   a. they involve the transfer of sulfate
   b. they are catalyzed by sulfotransferases
   c. the cofactor of the reaction is PAPS
   d. they are mainly excreted into the urine
Q.9 The number of UGT mammalian enzymes that have been identified is approximately
   a. 5
   b. 12
   c. 22
   d. 58
Q.10 In addition to cytoplasm, sulfotranferacss are present in mammals in the
   a. endoplasmic reticulum
   b. mitochondria
   c. plasma membrane
   d. Golgi apparatus

Answers
1. d; 2. d; 3. c; 4. b; 5. d; 6. a; 7. b; 8. a; 9. c; 10. d.

2.6.3 FILL IN THE BLANKS

Exercise 15

Q.1 The most common process of absorption of xenobiotics across the cell membrane is _____.

Q.2 The important route of excretion for xenobiotics is _____.

Q.3 The process of chemical transformation (conversion from one form to another) occurring in the body is known as _____.

Q.4 The major site for biotransformation of xenobiotics in body is _____.

Q.5 In a hepatocyte, metabolism of xenobiotics takes place in

_____.

Q.6 The most important among microsomal enzymes is _____ or

_____.

Q.7 The major biotransformation reaction occurring in phase I is _____ and in phase II is _____.

Q.8 Phase I oxidation reactions are mainly catalyzed by

_____.

Q.9 All phase II conjugation reactions are catalyzed by nonmicrosomal enzymes except for _____ which is catalyzed by microsomal enzymes.

Q.10 The ability of certain substances to increase the activity or synthesis of microsomal enzymes is known as _____.

Q.11 The metabolic reaction which is deficient in dogs is _____; cats are deficient in _____ and pigs are deficient in _____ reactions of biotransformation.

Q.12 The process of conversion of nontoxic substance into a toxic metabolite due to biotransformation is known as _____.

Answers

1. PASSIVE DIFFUSION; 2. RENAL EXCRETION; 3. BIOTRANSFORMATION; 4. LIVER (liver is the major site due to the presence of variety of metabolizing enzymes. Other important sites for biotransformation include lung, kidney, and intestines); 5. ENDOPLASMIC RETICULUMN (ER) or MICROSOMES; 6. MONOOXYGENASES or MIXED FUNCTION OXIDASES (MFO); 7. OXIDATION and CONJUGATION; 8. MICROSOMAL ENZYMES (MFO); 9. GLUCURONIDE CONJUGATION; 10. INDUCTION (nonmicrosomal enzymes which are present in cytosol are not inducible—microsomal enzymes which are present in cytosol are not inducible); 11. ACETYLATION, GLUCURONIDE CONJUGATION, and SULFATION (hence sulfonamides which undergo acetylation cause toxicity in dogs and similarly, paracetamol, which undergoes glucuronide conjugation, causes hepatotoxicity in cats); 12. LETHAL SYNTHESIS.

2.6.4 TRUE OR FALSE STATEMENTS (WRITE T FOR TRUE AND F FOR FALSE STATEMENT)

Exercise 16

Q.1 A water-soluble drug will pass across muscle membranes faster than across brain membranes (assume permeability-rate limitations).

Q.2 A neutral, lipophilic drug is likely to be absorbed faster in the intestines than in the stomach. Remember that stomach and intestine differ in their properties.

Q.3 Lipophilic drugs are generally taken up fast by highly perfused organs.

Q.4 Ionized and lipophilic drugs are most likely to cross most membrane barriers.

Q.5 Drugs with a high tissue binding always have a large volume of distribution.

Q.6 Compared to skin, liver would have a higher rate of uptake of perfusion-limited lipophilic drugs due to its higher blood flow rate.

Q.7 Distribution to a specific tissue for permeability-limited hydrophilic drugs depends on how much and how quickly the blood gets to the specific tissue.

Q.8 Perfusion-limited distribution is a type of drug distribution into tissue that occurs when the drug is able to cross membranes easily.

Q.9 Assume two drugs (identical molecular weight, same dose given): one neutral drug (Drug A) and one acidic drug ($pKa = 7.4$, Drug B). Drug A and the unionized form of drug B have the same partition coefficient. The fraction unbound in plasma and tissue is 0.5 for both drugs. Drug B will enter tissues somewhat slower than drug A.

Q.10 A weak acid whose unionized form shows a high partition coefficient is likely to cross most membrane barriers.

Answers

1. T; 2. T; 3. T; 4. F; 5. F; 6. T; 7. F; 8. T; 9. T; 10. T.

Exercise 17

Q.1 A volume of distribution of 41 L for a lipophilic drug suggest that the drug will not bind to tissue and plasma proteins.

Q.2 Transporters pumping the drug into the tissues are more active in babies.

Q.3 Compared to skin, liver would have a higher rate of uptake for small lipophilic drugs due to its higher blood flow rate.

Q.4 Free drug concentrations are always the same in plasma and tissues, when the distribution occurs instantaneously.

Q.5 Enzyme induction affects the hepatic clearance of a low and high extraction drugs.

Q.6 Enzyme induction affects the oral bioavailability of high extraction drugs.

Q.7 A fast absorption might allow less frequent dosing.

Q.8 A slower absorption might be advantageous for a drug with a narrow therapeutic window.

Q.9 Concentrations in plasma are of relevance for drug therapy as they generally correlate well with concentrations observed at the effect (target) site.

Q.10 When heparin is added to blood and the blood is centrifuged, the resulting supernatant is called serum.

Answers

1. F; 2. T; 3. T; 4. T; 5. F; 6. T; 7. F; 8. T; 9. T; 10. F.

Exercise 18
Part A

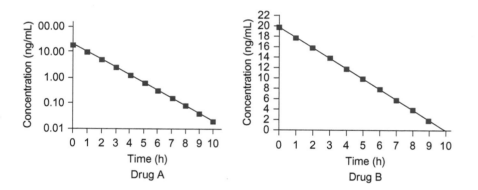

Q.1 In Figure A, Drug A's rate of elimination depends on the amount of drug in the body.

Q.2 In Figure B, Drug B's rate of elimination is constant.

Q.3 In Figure B, the fraction of drug eliminated per hour is constant.

Q.4 In Figure B, Drug B's behavior might be explained with saturated metabolic enzymes.

Q.5 In both the figures, for both drugs, the model assumes that drug distribution does not take any time.

Part B

Assume no active transport. Assume the same dose of penicillin G is given to patients as IV bolus injection (as solution in saline), intramuscular (IM) in oily injection or orally:

Q.6 Giving the drug IM injections will result in a much smaller AUC than after oral administration.

Q.7 Giving penicillin as an aqueous IV bolus injection will result in a higher maximum concentration.

Q.8 Oily IM injection allows a less frequent dosing.

Part C

Q.9 The rate with which hydrophilic compounds will move across well-built membranes will depend on the concentration gradient between total drug in plasma and total drug in tissue.

Q.10 Assuming that a protein drug does not bind to plasma and tissue component, the volume of distribution is likely to be 41 L.

Answers

1. T; 2. T; 3. F; 4. T; 5. T; 6. F; 7. T; 8. T; 9. F; 10. F.

Exercise 19

Assume a drug is a substrate of a specific transport protein. Which of the following statements are true or false?

Q.1 Transporters do not use energy.

Q.2 Transporters only eliminate drugs from the body.

Q.3 Transporters are only present in liver and kidney.

Q.4 Transporters are saturable.

Q.5 Transporters work often in conjunction with enzymes.
Assume passive diffusion as the driving force for distribution. Which of the following statements are true or false?

Q.6 The $T_{1/2}$ of a drug eliminated through a zero-order process is a drug-specific constant.

Q.7 A lipophilic drug of low molecular weight cannot have a volume of distribution that is smaller than V_T (apparent tissue volume).

Q.8 The fraction of the drug being eliminated per hour is increasing in a first-order process.

Q.9 Two drugs that have similar elimination half-lives will have similar volumes of distributions.

Q.10 The same dose of a drug is given orally either as a solution or in the form of as low dissolving crystal suspension. The solution will show higher maximum concentrations in plasma.

Answers

1. F; 2. F; 3. F; 4. T; 5. T; 6. F; 7. F; 8. F; 9. F; 10. T.

FURTHER READING

Ehrnebo, M., 2010. Kinetic analysis of. In: Gupta, P.K. (Ed.), Modern Toxicology: Basis of Organ and Reproduction Toxicity, vol. 1, second reprint. PharmaMed Press, Hyderabad, India, pp. 130–151.

Gupta, P.K., 2010. Absorption, distribution, & excretion of xenobiotics. In: Gupta, P.K. (Ed.), Modern Toxicology: Basis of Organ and Reproduction Toxicity, vol. 1, second reprint. PharmaMed Press, Hyderabad, India, pp. 71–92.

Gupta P.K., 2014. Essential concept in toxicology. BSP India (Chapter 7).

Gupta, P.K., 2016. Fundamental of Toxicology: Essential Concept and Applications. Elsevier/BSP, San Diego, USA (Chapters 8 and 9).

Krishnamurti, C.R., 2010. Biotransformation of xenobiotics. In: Gupta, P.K. (Ed.), Modern Toxicology: Basis of Organ and Reproduction Toxicity, vol. 1, second reprint. PharmaMed Press, Hyderabad, India, pp. 95–129.

Lehman-McKeeman, L.D., 2013. Absorption distribution and excretion of toxicants. In: Klaassen, C.D. (Ed.), Casarett and Doull's Toxicology: The Basic Science of Poisons, eighth ed. McGraw-Hill, New York, NY, pp. 153–184.

Merwe, van der D., Gehring, R., Buur, J.L., 2018. Toxicokinetics in Veterinary Toxicology. In: Gupta, R.C. (Ed.), Veterinary Toxicology: Basic and Clinical Principles, third ed. Academic Press/Elsevier, Amsterdam, pp. 133–144.

Patkinson, A., Ogilvie, B.W., 2013. Biotransformation of xenobiotics. In: Klaassen, C.D. (Ed.), Casarett and Doull's Toxicology: The Basic Science of Poisons, eighth ed. McGraw-Hill, New York, NY, pp. 185–366.

Renwick, A.G., 2008. Toxicokinetic. In: Hays, A.W. (Ed.), Principles and Methods of Toxicology, fifth ed. Taylor and Francis, Boca Raton, FL, pp. 179–230.

Rose, R.L., Hodgson, E., 2010. Metabolism of toxicants. In: Hodgson, E.A. (Ed.), A Textbook of Modern Toxicology, fourth ed. John Wiley, Hoboken, NJ, pp. 111–148.

Rose, R.L., Hodgson, E., 2010. Chemical and physiological influences on xenobiotic metabolism. In: Hodgson, E.A. (Ed.), A Textbook of Modern Toxicology, fourth ed. John Wiley, Hoboken, NJ, pp. 163–201.

Rose, R.L., Levi, P.E., 2010. Reactive metabolites. In: Hodgson, E.A. (Ed.), A Textbook of Modern Toxicology, 4th ed. John Wiley, New Jersey, pp. 149–161.

Shen, D.D., 2013. Toxicokinetics. In: Klaassen, C.D. (Ed.), Casarett and Doull's Toxicology: The Basic Science of Poisons, eighth ed. McGraw-Hill, New York, NY, pp. 367–390.

Timbrell, J.A., 2009. Factors affecting toxic responses: disposition. In: Timbrell, J.A. (Ed.), Principles of Biochemical Toxicology, fourth ed. Informa, New York, NY, pp. 35–74.

Mechanism of toxicity

3

CHAPTER OUTLINE

3.1 DEFINITIONS

Q. Define mechanism of toxicity.

Mechanism of toxicity is the study of how chemical or physical agents interact with living organisms to cause toxicity. Knowledge of the mechanism of toxicity of a substance enhances the ability to prevent toxicity and design more desirable chemicals; it constitutes the basis for therapy upon overexposure and frequently enables a further understanding of fundamental biological processes.

Q. Describe mechanism of action.

The term mechanism of action (MOA) refers to the specific biochemical interaction through which a drug substance produces its pharmacological effect or toxic response. An MOA usually includes mention of the specific molecular targets to which the drug binds, such as an enzyme or a receptor. Receptor sites have specific affinities for drugs based on the chemical structure of the drug, as well as the specific action that occurs there. Drugs that do not bind to receptors produce their corresponding therapeutic effect by simply interacting with chemical or physical properties in the body. Common examples of drugs that work in this way are antacids and laxatives.

Illustrated Toxicology. DOI: http://dx.doi.org/10.1016/B978-0-12-813213-5.00003-1

3.2 MODE OF ACTION

Q. What are the different types of mode of toxic actions?

There are two major types of modes of toxic action:

1. Nonspecific acting toxicants are those that produce narcosis.

2. Specific acting toxicants are those that are nonnarcotic and that produce a specific action at a specific target site.

Q. What is nonspecific type of mode of action?

Nonspecific acting modes of toxic action result in narcosis; therefore, narcosis is a mode of toxic action. Narcosis is defined as a generalized depression in biological activity due to the presence of toxicant molecules in the organism. The target site and mechanism of toxic action through which narcosis affects organisms are still unclear, but there are hypotheses that support that it occurs through alterations in the cell membranes at specific sites of the membranes, such as the lipid layers or the proteins bound to the membranes. Even though continuous exposure to a narcotic toxicant can produce death, if the exposure to the toxicant is stopped, narcosis can be reversible.

Q. What do you mean by specific type of mode of actions?

Toxicants that at low concentrations modify or inhibit some biological process by binding at a specific site or molecule have a specific acting mode of toxic action. However, at high enough concentrations, toxicants with specific acting modes of toxic actions can produce narcosis that may or may not be reversible. Nevertheless, the specific action of the toxicant is always shown first because it requires lower concentrations.

Q. What are the different specific modes of toxic actions?

- Uncouplers of oxidative phosphorylation: The action involves toxicants that uncouple the two processes that occur in oxidative phosphorylation: electron transfer and adenosine triphosphate (ATP) production.
- Acetylcholinesterase (AChE) inhibitors: AChE is an enzyme associated with nerve synapses that it is designed to regulate nerve impulses by breaking down the neurotransmitter acetylcholine (ACh). When toxicants bind to AChE, they inhibit the breakdown of ACh. This results in continued nerve impulses across the synapses, which eventually cause nerve system damage. Examples of AChE inhibitors are organophosphates and carbamates.
- Irritants: These are chemicals that cause an inflammatory effect on living tissue by chemical action at the site of contact. The resulting effect of irritants is an increase in the volume of cells due to a change in size (hypertrophy) or an increase in the number of cells (hyperplasia). Examples of irritants are benzaldehyde, acrolein, zinc sulfate, and chlorine.
- Central nervous system (CNS) seizure agents: CNS seizure agents inhibit cellular signaling by acting as receptor antagonists. They result in the

inhibition of biological responses. Examples of CNS seizure agents are organochlorine pesticides.

- Respiratory blockers: These are toxicants that affect respiration by interfering with the electron transport chain in the mitochondria. Examples of respiratory blockers are rotenone and cyanide.

3.3 MECHANISM OF TOXICITY

Q. What are the steps involved in the process of mechanisms of toxicity?

- Delivery: site of exposure to the target
- Reaction of the ultimate toxicant with the target molecule
- Cellular dysfunction and resultant toxicity
- Repair or dysrepair (Fig. 3.1).

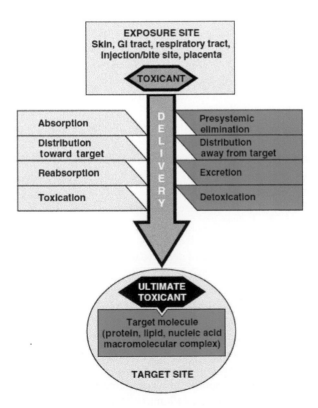

FIGURE 3.1

Mechanisms of toxicity.

nature.berkeley.edu/~dnomura/pdf/Lecture6Mechanisms3.pdf.

Q. What are the chemical factors that cause cellular dysfunction?

- Chemicals that cause DNA adducts can lead to DNA mutations which can activate cell death pathways; if mutations activate oncogenes or inactivate tumor suppressors, it can lead to uncontrolled cell proliferation and cancer (e.g., benzopyrene).
- Chemicals that cause protein adducts can lead to protein dysfunction which can activate cell death pathways; protein adducts can also lead to autoimmunity; if protein adducts activate oncogenes or inactivate tumor suppressors, it can lead to uncontrolled cell proliferation and cancer (e.g., diclofenac glucuronidation metabolite).
- Chemicals that cause oxidative stress can oxidize DNA or proteins leading to DNA mutations or protein dysfunction and all of the above (e.g., benzene, CCl4).
- Chemicals that specifically interact with protein targets chemicals that activate or inactivate ion channels can cause widespread cellular dysfunction and cause cell death and many physiological symptoms. For example, —Na^+, Ca^{2+}, K^+ levels are extremely important in neurotransmission, muscle contraction, and nearly every cellular function (e.g., tetrodotoxin closes voltage-gated Na^+ channels).
- Chemicals that inhibit cellular respiration—inhibitors of proteins or enzymes involved in oxygen consumption, fuel utilization, and ATP production will cause energy depletion and cell death (e.g., cyanide inhibits cytochrome c oxidase).
- Chemicals that inhibit the production of cellular building blocks, e.g., nucleotides, lipids, amino acids (e.g., amanitin from death cap mushrooms), that alter ion channels and metabolism (e.g., sarin inhibits AChE and elevates ACh levels to active signaling pathways and ion channels).

All of the above can also cause inflammation which can lead to cellular dysfunction.

Q. What are two forms of cell deaths?

1. Necrosis: unprogrammed cell death (dangerous)
   a. Passive form of cell death induced by accidental damage of tissue does not involve the activation of any specific cellular program.
   b. Early loss of plasma membrane integrity and swelling of the cell body followed by bursting of cell.
   c. Mitochondria and various cellular processes contain substances that can be damaging to surrounding cells and are released upon bursting and cause inflammation.
   d. Cells necrotize in response to tissue damage (injury by chemicals and viruses, infection, cancer, inflammation, ischemia (death due to blockage of blood to tissue)) (Fig. 3.2).

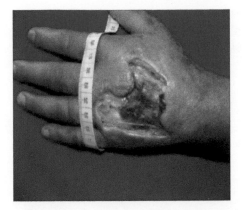

FIGURE 3.2

Extensive tissue necrosis of the dorsum of hand.

https://openi.nlm.nih.gov/imgs/512/94/2740528/PMC2740528_IJPS-41-145-g001.png?

keywords=necroses.

2. Apoptosis: one of the main forms of programmed cell death (not as dangerous to organism as necrosis).
   a. Active form of cell death enabling individual cells to commit suicide.
   b. Caspase dependent.
   c. Dying cells shrink and condense and then fragment, releasing small membrane-bound apoptotic bodies, which are phagocytosed by immune cells (i.e., macrophages).
   d. Intracellular constituents are not released where they might have deleterious effects on neighboring cells.

Q. What is necrosis of tissues?

Necrosis is caused by factors external to the cell or tissue, such as infection, toxins, or trauma which result in the unregulated digestion of cell components. Cell commits homicide is necrosis (Fig. 3.2).

Q. What is apoptosis?

Apoptosis is the term used to describe generally the normal death of the cell in living organisms. Since new cells regenerate, cell death is a normal and constant process in the body.

Q. What are the different stages of apoptosis?

Apoptosis has several distinct stages. In the first stage, the cell starts to become round as a result of the protein in the cell being eaten by enzymes that become active. Next, the DNA in the nucleus starts to come apart and

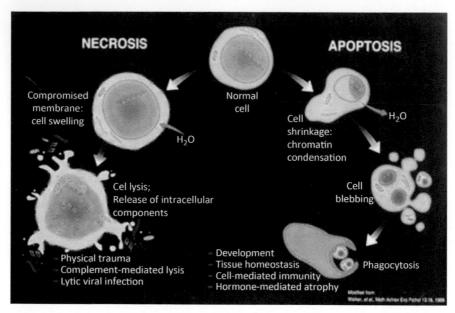

FIGURE 3.3

Different steps involved during the process of necrosis and apoptosis.

http://1.bp.blogspot.com/-ftJ7AFYXkmY/TW0q8cK4auI/AAAAAAAAC-o/AkM8Sgr65Z0/s1600/Necrosis%2BVs
%2BApoptosis.png.

shrink down. The membrane surrounding the nucleus begins to degrade and ultimately no longer forms the usual layer (Fig. 3.3). Cell commits suicide by apoptosis.

Q. Differentiate necrosis and apoptosis.

Table 3.1 highlights the major differences between necrosis and apoptosis.

Table 3.1 Difference Between Necrosis and Apoptosis

Necrosis	Apoptosis
• Cellular swelling	• Cell shrinkage
• Membranes are broken	• Membranes remain intact
• Cell lysis, eliciting an inflammatory reaction	• Cell is phagocytosed, no tissue reaction
• DNA fragmentation is random, pyknosia	• DNA fragmentation in to nucleosome size fragments
• Mechanism—ATP depletion, membrane injury, free radical damage	• Mechanism-caspase activation, endonuclease and proteases
• In vivo, whole areas of the tissue are affected	• In vivo, individual cells appear affected

3.4 QUESTION AND ANSWER EXERCISES

3.4.1 SHORT QUESTIONS AND ANSWERS

Exercise 1

Q.1 What are the possible toxic mechanisms for chemicals?

1. Produce reversible or irreversible bodily injury.
2. Have the capacity to cause tumors, neoplastic effects, or cancer.
3. Cause reproductive errors including mutations and teratogenic effects.
4. Produce irritation and sensitization of mucous membranes.
5. Cause a reduction in motivation, mental alertness, or capability.
6. Alter behavior or cause death of the organism.

Q.2 List the variety of processes of absorption including their characteristics.

1. Diffusion: molecules move from areas of high concentration to low concentration.
2. Facilitated diffusion: requires specialized carrier proteins, no high energy phosphate bonds are required.
3. Active transport: ATP is required in conjunction with special carrier proteins to move molecules through a membrane against a concentration gradient.
4. Endocytosis: particles and large molecules that might otherwise be restricted from crossing a plasma membrane can be brought in or removed by this process.

Q.3 How do toxic substances enter the body?

There are several ways in which toxic substances can enter the body. They may enter through the lungs by inhalation, through the skin, mucous membranes or eyes by absorption, or through the gastrointestinal tract by ingestion.

Q.4 What are the major functions of the skin?

The skin can help to:

1. regulate body temperature through sweat glands;
2. provide a physical barrier to dehydration, microbial invasion, and some chemical insults;
3. excrete salts, water, and organic compounds;
4. serve as a sensory organ for touch, temperature, pressure, and pain;
5. provide some important components of immunity.

Q.5 What are the three major mechanisms for the harmful effects of environmental toxins?

1. The toxins influence on enzymes.
2. Direct chemical combination of the toxin with a cell constituent.
3. Secondary action as a result of the toxins present in the system.

Q.6 List the four major types of hypersensitivity reactions.

1. Cytotoxic
2. Cell-mediated

   3. Immune complex
   4. Anaphylactic.

Q.7 What is the difference between mode of action and mechanism of toxicity?

   A mode of action should not be confused with mechanism of action, which refers to the biochemical processes underlying a given mode of action. Modes of toxic action are important, and are the widely used tools in ecotoxicology and aquatic toxicology because they classify toxicants or pollutants according to their type of toxic action.

Q.8 Define mode of toxic action.

   A mode of toxic action is a common set of physiological and behavioral signs that characterize a type of adverse biological response.

Q.9 What is cytotoxicity?

   Cytotoxicity is the quality of being toxic to cells. Treating cells with the cytotoxic compound can result in a variety of cell fates. The cells may undergo necrosis, in which they lose membrane integrity and die rapidly as a result of cell lysis. The cells can stop actively growing and dividing (a decrease in cell viability), or the cells can activate a genetic program of controlled cell death (apoptosis). Examples of toxic agents are an immune cell or some types of venom, e.g., from the puff adder (*Bitis arietans*) or brown recluse spider (*Loxosceles reclusa*).

Q.10 What is anaphylaxis?

   Anaphylaxis is a serious allergic reaction that is rapid in onset and may cause death. It typically causes more than one of the following: an itchy rash, throat or tongue swelling, shortness of breath, vomiting, lightheadedness, and low blood pressure. These symptoms typically come on over minutes to hours. Common causes include insect bites and stings, foods, and medications.

3.4.2 MULTIPLE CHOICE QUESTIONS (CHOOSE THE BEST STATEMENT, IT CAN BE ONE, TWO OR ALL OR NONE)

Exercise 2

Q.1 A possible reason for the selective embryo/fetal toxicity of DES is
   a. higher concentration of free DES in embryo/fetal compared to adults
   b. binding to retinoic acid receptors
   c. lack of placental drug metabolism
   d. all of the above

Q.2 The liver and kidney are the major target organs of toxicity because
   a. they both receive a high percentage of cardiac output
   b. they both have substantial xenobiotic metabolizing capacity
   c. they both have transport systems that can concentrate xenobiotics
   d. all of the above

Q.3 Acyl glucuronides are particularly toxic to the liver because
    a. they selectively interact with macrophages releasing active oxygen
    b. active transport systems in the hepatocyte and bile duct system can greatly concentrate them.
    c. they are resistant to glucuronidase
    d. they are suitable inhibitors of UGT2B7

Q.4 The selective renal toxicity of cephaloridine over cephalothin is due to
    a. selective uptake by the organic cation transporter
    b. selective inhibition of P-glycoprotein
    c. selective uptake by the organic anion transporter
    d. significantly less plasma protein binding of cephaloridine

Q.5 All of the following are of α-amanitin except
    a. it is less orally available than phalloidin
    b. it inhibits RNA polymerase II
    c. it is transported into the hepatocyte by a bile acid transporter
    d. it is a mushroom toxin

Q.6 All of the following are true of the toxic mechanism of paraquat except
    a. lungs accumulate paraquat in an energy-dependent manner
    b. its energy into the lungs is assumed to be via the polyamine transport system
    c. similar molecules with smaller distances between nitrogen atoms do not enter lungs as readily
    d. cytotoxicity to alveolar cells is caused by interference with calcium channels

Q.7 Enzyme induction of phenobarbital is mediated through
    a. aryl hydrocarbon receptor
    b. Peroxisome proliferator-activated receptor (PPAR)-α receptor
    c. constitutively active receptor (CAR)
    d. estrogen receptor

Q.8 CAR is downregulated by
    a. hypericum extracts
    b. acetaminophen
    c. aspirin
    d. proinflammatory cytokines

Q.9 The pregnane X receptor
    a. is a cytosolic receptor
    b. is involved in induction of CYP3A4
    c. is primarily expressed in skin
    d. all of the above

Q.10 Xenobiotic toxicity that occurs after repair and adaptive processes are overwhelmed include all of the following except
    a. fibrosis
    b. apoptosis
    c. necrosis
    d. carcinogenesis

Answers

1. a; 2. d; 3. b; 4. c; 5. a; 6. d; 7. c; 8. d; 9. b; 10. b.

Exercise 3

Q.1 Amphipathic xenobiotics that can become trapped in lysosomes and cause phospholipidosis include all of the following except
  a. ethylene glycol
  b. amiodarone
  c. amitriptyline
  d. fluoxetine

Q.2 Which of the following parent toxicant-electrophilic metabolite pairs is incorrect?
  a. Halothane—phosgene
  b. Bromobenzene—bromobenzene 3,4-oxide
  c. Benzene—muconic aldehyde
  d. Allyl alcohol—acrolein

Q.3 All of the following are capable of accepting the electrons from reductases and forming radicals except
  a. paraquat
  b. doxorubicin
  c. n-hexane
  d. nitrofurantoin

Q.4 An example of the formation of an electrophilic toxicant from an inorganic chemical is
  a. CO to CO_2
  b. AsO_4
  c. NO to NO_2
  d. hydroxide ion to water

Q.5 The general mechanism for detoxification of electrophiles is
  a. conjugation with glucuronic acid
  b. conjugation with acetyl CoA
  c. conjugation with glutathione
  d. conjugation with sulfate

Q.6 The most common nucleophilic detoxification reaction that amines undergo is
  a. acetylation
  b. sulfation
  c. methylation
  d. amino acid conjugation

Q.7 Detoxification mechanisms fail because
  a. toxicants may overwhelm the detoxification process
  b. a reactive toxicant may inactivate a detoxicating enzyme
  c. detoxication may produce toxic by-product
  d. all of the above

Q.8 The most potent carcinogen derived from nicotine is
  a. naphthene
  b. styrene
  c. nicotine-derived nitrosamine ketone (NNK)
  d. methyl tert-butyl ketone
Q.9 Hydroxyl radical can be produced by all of the following except
  a. the action of nitric oxide synthetase on water
  b. interaction of ionizing radiation and water
  c. reductive homolytic fission of hydrogen peroxide
  d. interaction of silica with surface iron ions in lung tissue
Q.10 If an electrophile is covalently bound to a protein that does not play a critical function, the result is considered a
  a. toxication reaction
  b. detoxication reaction
  c. MNA-adduct formation
  d. Fenton reaction

Answers
1. a; 2. a; 3. c; 4. b; 5. c; 6. a; 7. d; 8. c; 9. a; 10. b.

Exercise 4

Q.1 Which of the following receptor-exogenous ligand pairs is incorrect?
  a. Estrogen receptor—zearalenone
  b. Glucocorticoid receptor—dexamethasone
  c. Aryl hydrocarbon receptor—rifampicin
  d. PPAR—clofibrate
Q.2 Which of the following receptor-agonist pairs incorrect?
  a. Glutamate receptor—kainate
  b. Glycine receptor—strychnine
  c. Gamma-aminobutyric acid (GABA) (A) receptor—muscimol
  d. Opioid receptor—meperidine
Q.3 Which of the following receptor-antagonist pairs is incorrect?
  a. Adrenergic beta I receptor—metoprolol
  b. Serotonin (2) receptor—ketanserin
  c. Glutamate receptor—ketamine
  d. GABA (A) receptor—avermectins
Q.4 Clonidine overdose mimics poisoning with
  a. morphine
  b. cocaine
  c. phencyclidine
  d. amphetamine
Q.5 All of the following act as inhibitors of the citric acid cycle except
  a. 4-pentenoic acid
  b. fluoroacetate

     c. DCVC (*S*-(1,2-dichlorovinyl)-L-cysteine)

     d. malonate

Q.6 All of the following are inhibitors of ADP phosphorylation except
     a. oligomycin
     b. dichlorodiphenyltrichloroethane (DDT)
     c. ethanol
     d. *N*-ethylmaleimide

Q.7 All of the following cause calcium influx into the cytoplasm except
     a. capsaicin
     b. formate
     c. domoate
     d. amphotericin B

Q.8 All of the following inhibit calcium export from the cytoplasm except
     a. vanadate
     b. methyl mercury
     c. bromobenzene
     d. carbon tetrachloride

Q.9 Hydroxyl radical is enzymatically detoxified by
     a. catalase
     b. glutathione peroxide
     c. glutathione reductase
     d. none of the above

Q.10 Which of the following regarding cell death is true?
     a. Necrosis requires ATP.
     b. Release of cytochrome c usually triggers necrosis.
     c. Toxicants at low doses usually cause apoptosis and necrosis at higher doses.
     d. Apoptosis is never a desirable effect

Answers

1. c; 2. b; 3. d; 4. a; 5. a; 6. c; 7. b; 8. b; 9. d; 10. c.

Exercise 5

Q.1 Major target molecules for toxicants include all of the following except
     a. proteins
     b. vitamins
     c. DNA
     d. lipids

Q.2 All of the following toxins act by enzymatic reaction except
     a. ricin
     b. anthrax
     c. tetrodotoxin
     d. botulinum

Q.3 Apoptotic pathways can be initiated by
  a. DNA damage
  b. mitochondrial insult
  c. death-receptor stimulation
  d. all of the above

Q.4 The enzyme that repairs oxidized protein thiols is called
  a. HMG-coenzyme A reductase
  b. adenylyl cyclase
  c. phospholipase
  d. none of the above

Q.5 The MOA for bleomycin-induced lung injury is presumed to include
  a. DNA-adduct formation
  b. generation of reactive oxygen species
  c. inhibition of cytochrome oxidase
  d. none of the above

Q.6 All of the following are true of oxidative DNA damage except
  a. mitochondrial DNA is much more resistant to damage than nuclear DNA
  b. 8-hydroxy-deoxyguanosine in the urine is a marker
  c. it can lead to base pair transversions
  d. it can lead to a point mutation

Q.7 An example of a denatured protein is
  a. Golgi complex
  b. micronuclei
  c. Heinz body
  d. histone

Q.8 An important feature of lipid peroxidation is
  a. it cannot be blocked by antioxidants
  b. damage can be propagated in a chain reaction-like manner
  c. it never involves the Fenton reaction
  d. the end products are different from the end products of the reaction of lipids with ozone

Q.9 All of the following are true regarding mechanisms of immune system toxicology except
  a. 2,3,7,8-Tetrachlorodibenzo-p-dioxin (TCDD)-induced thymic atrophy may be mediated by the aryl hydrocarbon receptor
  b. the addition of a hapten to a protein may cause a conformational change that displays previously hidden antigenic regions
  c. oral exposure of a xenobiotic is associated with a much greater chance of an immune reaction than by other routes
  d. the "danger hypothesis" refers to a break in immune tolerance to an antigen triggered by signals initiated by cellular or systemic stress

Q.10 Which statement is true regarding the PPAR-α receptor?
  a. Stimulation causes peroxisome proliferation in humans
  b. They are present in adipose tissues

    c. They are involved in fatty acid β-oxidation
    d. Thiazolidinediones act as ligands

Answers

1. b; 2. c; 3. d; 4. d; 5. b; 6. a; 7. c; 8. b; 9. c; 10. c.

Exercise 6

Q.1 Alterations in retinoic acid receptor function been associated with
    a. cardiac and vascular toxicity
    b. CNS and peripheral nerve toxicity
    c. hepatic and renal toxicity
    d. embryo and testicular toxicity

Q.2 Proteins present in brown adipose tissue act mechanically like
    a. pentachlorophenol
    b. rotenone
    c. cyanide
    d. doxorubicin

Q.3 Which of the following regarding glutathione is false?
    a. It can act nonenzymatically as a radical scavenger.
    b. It is a dipeptide.
    c. Its levels can be upregulated in response to a need.
    d. It is a substrate for glutathione peroxidase.

Q.4 All of the following are associated with necrosis except
    a. requirement of ATP
    b. cell swelling
    c. association with an inflammatory response
    d. initiation by plasma membrane permeability changes

Q.5 Another name for apoptosis is
    a. passive cell death
    b. accidental cell death
    c. programmed cell death
    d. immune cell death

Q.6 All of the following are true of apoptosis except
    a. cell membrane remains intact
    b. early in the process, caspases are activated
    c. oxidative stress can initiate it
    d. it can lead to carcinogenesis

Q.7 A mitochondrial factor involved in the process of apoptosis is
    a. cytochrome a3
    b. cytochrome b6
    c. cytochrome c
    d. cytochrome a1

Q.8 A class of drugs that can induce apoptosis in certain cancer cells is
    a. barbiturates
    b. digitalis glycosides

    c. protein pump inhibitors

    d. cyclooxygenase-2 (COX-2) inhibitors

Q.9 Which of the following signals-transduction pathway effect pairs is correct?

    a. ras/ERK—suppression of apoptosis

    b. JNK—mediate apoptosis

    c. p38—production of inflammatory cytokines

    d. All of the above

Q.10 A drug that works by disrupting mitosis is

    a. paclitaxel

    b. doxorubicin

    c. methotrexate

    d. cyclophosphamide

Answers

1. d; 2. a; 3. b; 4. a; 5. c; 6. d; 7. c; 8. d; 9. d; 10. a.

Exercise 7

Q.1 Galactosamine causes

    a. proximal tubular damage

    b. focal liver necrosis

    c. peripheral neuropathy

    d. all of the above

Q.2 Practolol was withdrawn from use because of

    a. unpredictable beta blockade

    b. rebound hypertension

    c. teratogenicity

    d. oculomucocutaneous syndrome

Q.3 All of the following can inhibit opening of the mitochondrial permeability transition pore except

    a. cyclosporine A

    b. hydrophobic bile ducts

    c. L-deprenyl

    d. bongkrekic acid

Q.4 Microcystins target

    a. adenylyl cyclase

    b. phosphodiesterase

    c. protein phosphatase

    d. guanyl cyclase

Q.5 All of the following are true of cytokines except

    a. short half-life

    b. act locally

    c. produced in specialized organs

    d. have complex interactions

Q.6 Molecular chaperones
  a. repair denatured proteins
  b. repair damaged DNA
  c. repair damaged transfer RNA
  d. act as a catalyst for new protein synthesis

Q.7 Lipid repair
  a. cannot occur
  b. requires Nicotinamide adenine dinucleotide phosphate (NADPH)
  c. may involve catalase
  d. none of the above

Q.8 In peripheral neurons with damaged axons, repair
  a. can only occur until approximately age 3
  b. follows the same mechanism as CNS repair
  c. requires activated neutrophils and astrocytes
  d. requires macrophages and Schwann cells

Q.9 Apoptosis is most advantageous in
  a. neoplastic prostate cells
  b. female germ cells
  c. cardiac myocytes
  d. CNS neurons

Q.10 The principal factor leading to fibrogenesis is
  a. interleukin-8 (IL-8)
  b. interferon-α (INF-α)
  c. transforming growth factor-β (TGF-β)
  d. interleukin-1 (IL-1)

Answers
1. b; 2. d; 3. b; 4. c; 5. c; 6. a; 7. b; 8. d; 9. a; 10. c.

Exercise 8

Q.1 Fibrosis is harmful because
  a. it may compress blood cells
  b. it may contribute to tissue malnutrition
  c. it may interfere with mechanical organ function
  d. all of the above

Q.2 All of the following are true regarding idiosyncratic drug reactions except
  a. they are rare
  b. they are predictable from the pharmacology of the drug
  c. the reaction can be dose dependent
  d. they involve genetic or acquired factors that increase susceptibility

Q.3 All of the following would indicate initiation of a cellular stress response except
  a. downregulation of DNA repair enzymes
  b. induction of apoptosis

   c. upregulation of antioxidant mechanisms
   d. stimulation of an immune response
Q.4 All of the following contribute to organ-selective toxicity except
   a. organ-selective uptake
   b. tissue-specific expression of transcription factors
   c. number of chromosomes in nucleus
   d. tissue-specific receptors
Q.5 The nephrotoxic effect of mercury on the kidney is thought to be mediated by
   a. blocking the effect of ADH on the collecting duct
   b. interfering with ionic charges on the glomerulus
   c. a dicysteinyl−mercury complex mimicking endogenous cysteine
   d. interfering with chloride transport in the loop of Henle
Q.6 An example of a soft neutrophil is
   a. sulfur in glutathione
   b. phosphate oxygen in nucleic acids
   c. mercuric ion
   d. carboxylate anion
Q.7 The Fenton reaction produces
   a. phosgene from chloroform
   b. formic acid from formaldehyde
   c. nitrogen dioxide from ozone and nitrogen
   d. hydroxyl radical and hydroxyl ions from hydrogen peroxide
Q.8 Which is the most likely process of absorption for amino acids?
   a. Diffusion
   b. Facilitated diffusion
   c. Active transport
   d. Endocytosis
   e. None of the above
Q.9 Which of the following sites in the respiratory system is the most likely place for the carbon dioxide and oxygen to exchange in the blood?
   a. Nose
   b. Pharynx
   c. Larynx
   d. Trachea
   e. Alveoli
Q.10 Which of the following processes, when prolonged and severe, can be life threatening such as in asthmatic attacks?
   a. Mucociliary streaming
   b. Coughing
   c. Sneezing
   d. Bronchoconstriction
   e. None of the above

Answers

1. d; 2. b; 3. a; 4. c; 5. c; 6. a; 7. d; 8. b; 9. e; 10. d.

Exercise 9

Q.1 What is the best estimate for the area of skin coverage in the average adult?

   a. 2500 in^2
   b. 3000 in^2
   c. 3500 in^2
   d. 4000 in^2
   e. 4500 in^2

Q.2 By which absorptive process does hexane pass through the skin?

   a. Passive diffusion
   b. Facilitated diffusion
   c. Active transport
   d. Endocytosis
   e. None of the above

Q.3 How long is the average adult human gastrointestinal tract?

   a. 20 ft
   b. 22 ft
   c. 30 ft
   d. 41 ft
   e. 52 ft

Q.4 Where is the most likely site for the absorption of toxic agents in the gastrointestinal tract?

   a. Between the stomach and the upper portion of the intestine
   b. Stomach
   c. Small intestine
   d. Large intestine
   e. The lower portion of large intestine

Q.5 What is the mechanism for the harmful effects of CO (carbon monoxide)?

   a. Interferes with or blocks the active sites of some important enzymes.
   b. Direct chemical combination with a cell constituent.
   c. Secondary action as a result of its presence in the system.
   d. Competes with the cofactors for a site on an important enzyme.
   e. None of the above.

Q.6 What is the major organ responsible for detoxification in the body?

   a. Lung
   b. Intestines
   c. Kidney
   d. Liver
   e. Skin

Q.7 What is the major toxic mechanism for hydrogen cyanide?
   a. Interferes with or blocks the active sites of the enzyme.
   b. Inactivates or removes the cofactor.
   c. Competes with the cofactor for a site on the enzyme.
   d. Alters the enzyme structure directly, thereby changing the specific three-dimensional nature of the active site.
   e. None of the above.

Q.8 What is the major mechanism for toxicity of dithiocarbamate during alcohol consumption?
   a. Interferes with or blocks the active sites of the enzyme.
   b. Inactivates or removes the cofactor.
   c. Competes with the cofactor for a site on the enzyme.
   d. Alters the enzyme structure directly, thereby changing the specific three-dimensional nature of the active site.
   e. None of the above.

Q.9 Which of the following substances can cause a syndrome in infants referred to as "blue baby"?
   a. Carbon monoxide
   b. Chlorine gas
   c. Ozone
   d. Sulfuric oxides
   e. Nitrogen compounds

Q.10 Which of the following refers to a substance that is attached to an antigen and promotes an antigenic response?
   a. Light chain
   b. Heavy chain
   c. Leukocyte
   d. Helper cell
   e. Hapten

Answers

1. b; 2. a; 3. c; 4. a; 5. b; 6. d; 7. b; 8. b; 9. e; 10. e.

Exercise 10

Q.1 Which kind of cells are the primary targets of the AIDS virus?
   a. Cytotoxic (killer) cell
   b. Helper T-cells (e.g., CD4)
   c. Memory cells
   d. Suppressor T-cells
   e. Delayed hypersensitivity T-cells

Q.2 The largest percent of antibodies belong to the _____ class.
   a. IgG
   b. IgE
   c. IgM

    d. IgA

    e. IgD

Q.3 Which of the following hypersensitivity reactions is most often seen in transfusion reactions?

    a. Cytotoxic

    b. Cell-mediated

    c. Immune complex

    d. Anaphylactic

    e. None of the above

Q.4 Which kind of hypersensitivity is associated with asthma?

    a. Cytotoxic

    b. Cell-mediated

    c. Immune complex

    d. Anaphylactic

    e. None of the above

Q.5 Which kind of the following interactions is a characteristic of that for caffeine and sleeping pills?

    a. Additive

    b. Synergistic

    c. Antagonistic

    d. None of the above

    e. They do not interact with each other

Q.6 Yu-Cheng disease in Taiwan is due to the toxic effect of

    a. lead

    b. polychlorinated biphenyls (PCBs)

    c. dioxin

    d. asbestos

    e. mercury

Q.7 When were both federal regulatory and legislative efforts begun to reduce lead hazards, including the limitation of lead in paint and gasoline?

    a. 1970s

    b. 1980s

    c. 1990s

    d. 2000s

    e. 2015

Q.8 Cytochrome P450 activity can be affected by

    a. foods

    b. social habits

    c. thyroid disease

    d. all of the above

Q.9 An example of oxidative desulfurization is

    a. parathion to paraoxon

    b. imipramine to desipramine

    c. codeine to morphine

    d. enalapril to enalaprilat

Q.10 CYP3A7 is present mostly in

    a. adult human liver

    b. fetal human liver

    c. rodent liver

    d. human lymphoma cells

Answers

1. b; 2. a; 3. a; 4. d; 5. c; 6. b; 7. a; 8. d; 9. a; 10. b.

3.4.3 TRUE OR FALSE STATEMENTS (WRITE T FOR TRUE AND F FOR THE FALSE STATEMENT)

Exercise 11

Q.1 When lead covalently bonds to an enzyme, its inhibition of enzymes is considered to be irreversible.

Q.2 The exposure of allergens can trigger a diminished immune response in some people.

Q.3 Chemical pollutants such as ozone can depress the immune response by inactivating alveolar macrophages.

Q.4 B-cells are the principle agents in cell-mediated immunity.

Q.5 Humoral immune responses are characterized by subcutaneous bleeding.

Q.6 The environmental pollutants such as ozone and fine particulates contribute to the significant rise in the numbers and severity of asthma cases.

Q.7 If absorbed, lead tends to be stored mostly in fatty tissue.

Q.8 Dioxin is considered to be one of the most toxic natural chemicals.

Q.9 The US Environmental Protection Agency (EPA) has listed 20 µg/dL as the maximum acceptable blood lead level for fetuses and young children.

Q.10 Lead may impair fertility in both men and women when blood lead levels approach 50 µg/dL.

Answers

1. T; 2. F; 3. T; 4. F; 5. T; 6. T; 7. F; 8. F; 9. F; 10. T.

Exercise 12

Q.1 Lead has been recognized as a hazard since early civilization when it was used to store wine, to pipe water, and even as vessels in which to cook food.

Q.2 Once a potential toxic substance goes into our society, it automatically produces an adverse effect.

Q.3 External respiration refers to the exchange of gases between blood and individual cells.

Q.4 Sulfur oxides tend to reach deep into lung tissue while nitrogen dioxides tend to act in the upper moist airways of the respiratory tree.

Q.5 The skin is the body's largest organ and consists of many interconnected tissues.

Q.6 Epidermis is the outer, thinner layer of the skin and dermis is the inner and much thicker layer of the skin.

Q.7 The gastrointestinal tract is a major route of absorption for many toxic agents including mercury, lead, and cadmium.

Q.8 A toxin can produce a harmful effect upon an organ only by stimulating the normal metabolic actions of that particular organ.

Q.9 Many enzymes require a nonprotein component called apoenzyme and a protein component called cofactor to become active.

Q.10 Cadmium and beryllium are believed to inactivate enzymes by blocking the sites on the enzyme where such cofactors as iron normally attach.

Answers

1. T; 2. F; 3. F; 4. F; 5. T; 6. T; 7. T; 8. F; 9. F; 10. F.

3.4.4 MATCH THE STATEMENTS

Exercise 13

Q. Match the following statements in Columns A and B.

Column A	Column B
1. Muscimol	a. Serotonin agonist
2. Benzodiazepines	b. Prevents vesicle dopamine uptake
3. Clonidine	c. Inhibits norepinephrine uptake
4. Baclofen	d. Direct nicotine antagonist
3. Bicuculline	e. Direct dopamine agonist
6. Theophylline	f. Direct serotonin antagonist/glycine uptake inhibitor
7. Nicotine	g. Direct GABA (A) agonist
8. Clozapine	h. Indirect GABA (A) agonist
9. Recadenoson	i. α-2 Adrenoceptor agonist
10. Yohimbine	j. Dopamine antagonist
11. Cocaine	k. Direct GABA (B) agonist
12. α-Bungarotoxin	l. Adenosine antagonist
13. Botulinum toxin	m. Direct adenosine agonist
14. Bromocriptine	n. α-2 Adrenoceptor antagonist
13. Haloperidol	o. Direct GABA (A) antagonist
16. Reserpine	p. Agonist at neuromuscular junction
17. Ergonovine	q. Inhibits ACh release

Answers

Column A	Column B
1. Muscimol	g. Direct GABA (A) agonist
2. Benzodiazepines	h. Indirect GABA (A) agonist
3. Clonidine	i. α-2 Adrenoceptor agonist
4. Baclofen	k. Direct GABA (B) agonist
3. Bicuculline	o. Direct GABA (A) antagonist
6. Theophylline	l. Adenosine antagonist
7. Nicotine	p. Agonist at neuromuscular junction
8. Clozapine	f. Direct serotonin antagonist/glycine uptake inhibitor
9. Recadenoson	m. Direct adenosine agonist
10. Yohimbine	n. α-2 Adrenoceptor antagonist
11. Cocaine	c. Inhibits norepinephrine uptake
12. α-Bungarotoxin	d. Direct nicotine antagonist
13. Botulinum toxin	q. Inhibits ACh release
14. Bromocriptine	e. Direct dopamine agonist
13. Haloperidol	j. Dopamine antagonist
16. Reserpine	b. Prevents vesicle dopamine uptake
17. Ergonovine	a. Serotonin agonist

FURTHER READING

Boelsterli, U.A., 2007. Mechanistic Toxicology: The Molecular Basis of How Chemicals Disrupt Biological Targets, second ed. CRC Press, Taylor and Francis, pp. 1−416.

Curry, S.C., 2011. Neurotransmitters and neuromodulators. In: Nelson, L.S. (Ed.), Goldfrank's Toxicologic Emergencies, ninth ed. McGraw-Hill, New York, NY, pp. 189−220.

Gregus, Z., 2013. Mechanisms of toxicity. In: Klaassen, C.D. (Ed.), Casarett and Doull's Toxicology: The Basic Science of Poisons, eighth ed. McGraw-Hill, New York, NY, pp. 49−122.

Timbrell, J.A., 2009. Biochemical mechanisms of toxicity: specific examples. In: Timbrell, J.A. (Ed.), Principles of Biochemical Toxicology, fourth ed. Informa, New York, NY, pp. 221−250.

Target organ toxicity

CHAPTER OUTLINE

4.1 INTRODUCTION

There are several thousands of chemicals used in day-to-day life. The chemical industry introduces about 200–1000 new chemicals each year. Because of this, we are exposed to a number of chemicals in our home, at work, and in the general environment. Trace amounts of toxic chemicals are present in the food, the air, and the drinking water. Exposure to toxic substances occurs through four major routes listed as follows. The major target organs are shown in Fig. 4.1.

1. Inhalation
2. Injections
3. Oral exposure
4. Dermal.

Illustrated Toxicology. DOI: http://dx.doi.org/10.1016/B978-0-12-813213-5.00004-3

Target organs

- Nervous system
- Skin
- Lung
- Liver
- Kidney
- Reproduction

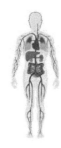

FIGURE 4.1

Major target organs of body.

https://media.licdn.com/mpr/mpr/shrinknp_800_800/
AAEAAQAAAAAAAYhAAAAJGNjNTlyNDY0LTBlZDctNGQwMi04YTI3LWQxZTdjNWVkNjVhZg.png.

4.2 DEFINITIONS

Q. Define an organ.

An organ is a part of your body that has a particular purpose or function, e.g., heart or lungs, muscles and internal organs, and the reproductive organs.

Q. Define organ toxicity.

Toxicity is the degree to which a substance can damage an organism. Toxicity can refer to the effect on a whole organism, such as an animal, bacterium, or plant, as well as the effect on a substructure of the organism, such as a cell (cytotoxicity) or an organ such as the liver (hepatotoxicity).

Q. What do you mean by target organ toxins?

Target organ toxins are chemicals that can cause adverse effects or disease states manifested in specific organs of the body. Toxins do not affect all organs in the body to the same extent due to their different cell structures.

4.3 HEPATOTOXICITY

Q. What is hepatotoxicity (liver)?

Hepatotoxicity is damage produced to liver such as liver enlargement, and even cirrhosis. Prescription medications, herbal remedies, and natural chemicals or any toxicant/toxin can lead to hepatotoxicity. Approximately half of all cases of acute liver failure are related to hepatotoxicity. The type of liver damage caused by toxic substances/medications varies widely and depends upon the type of drug being taken, the dosage, and the overall health of the patient. The most common over-the-counter medication associated with the development of liver damage is acetaminophen. Other types of drugs which have been linked to high rates of hepatotoxicity include chemotherapy drugs, carbon tetrachloride, alcohol (Fig. 4.2), nitrosamines, chloroform, toluene, perchloroethylene, cresol, and dimethylsulfate.

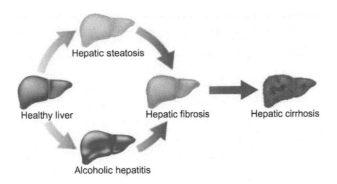

FIGURE 4.2

Alcoholic liver disease.

http://images.wisegeek.com/alcoholic-liver-disease-diagram.jpg.

4.4 NEPHROTOXICITY (KIDNEY)

Q. What is nephrotoxicity?

Nephrotoxicity is a toxic/poisonous effect of any substance on renal function. The nephrotoxic effect of most drugs is more profound in individuals already suffering from kidney failure. Acute ethylene glycol poisoning is serious with a fatal outcome in more than 88% of cases (Fig. 4.3). Several other chemicals are known to cause edema, proteinuria, and other kidney problems. Some of these chemicals include halogenated hydrocarbons, uranium, chloroform, mercury, and dimethyl sulfate.

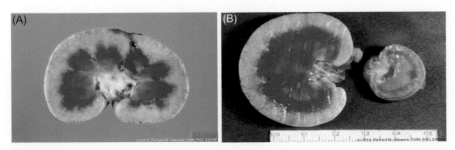

FIGURE 4.3

Feline kidney granular cortex (ethylene glycol poisoning) (A) and canine kidneys unilateral hypoplasia (ethylene glycol toxicity) (B).

(A) http://ocw.tufts.edu/Content/72/imagegallery/1362318/1368971/1377332 and
(B) http://ocw.tufts.edu/Content/72/imagegallery/1362318/1368971/1377322

4.5 NEUROTOXICITY (NERVOUS SYSTEM)

Q. What is neurotoxicity?

Neurotoxicity refers to damage/or toxic effect to nervous system. Neurotoxins are an extensive class of exogenous chemical neurological insults that can adversely affect function in both developing and mature nervous tissue. These toxins may cause narcosis, behavioral changes, and decreased muscle coordination. The term can also be used to classify endogenous compounds, which, when abnormally contact, can prove neurologically toxic. Common examples of neurotoxins include lead, ethanol (drinking alcohol), manganese, glutamate, nitric oxide (NO), botulinum toxin (e.g., Botox) (Fig. 4.4), tetanus toxin, and tetrodotoxin, mercury, carbon disulfide, benzene, carbon tetrachloride, lead, mercury, and nitrobenzene.

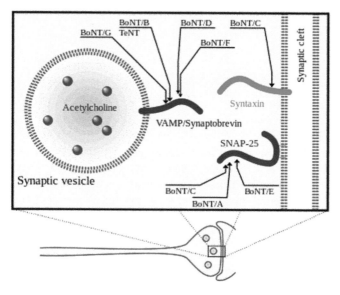

FIGURE 4.4

Mechanism of action of botulinum toxin.

Reproduced from Wikipedia (https://upload.wikimedia.org/wikipedia/commons/thumb/8/8b/
Presynaptic_CNTs_targets.svg/425px-Presynaptic_CNTs_targets.svg.png).

4.6 HEMATOPOIETIC (BLOOD) TOXICITY

Q. What is hematopoietic toxicity?

The hematopoietic system includes bone marrow, thymus, lymph nodes, and spleen. Hematopoietic system produces the cellular components of the blood. Several toxicants such as copper deficiency, vitamin B12 deficiency, cobalt and folic acid deficiencies, toxins and toxicants (snake venoms, potassium and sodium chlorate, chronic lead poisoning, carbon monoxide, cyanides, nitrobenzene, aniline, arsenic, benzene, toluene) are known to cause toxicity to hematopoietic system (Fig. 4.5).

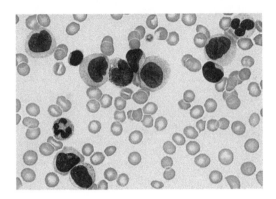

FIGURE 4.5

Blood smear of the patient with chronic lymphocytic leukemia.

Reproduced from https://upload.wikimedia.org/wikipedia/commons/6/6f/AML-M4.jpg.

4.7 PULMONARY TOXICITY

Q. What is pulmonary toxicity?

Damage to the lungs is known as pulmonary toxicity. Lung damage often presents as inflammation, also called pneumonitis. Problems due to lung system include cough, tightness in chest, and shortness of breath. For example, in cystic fibrosis patients (Fig. 4.6), mucus buildup impairs lung function by blocking airways. The mucus also traps pathogens that we inhale instead of clearing them out of the lungs, causing frequent lung infections. Other substances known to damage lungs include paraquat herbicides, silica asbestos, nitrogen dioxide, ozone, hydrogen sulfide chromium, nickel, and alcohol.

4.8 DEVELOPMENTAL AND REPRODUCTIVE TOXICITY

Q. Define reproductive toxicology.

Reproductive toxicology is the study of occurrence of adverse effects on the male and female reproductive system due to exposure to chemicals or physical agents.

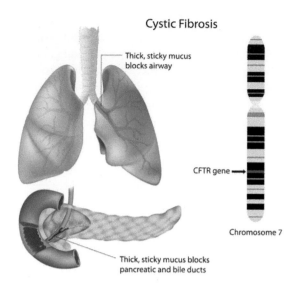

FIGURE 4.6

Cystic fibrosis of lungs.

Reproduced from Genetics Home Reference (https://ghr.nlm.nih.gov/art/large/cystic-fibrosis-overview.jpeg?ow).

Q. Define development toxicology.

Development toxicology deals with the study of harmful effects of chemicals and drugs on the development of an organism, and manifestations of development toxicity include structural malformations, growth retardation, functional impairment, and/or death of an organism.

Q. Define teratology.

Teratology is the study of malformations induced by the toxic agents during development between conception and birth.

Q. Define genetic toxicology.

It deals with the study of interaction of toxicants with the process of hereditary.

Q. What is reproductive toxicity?

Reproductive toxicity is a hazard associated with some chemical substances that interfere in some way with normal reproduction; such substances are called reprotoxic. It includes adverse effects on sexual function and fertility in adult males and females, as well as developmental toxicity in the offspring such as birth defects and sterility. Chemicals such as dibromo dichloropropane, (*S*)-thalidomide, endocrine disruptors, and many other toxicants including metals and pesticides are known to have adverse effects on the development and reproduction in human beings and animals. For example, a rare congenital deformity in which the hands or feet are attached close to the trunk, and the limbs are grossly underdeveloped or absent has been reported as a side effect of the drug thalidomide taken during early pregnancy.

4.9 DERMAL TOXICITY

Q. What is dermal toxicity?

Dermal toxicity is the ability of a substance or poison to adversely affect the skin. Defatting of skin, rashes, and irritation are common with various toxins, drugs, ketones, chlorinated compounds, alcohols, nickel, phenol, trichloroethylene, zinc deficiency, etc. (Acneiform eruptions, or folliculitis (Fig. 4.7), often begin as facial erythema that progresses to papules and pustules and spreads to the upper trunk. Causes of folliculitis in cancer patients include actinomycin-D (Cosmegen)—the most common—as well as epidermal growth factor receptor inhibiting agents, such as gefitinib (Iressa) and cetuximab (Erbitux).)

FIGURE 4.7

Folliculitis.

Reproduced from Shutterstock (https://www.shutterstock.com/th/image-photo/human-skin-texture-309950684?src=FO-zYRAZyO5sVoVCVLOnyg-1-17).

4.10 OCULAR TOXICITY

Q. What is ocular toxicity?

Ocular toxicity results from direct contact or after exposure to any toxicant that leads to conjunctivitis, corneal damage, etc. Some of the common toxicants include organic solvents, acids, cresol, quinone, hydroxycholoroquine (Fig. 4.8), benzyl chloride, butyl alcohol, and bases.

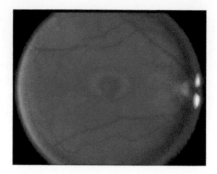

FIGURE 4.8

Retinal photograph showing classic "bull's eye" retinopathy of hydroxychloroquine toxicity, which represents atrophy of the retinal pigment epithelium.

http://www.the-rheumatologist.org/wp-content/uploads/springboard/image/THR_May_2011_pp50_02.jpg.

4.11 TARGET ORGAN TOXICITY END POINTS

Q. Why are toxins often selective to tissues? Give suitable examples.

1. Preferential accumulation: Toxicant may accumulate in only certain tissues and cause toxicity to that particular tissue, e.g., Cd in kidney, paraquat in lung.
2. Selective metabolic activation: Enzymes needed to convert a compound to the active form may be present in highest quantities in a particular organ, e.g., CCl_4, nitrosamines in liver.
3. Characteristics of tissue repair: Some tissues may be protected from toxicity by actively repairing toxic damage; some tissues may be susceptible because they lack sufficient repair capabilities, e.g., nitrosamines in liver.
4. Specific receptors and/or functions: Toxicant may interact with receptors in a given tissue, e.g., curare—a receptor-specific neuromuscular blocker.
5. Physiological sensitivity: The nervous system is extremely sensitive to agents that block utilization of oxygen, e.g., nitrite, oxidizes hemoglobin (methemoglobinemia), cyanide, inhibits cytochrome oxidase (cells not able to utilize oxygen), and barbiturates, interfere with sensors for oxygen and carbon dioxide content in blood.

Q. What are the main target organs most frequently affected by toxicants?

1. Central nervous system (CNS)
2. Circulatory system (blood, blood-forming system)
3. Visceral organs (liver, kidneys, lung)
4. Muscle and bone.

   Table 4.1 presents only examples of toxicological end points and examples of agents of concern in humans. It is not an exhaustive or inclusive list of organs, end points, or agents. Absence from this list does not indicate a relative lack of evidence for a causal relation as to any agent of concern.

Table 4.1 Sample of Selected Toxicological End Points and Examples of Agents of Concern in Humans

Organ System	Examples of End Points	Examples of Agents of Concern
Skin	Allergic contact dermatitis	Nickel, poison ivy, cutting oils
	Chloracne	Dioxins
	Cancer	Polycyclic aromatic hydrocarbons
Respiratory tract	Nonspecific irritation (reactive airway disease)	Formaldehyde, acrolein, ozone
	Asthma	Toluene diisocyanate
	Chronic obstructive pulmonary disease	Cigarette smoke
	Fibrosis, pneumoconiosis, cancer	Silica, mineral dusts, cotton dust cigarette smoke, arsenic, asbestos, nickel
Blood and the immune system	Anemia	Arsine, lead, methyldopa
	Secondary polycythemia	Cobalt
	Methemoglobinemia	Nitrites, aniline dyes, dapsone
	Pancytopenia	Benzene, radiation, chemotherapeutic agents
	Secondary lupus erythematosus	Hydralazine
	Leukemia	Benzene, radiation, chemotherapeutic agents
Liver and gastrointestinal tract	Hepatic damage (hepatitis)	Acetaminophen, ethanol, carbon tetrachloride, vitamin A
	Cancer	Aflatoxin, vinyl chloride
Urinary tract	Kidney toxicity	Ethylene and diethylene glycols, lead, melamine, aminoglycoside antibiotics
	Bladder cancer	Aromatic amines
Nervous system	Nervous system toxicity	Cholinesterase inhibitors, mercury, lead, n-hexane, bacterial toxins (botulinum, tetanus)
	Parkinson's disease	Manganese
Reproductive and developmental toxicity	Fetal malformations	Thalidomide, ethanol
Endocrine system	Thyroid toxicity	Radioactive iodine, perchlorate
Cardiovascular system	Heart toxicity	Anthracyclines, cobalt
	Arrhythmias	Plant glycosides (e.g., digitalis)

Q. What are the pathways through which acetaminophen is metabolized?

There are three pathways:

- Sulfonation (about 52%)
- Glucuronidation (about 42%)
- P450 1A, 3A, and 2E1 (about 4%) (about 2% is excreted unchanged).

Explanation: The P450-mediated pathway creates a reactive intermediate that can react with electrophilic sites in the cell. This reactive intermediate is detoxified by glutathione.

When glutathione become depleted, the reactive intermediate becomes available for covalent binding to hepatic cells and hepatic necrosis ensues. Acetaminophen causes centrilobular liver injury. However, if a person is taking an inducer of P450 (e.g., phenobarbital), they are expected to produce more of the toxic metabolite and suffer greater liver damage. Conversely, if a person is taking a P450 inhibitor (e.g., piperonyl butoxide), they are expected to produce less of the toxic metabolite and suffer reduced toxicity.

Q. What is/are the most likely mechanism(s) by which glomerular nephrotoxicants such as antibiotics induce proteinuria?

The glomerulus is responsible for ultrafiltration of the plasma. The glomerular basement membrane contains anionic proteins which produce an electrostatic barrier that retards the passage of anionic macromolecules. Neutral molecules will pass through the glomerulus better than anionic molecules of the same size. The plasma protein concentration in the glomerular filtrate is low.

Some toxicants reduce the anionic charge on the glomerular elements, resulting in proteinuria. Since albumin is anionic, one often sees albuminuria if the charge-selective properties of the filtration barrier are decreased.

The proximal tubule is often the site of toxicity; the tubule has a high rate of blood flow. The proximal tubule absorbs the bulk of the water and solute filtered at the glomerulus. The proximal tubule reabsorbs Na, K, Ca, Mg, Cl, PO_4, and HCO_3. Filtered sugar, amino acids, and some small organic acids are reabsorbed. The proximal tubule reabsorbs peptides and proteins which are filtered at the glomerulus. If the energy for sodium transport or other transport functions is decreased, the reabsorption rate in the proximal tubule can decline, producing glycosuria and proteinuria.

The osmolality of urine is controlled in the collecting duct.

4.12 QUESTION AND ANSWER EXERCISES

4.12.1 SHORT QUESTIONS AND ANSWERS

Exercise 1

Q.1 What is the target where a toxicant produces its effect?

Location-target site (molecular, subcellular organelle).

Q.2 What are the target organs on which toxic substance affect(s)?

1. Localized
2. Multiple organs.

Q.3 How glomerulus is responsible for ultrafiltration of the plasma?

The glomerular basement membrane of kidney contains anionic proteins which produces an electrostatic barrier that retards the passage of anionic macromolecules. Neutral molecules will pass through the glomerulus better than anionic molecules of the same size. The plasma protein concentration in the glomerular filtrate is low.

Some toxicants reduce the anionic charge on the glomerular elements, resulting in proteinuria. Since albumin is anionic, one often sees albuminuria if the charge-selective properties of the filtration barrier are decreased.

Q.4 Which area of kidney is the site of toxicity?

The proximal tubule is often the site of toxicity.

Q.5 Why proximal tubule is often the site of toxicity?

The proximal tubule has a high rate of blood flow. The proximal tubule absorbs the bulk of the water and solute filtered at the glomerulus. The proximal tubule reabsorbs Na, K, Ca, Mg, Cl, PO_4, and HCO_3. Filtered sugar, amino acids, and some small organic acids are reabsorbed. The proximal tubule reabsorbs peptides and proteins which are filtered at the glomerulus. If the energy for sodium transport or other transport functions is decreased, the reabsorption rate in the proximal tubule can decline, producing glycosuria and proteinuria.

Q.6 In which tissues arsenic tends to accumulate and why?

Arsenic accumulates in keratin-rich tissues such as hair and nails because arsenic has high affinity for sulfhydryl groups ($-SH$). Since hair and nails contain $-SH$-rich keratin, arsenic accumulates in them.

Q.7 What are the predominant symptoms of organic mercury poisoning?

The predominant symptoms of organic mercury poisoning are neurological such as ataxia, incoordination, convulsions, and abnormal behavior.

Q.8 Name at least three chemicals known to cause pancytopenia.

1. Benzene

2. Radiation

3. Chemotherapeutic agents.

Q.9 Name at least five chemicals/agents responsible for lung toxicity.

Substances known to damage lungs include paraquat herbicides, silica asbestos, nitrogen dioxide, ozone, hydrogen sulfide chromium, and nickel.

Q.10 What is hepatotoxicity?

Hepatotoxicity (from *hepatic toxicity*) implies chemical-driven liver damage. For example, drug-induced liver injury is a cause of acute and chronic liver disease.

Exercise 2

Q.1 What is the function of liver?

In the liver three main functions occur: storage, metabolism, and biosynthesis. Glucose is converted to glycogen and stored; when needed for energy, it is converted back to glucose. Fat, fat-soluble vitamins, and other nutrients are also stored in the liver. Fatty acids are metabolized and converted to lipids, which are then conjugated with proteins synthesized in the liver and released into the bloodstream as lipoproteins. The liver also synthesizes numerous functional proteins, such as enzymes and blood-coagulating factors.

In addition the liver, which contains numerous xenobiotic metabolizing enzymes, is the main site of xenobiotic metabolism.

Q.2 What is cholestasis?

Cholestasis is the suppression or stoppage of bile flow and may have either intrahepatic or extrahepatic causes. Inflammation or blockage of the bile ducts results in retention of bile salts as well as bilirubin accumulation, an event that leads to jaundice. Other mechanisms causing cholestasis include changes in membranes permeability of either hepatocytes or biliary canaliculi.

Q.3 What is cirrhosis?

Cirrhosis is a progressive disease that is characterized by the deposition of collagen throughout the liver. In most cases cirrhosis results from chronic chemical injury. The accumulation of fibrous material causes severe restriction in blood flow and in the liver's normal metabolic and detoxication processes. This situation can in turn cause further damage and eventually lead to liver failure. In humans, chronic use of ethanol is the single most important cause of cirrhosis.

Q.4 What is hepatitis?

Hepatitis is an inflammation of the liver and is usually viral in origin; however, certain chemicals, usually drugs, can induce a hepatitis that closely resembles that produced by viral infections.

Q.5 What is the mechanism of hepatotoxicity?

Chemically induced cell injury can be thought of as involving a series of events occurring in the affected animal and often in the target organ itself:

1. The chemical agent is activated to form the initiating toxic agent.
2. The initiating toxic agent is either detoxified or causes molecular changes in the cell.
3. The cell recovers or there are irreversible changes.
4. Irreversible changes may culminate in cell death.

Q.6 Give four examples of hepatotoxicants

Carbon tetrachloride
Ethanol
Bromobenzene
Acetaminophen.

Q.7 What is nephrotoxicity?

Nephrotoxicity is toxicity in the kidneys. It is a poisonous effect of some substances, both toxic chemicals and medications, on renal function.

The nephrotoxic effect of most drugs is more profound in patients already suffering from kidney failure. Nephrotoxins are substances displaying nephrotoxicity.

Q.8 What is the function of the renal system?

The primary function of the renal system is the elimination of waste products, derived either from endogenous metabolism or from the metabolism of xenobiotics. The latter function is discussed in detail in Chapter 10, Poisonous Foods and Food Poisonings. The kidney also plays an important role in the regulation of body homeostasis, regulating extracellular fluid volume, and electrolyte balance.

Q.9 Give some examples of nephrotoxins.

Many heavy metals are potent nephrotoxicants. They interfere with enzymes of energy metabolism.

Certain antibiotics, most notably the aminoglycosides, are known to be nephrotoxic in humans, especially in high doses or after prolonged therapy. The group of antibiotics includes streptomycin, neomycin, kanamycin, and gentamycin.

Aristolochic acid, found in some plants and in some herbal supplements derived from those plants, has been shown to have nephrotoxic effects on humans.

Rhubarb contains some nephrotoxins which can cause inflammation of the kidneys in some people.

Q.10 What are neurotoxicants?

Neurotoxicants are substances capable of causing adverse effects in the central and peripheral nervous system, and in sense organs. These effects include narcosis, nausea, dizziness, vertigo, irritability, euphoria, movement coordination problems, impaired memory and behavior, and alterations of the peripheral nerves.

Exercise 3

Q.1 What is neuronopathy?

Neuronopathy refers to generalized damage to nerve cells, with the primary damage occurring at the nerve cell body. Axonal and dendritic processes die secondarily in response to loss of the cell body. Like other cells in the body, neurons die by one of two processes distinguished by their morphological and molecular features: apoptosis and necrosis.

Q.2 Name at least three agents which can lead to neurotoxicity.

1. β-Amyloid (Aβ)
2. Glutamate
3. Oxygen radicals.

Q.3 What does the endocrine system do?

The endocrine system is the collection of glands that produce hormones that regulate metabolism, growth and development, tissue function, sexual function, reproduction, sleep, and mood, among other things.

Q.4 What are the major endocrine glands in our body?

The major glands of the endocrine system are the hypothalamus, pituitary, thyroid, parathyroids, adrenals, pineal body, and the reproductive organs (ovaries and testes). The pancreas is also a part of this system; it has a role in hormone production as well as in digestion.

Q.5 What is endocrine disruption?

Xenobiotics have the ability to disrupt hormone activity through a variety of mechanisms, though the predominant mechanisms appear to involve binding to the hormone receptor, either as an agonist or antagonist, or by modulating endogenous steroid hormone levels.

Q.6 What are the main causes of pulmonary diseases?

Pulmonary diseases caused by agents in the environment have been known for centuries and have been associated with occupations such as stone quarrying, coal mining, and textiles. The problem is more complex and widespread today because new agents are constantly being added to the environment.

Q.7 What are inhalant toxicants?

They include all types of inhalant toxicants, gases, vapors, fumes, aerosols, organic and inorganic particulates, and mixtures of any or all of these. Gasoline additives and exhaust particles, pesticides, plastics, solvents, deodorant and cosmetic sprays, and construction materials are all included.

Q.8 What is immunotoxicity?

Immunotoxicology (sometimes abbreviated as ITOX) is the study of immune dysfunction resulting from exposure of an organism to a xenobiotic. The immune dysfunction may take the form of immunosuppression or alternatively, allergy, autoimmunity, or any number of inflammatory-based diseases or pathologies.

Q.9 What is allergic contact dermatitis?

Allergic contact dermatitis is an itchy skin condition caused by an allergic reaction to material (the allergen) in contact with the skin. It arises some hours after contact with the responsible material and settles down over some days providing the skin is no longer in contact with it. In severe cases contact allergic dermatitis may be followed by generalized autoeczematization (id reaction). Ingestion of a contact allergen is usually safe, but rarely may lead to baboon syndrome or generalized systemic contact dermatitis.

Q.10 What is reproductive toxicity

Reproductive toxicity is a hazard associated with some chemical substances that they will interfere in some way with normal reproduction; such substances are called reprotoxic. It includes adverse effects on sexual function and fertility in adult males and females, as well as developmental toxicity in the offspring.

4.12.2 MULTIPLE CHOICE QUESTIONS (CHOOSE THE BEST STATEMENT, IT CAN BE ONE, TWO OR ALL OR NONE)

Exercise 4

Q.1 Which of the following statements is NOT correct?

   a. Many nephrotoxicants appear to have the primary site of action on (in) the proximal tubule.

   b. The proximal convoluted tubule is the primary site of reabsorption of glucose and amino acids.

   c. The pars recta (S3) has a greater capacity to absorb organic compounds than the distal tubule.

   d. The loop of Henle is the site of damage produced by chronic administration of analgesic mixtures.

   e. The collecting duct appears relatively insensitive to most nephrotoxicants.

Q.2 Acetaminophen-induced liver injury is

   a. periportal

   b. midzonal

   c. centrilobular

   d. biliary

   e. diffuse

Q.3 The grayanotoxins found in many species of Rhododendron produce effects similar to

   a. cyanogenic glycosides

   b. veratrum alkaloids

   c. lycopenes

   d. disulfiram

   e. taxol

Q.4 What is/are the most likely mechanism(s) by which glomerular nephrotoxicants such as antibiotics induce proteinuria?

   a. By increasing the diameter of pores in the glomerular basement membrane

   b. By enhancing the carrier-mediated transport of protein across the glomerular membrane

   c. By inhibiting the lysosomal protease activity

   d. By reducing the number of fixed anionic charges on glomerular structural elements

Q.5 Which of the following is/are difference(s) in the chronic toxicity of inhaled elemental mercury and the toxicity of ingested mercurous salts?

   a. Elemental mercury causes tremors, gingivitis, and increased excitability, whereas mercurous salts cause acrodynia, fever, and increased activity of sweat glands.

   b. Mercurous salts produce renal toxicity similar to mercuric salts, whereas elemental mercury does not produce any renal toxicity.

     c. Hypersensitivity reactions are more commonly associated with mercurous compounds than with mercury vapor.

     d. Both compounds produce very similar chronic toxicity syndromes.

Q.6 Which of the following is NOT a characteristic of active transport?

     a. Blocked by saxitoxin

     b. Movement against a concentration gradient

     c. Exhibits a transport maximum

     d. Energy dependent

     e. Selectivity

Q.7 Which of the following is NOT an initiating event in carcinogenesis?

     a. DNA adduct formation

     b. DNA strand breakage

     c. Mutation of proto-oncogenes

     d. Oxidative damage of DNA

     e. Mitogenesis

Q.8 Reabsorption of toxicants does NOT occur through

     a. enterohepatic recirculation

     b. glomerular filtration

     c. diffusion

     d. active transport

     e. carriers for physiological oxyanions

Q.9 Which of the following does NOT uncouple oxidative phosphorylation?

     a. Pentachlorophenol

     b. Dinitrophenol

     c. Aconitase

     d. Salicylate

     e. Gramacidin

Q.10 Which of the following is NOT true regarding peroxisome proliferators?

     a. They are a structurally diverse group of chemicals.

     b. They cause marked induction of lipid metabolizing enzymes.

     c. They often are nongenotoxic hepatocarcinogens in rodents.

     d. They induce hepatic CYP1A which is indicative of peroxisome proliferation.

     e. They operate via the peroxisome proliferator activated receptor.

Answers

1. c; 2. c; 3. b; 4. d; 5. b; 6. a; 7. e; 8. b; 9. c; 10. d.

Exercise 5

Q.1 The percentage of mating resulting in pregnancy is called

     a. fertility index

     b. gestation index

     c. viability index

     d. survival index

Q.2 The percentage of pregnancies resulting in live litters is
  a. fertility index
  b. gestation index
  c. viability index
  d. survival index

Q.3 The lactation index in rats is the
  a. number of live births that breast-feed
  b. number of days an animal breast-feeds
  c. calories lost per day by a mother who breast-feeds
  d. percentage of animals alive at 4 days that survive the 21-day lactation period

Q.4 Which of the following statement is false?
  a. There is good concordance between human and animal neurotoxicity assessment.
  b. The developing nervous system is insensitive to toxicant exposure
  c. Monkeys can be used to test low-level effects of neurotoxic cells
  d. In vitro B cell cultures can be used in neurotoxicity evaluation.

Q.5 A severe cytokine response that progressed in systemic organ failure occurred in a phase 1 study involving the use of
  a. an uncoupler of oxidative phosphorylation
  b. a cyclooxygenase-2 (COX-2) inhibitor
  c. a CD28 monoclonal antibody
  d. a microtubule assembly inhibitor

Q.6 It has been postulated that within the human genome, how much variability in DNA sequence exists between any two individuals?
  a. 0.01%
  b. 0.1%
  c. 0.5%
  d. 1.0%

Q.7 Methyl bromide (CH_3Br)
  a. is a liquid used primarily as a fumigant
  b. has essentially no warning properties, even at physiologically hazardous concentrations
  c. is extremely flammable
  d. is of greater concern from its oral toxicity than from its inhalation toxicity
  e. would not be expected to be readily absorbed through the lungs

Q.8 The chloronicotinyl compound imidacloprid demonstrates a high insecticidal potency and exceptionally low mammalian toxicity due to
  a. its high affinity for insect nicotinic acetylcholine receptors and low affinity for mammalian nicotinic acetylcholine receptors
  b. the blood—brain barrier in mammals
  c. the first-pass effect in the liver in mammals
  d. the low pH in the stomach of monogastric mammals
  e. the presence of true acetylcholinesterase in mammals

Q.9 The most commonly used pyrethroid synergist is
    a. silica
    b. piperonyl butoxide
    c. methyl butyl ether
    d. n-octyl bicycloheptene dicarboximide
    e. toluene
Q.10 Paraquat and diquat differ substantially in their
    a. metabolism to a free radical
    b. ability to initiate lipid peroxidation in vivo
    c. uptake by the lung
    d. generation of superoxide anion in vivo
    e. mechanism of cytotoxicity

Answers

1. a; 2. b; 3. d; 4. b; 5. c; 6. b; 7. b; 8. a; 9. b; 10. c.

Exercise 6

Q.1 Which of the following assumptions is NOT correct regarding risk assessment for male reproductive effects in the absence of mechanistic data?
    a. An agent that produces an adverse reproductive effect in experimental animals is assumed to pose a potential reproductive hazard to humans.
    b. In general, a nonthreshold is assumed for the dose−response curve for male reproductive toxicity.
    c. Effects of xenobiotics on male reproduction are assumed to be similar across species unless demonstrated otherwise.
    d. The most sensitive species should be used to estimate the human risk.
    e. Reproductive processes are similar across mammalian species.
Q.2 The most serious consequence of crude oil or kerosene ingestion by cattle is
    a. liver damage
    b. kidney damage
    c. aspiration pneumonia
    d. CNS stimulation
    e. leukemia
Q.3 Toxic injury to the cell body, axon, and surrounding Schwann cells of peripheral nerves are referred to, respectively, as
    a. neuropathy, axonopathy, and myelopathy
    b. neuronopathy, axonopathy, and myelinopathy
    c. neuropathy, axonopathy, and gliosis
    d. neuronopathy, dying-back neuropathy, and myelopathy
    e. chromatolysis, axonopathy, and gliosis
Q.4 The conceptus is considered preferentially vulnerable to chemical insult due to all of the following EXCEPT
    a. rapid rate of cell proliferation

    b. requirement for precise temporal and spatial localization of cells and cell products

    c. rapid blood flow (heart rate) and increased tissue distribution of the chemical

    d. limited drug metabolism capability

    e. immaturity of the immune system

Q.5 Which of the following is a nongenotoxic liver carcinogen in rats?

    a. Aflatoxin

    b. Vinyl chloride

    c. Pyrrolizidine alkaloids

    d. Clofibrate

    e. Tamoxifen

Q.6 Suppression of NK (natural killer) cell activity produces adverse effects in animals because

    a. NK cells play a role in the immune surveillance of tumors and the inhibition of metastases.

    b. NK cells are precursors to pulmonary macrophages, and suppression of activity results in a decreased ability to combat pulmonary infections.

    c. NK cells function as a helper cell in erythropoiesis, and suppression of NK cell activity results in anemia.

    d. NK cells function in the complement-fixation cascade, and reduced NK cell activity causes loss of blood clotting.

    e. NK cells function directly by phagocytosis of pathogens to protect the host from pathogenic bacteria (acquired cell-mediated immunity).

Q.7 Which of the following is NOT true about arsine?

    a. It is a gas at room temperature

    b. It produces acute intravascular hemolysis

    c. It has a garlic-like odor

    d. Acute renal failure is a common manifestation of arsine poisoning

    e. Significant hepatotoxicity often occurs as part of arsine poisoning

Q.8 No specific antidote is available for poisoning by

    a. sodium fluoroacetate

    b. warfarin

    c. chlorinated hydrocarbon insecticides

    d. rotenone

    e. cyanide

Q.9 Which of the following is NOT commonly associated with mercury vapor poisoning?

    a. Acute, corrosive bronchitis

    b. Interstitial pneumonitis

    c. Tremor

    d. Increased excitability

    e. Vomiting and bloody diarrhea

Q.10 Compounds containing beryllium are NOT readily absorbed from the gastrointestinal tract because

    a. they form insoluble phosphate precipitates at the pH of the intestinal tract

    b. they are chelated by bile salts in the small intestine

    c. their size prevents passage through cell membranes

    d. they are converted to an oxide form

    e. exposures rarely occur to the soluble metallic form

Answers

1. b; 2. c; 3. b; 4. c; 5. d; 6. a; 7. e; 8. c; 9. e; 10. a.

Exercise 7

Q.1 An individual exposed to 10 rads (0.1 Gy) of whole body x-irradiation would be expected to

    a. have a severe bone marrow depression

    b. die

    c. be permanently sterilized

    d. exhibit no symptoms

    e. vomit

Q.2 Benzene is similar to toluene

    a. in its metabolism to redox active metabolites

    b. regarding covalent binding of its metabolites to proteins

    c. in its ability to produce CNS depression

    d. in its ability to produce acute myelogenous leukemia

    e. in its ability to be metabolized to benzoquinone

Q.3 Consumption of milk from goats which have grazed on lupine plants containing the alkaloid, anagyrine, may cause

    a. birth defects when ingested by women during early pregnancy

    b. severe liver damage characterized by centrilobular necrosis

    c. dizziness, nausea, headaches, and hallucinations

    d. numbness of the extremities

    e. aphrodisia and a general increase in sexual awareness

Q.4 Sorbitol and other sugar alcohols have been associated with

    a. respiratory distress syndrome

    b. osmotic diarrhea

    c. hepatotoxicity

    d. immediate hypersensitivity reaction

    e. CNS depression

Q.5 Which of the following is NOT true regarding *Amanita phalloides* mushrooms?

    a. Toxic components are phalloidin and amatoxins.

    b. Produces liver and gastrointestinal toxicity.

    c. Cardiovascular toxicity is responsible for mortality.

d. Common name is "death cap."

e. No specific antidotal treatment of poisoning is available.

Q.6 Chloroform is NOT

a. a CNS depressant

b. hepatotoxic

c. metabolized to phosgene

d. a peroxisome proliferator

e. a contaminant of chlorinated water

Q.7 Increasing the casein content of a partially purified diet up to a level of 36%

a. reduces the spontaneous hepatoma incidence below background in mice

b. increases the spontaneous hepatoma incidence above background in mice

c. has no effect on the incidence of mouse hepatomas

d. reduces the spontaneous incidence of kidney tumors below background in mice

e. reduces the spontaneous incidence of lung tumors below background in mice

Q.8 All of the following may cause metabolic acidosis EXCEPT

a. renal failure

b. salicylates

c. methanol

d. diuretics

e. diarrhea

Q.9 A patient is admitted to the emergency room with the following symptoms: dry mouth and skin; weak, rapid pulse (130 beats/min); elevated body temperature (103°F); and mydriasis. He is excited and disoriented. In his pocket is a bottle of pills labeled: "take one as necessary for stomach pain." This patient is most likely to be suffering from an overdose of

a. a narcotic analgesic

b. a nonnarcotic analgesic

c. an antacid

d. an antimuscarinic agent

e. a benzodiazepine tranquilizer

Q.10 Each of the following solvents is paired with a correct target organ of toxicity EXCEPT

a. methanol:retina

b. ethylene glycol:kidney

c. ethylene glycol monomethyl ether:kidney

d. dichloromethane:CNS system

e. carbon tetrachloride:liver

Answers

1. a; 2. c; 3. a; 4. b; 5. c; 6. d; 7. b; 8. d; 9. d; 10. c.

Exercise 8

Q.1 A person was brought by police from the railway platform. He is talking irrelevant. He is having dry mouth with hot skin, dilated pupils, staggering gait, and slurred speech. The most probable diagnosis is
   a. alcohol intoxication
   b. carbamates poisoning
   c. organophosphorus poisoning
   d. *Datura* poisoning

Q.2 Regarding methanol poisoning
   Assertion: Administration of ethanol is one of the treatment modalities
   Reason: Ethanol inhibits alcohol dehydrogenase.
   Please select the most correct option from the following:
   a. Both assertion and reason are true, and the reason is the correct explanation for the assertion.
   b. Both assertion and reason are true, and the reason is not the correct explanation for the assertion.
   c. Assertion is true, but the reason is false.
   d. Assertion is false, but the reason is true.

Q.3 In methyl alcohol poisoning, there are CNS depression, cardiac depression, and optic nerve atrophy. These effects are produced due to:
   a. formaldehyde and formic acid
   b. acetaldehyde
   c. pyridine
   d. acetic acid

Q.4 A 39-year-old carpenter has taken two bottles of liquor from the local shop. After about an hour, he develops confusion, vomiting, and blurring of vision. He has been brought to the emergency department. He should be given
   a. naloxone
   b. diazepam
   c. flumazenil
   d. ethyl alcohol

Q.5 Phosphine liberated in the stomach in aluminum phosphide poisoning is toxic to all except
   a. lungs
   b. kidneys
   c. liver
   d. heart

Q.6 Paraquat poisoning causes
   a. renal failure
   b. cardiac failure
   c. respiratory failure
   d. multiple organ failure

Q.7 Ecstasy toxicity causes
    a. hypereflexia
    b. trismus
    c. dilated pupils
    d. visual hallucinations
    e. all of the above

Q.8 A housewife ingests a rodenticide white powder accidentally. She is brought to hospital where the examination shows generalized, flaccid paralysis and an irregular pulse. Electrocardiogram (ECG) shows multiple ventricular ectopics, generalized changes with ST−T. Serum potassium is 2.5 mEq/L. The most likely ingested poison is:
    a. barium carbonate
    b. super warfarins
    c. zinc phosphide
    d. aluminum phosphide

Q.9 All of the following are treatment options for toxic alcohol poisoning except
    a. fomepizole
    b. hydroxycobalamin
    c. thiamine
    d. folic acid
    e. pyridoxine

Q.10 Hyperthermia in a patient of poisoning is a pointer to all except
    a. ecstasy
    b. selective serotonin reuptake inhibitor
    c. salicylates
    d. chlorpromazine

Answers

1. d; 2. a; 3. a; 4. d; 5. b; 6. d; 7. e; 8. a; 9. b; 10. d.

Exercise 9

Q.1 Which of the following is NOT associated with spermatotoxicity in rats?
    a. Ethylene glycol monomethyl ether
    b. Ethylene glycol monoethyl ether
    c. Ethoxy acetic acid
    d. Methoxy acetic acid
    e. Propylene glycol monomethyl ether

Q.2 Which form of mercury was the predominant cause of Minamata Bay disease?
    a. Metallic mercury
    b. Mercuric salts
    c. Mercurous salts
    d. Organic mercury compounds
    e. Mercury was not the causative agent

Q.3 Ophitoxaemia refers to
    a. organophosphorus poisoning
    b. heavy metal poisoning
    c. scorpion venom poisoning
    d. snake venom poisoning

Q.4 Elapidaes are
    a. vasculotoxic
    b. neurotoxic
    c. musculotoxic
    d. nontoxic

Q.5 The most useful bedside test to suggest snake bite envenomation is
    a. prothrombin time
    b. 20-minute whole blood clotting time
    c. international normalized ratio
    d. platelet count

Q.6 A 12-year-old boy had an alleged history of snake bite and presented to the hospital with an inability to open eyes well and difficulty in breathing. He is very anxious and is having tachycardia and tachypnea. On examination bite mark cannot be visualized and there is no swelling of the limb. He has bilateral ptosis. His 20-minute whole blood clotting test is good quality. What is the next course of action?
    a. Do not give antisnake venom (ASV), but observe the patient.
    b. Give ASV and keep the patient in observation.
    c. Give ASV, and give neostigmine and observe the patient.
    d. Reassure the patient and send him home with anxiolytic.

Q.7 Magnan's symptoms are characteristic symptoms with which poisoning?
    a. Alcohol
    b. Charas
    c. Cocaine
    d. Ecstasy

Answers
1. e; 2. d; 3. d; 4. b; 5. b; 6. c; 7. c.

Exercise 10

Q.1 The Food and Drug Administration (FDA) protocol that primarily examines fertility and preimplantation and postimplantation viability is
    a. segment I
    b. segment II
    c. segment III
    d. segment IV

Q.2 The FDA protocol that primarily examines postnatal, survival, growth, and external morphology is
    a. segment I
    b. segment II

    c. segment III

    d. segment IV

Q.3 All of the following maternal diseases have been assumed with adverse pregnancy outcomes except

    a. allergic rhinitis

    b. febrile illness during the first trimester

    c. hypertension

    d. diabetes mellitus

Q.4 All of the following are true of the development toxicity of cadmium except

    a. it appears to involve placental toxicity

    b. it appears to involve inhibition of nutrient transport across the placenta

    c. zinc can affect the developmental toxicity of cadmium

    d. cadmium induces transferrin, which binds zinc in the placenta

Q.5 All of the following are necessary for a normally developing embryo except

    a. apoptosis

    b. cell proliferations

    c. cell differentiation

    d. necrosis

Q.6 The fetal period is characterized by all of the following except

    a. beginning organ development

    b. tissue differentiation

    c. growth

    d. physiological maturation

Q.7 Toxic exposure during the fetal period is likely to cause effects on

    a. organogenesis

    b. implantation

    c. growth and maturation

    d. all of the above

Q.8 Approximately what percentage of marked drugs belongs to FDA pregnancy category?

    a. 1%

    b. 10%

    c. 20%

    d. 30%

Answers

1. a; 2. c; 3. a; 4. d; 5. d; 6. a; 7. c; 8. a.

Exercise 11

Q.1 All of the following are features of megaloblastic anemia except

    a. low serum B12 or folate

    b. microcytosis (decreased mean corpuscular volume (MCV))

    c. pancytopenia

    d. hypersegmented neutrophils

Q.2 All of the following are associated with megaloblastic anemia except
   a. phenytoin
   b. ethanol
   c. aspirin
   d. methotrexate

Q.3 All of the following are characteristics of aplastic anemia except
   a. causation of radiation exposure
   b. peripheral blood pancytopenia
   c. bone marrow hypoplasia
   d. reticulocytosis

Q.4 All of the following have been associated with anemia except
   a. gold
   b. chloramphenicol
   c. acetone
   d. felbamate

Q.5 All of the following are associated with an increase of bleeding except
   a. aspirin
   b. ibuprofen
   c. vitamin B6
   d. N-methylthiotetrazole cephalosporins

Q.6 All of the following are true of heparin except
   a. unfractionated heparin causes higher incidence of thrombocytopenia
   b. it causes osteoporosis
   c. it crosses the placenta
   d. it causes transaminase elevations

Q.7 A grading system for hematological toxicity was established in 1979 by
   a. World Health Organization (WHO)
   b. Food and Drug Administration (FDA)
   c. US Environmental Protection Agency (EPA)
   d. Occupational Safety and Health Administration (OSHA)

Q.8 Serial blood and bone marrow sampling is best done in
   a. hamster
   b. rat
   c. dog
   d. mouse

Q.9 A chemical causing nonoxidative chemical-induced hemolysis of red blood cells is
   a. hydrogen sulfide
   b. arsine
   c. ozone
   d. xylene

Q.10 All of the following have been associated with warfarin except
   a. hepatitis
   b. congenital abnormalities

    c. bone demineralization

    d. skin necrosis

Answers

1. b; 2. c; 3. d; 4. c; 5. c; 6. c; 7. a; 8 c; 9. b; 10. a.

Exercise 12

Q.1 Which of the following is thought to be an important factor in the pathology of alcohol-induced liver disease?

    a. Inflammatory response

    b. Lipid peroxidation

    c. Oxidative stress

    d. All of the above

Q.2 Allyl alcohol is metabolized by ADH to

    a. benzaldehyde

    b. acrolein

    c. acetic anhydride

    d. butyraldehyde

Q.3 All of the following statements are true regarding idiosyncratic drug-induced hepatotoxicity except

    a. it probably involves failure to adapt to a mild drug adverse effect combined with a genetic defect

    b. traditional animal toxicology studies may not detect it

    c. carbon tetrachloride is an example

    d. preclinical studies may need to be done in genetically deficient animals to detect some examples

Q.4 Ethyl alcohol is metabolized in humans by all of the following except

    a. CYP3A4

    b. CYP2E1

    c. ADH

    d. peroxisomal catalase

Q.5 Idiosyncratic liver injury is characterized by all of the following except

    a. it can be immune or nonimmune mediated

    b. it has a clear dose—response relationship

    c. it is relatively rare

    d. it has a probable genetic basis

Q.6 The liver cell process associated with cell swelling leakage of cell contents and an influx of inflammatory cells is

    a. apoptosis

    b. fibrosis

    c. necrosis

    d. steatosis

Q.7 All of the following are true regarding the hepatotoxicity of carbon tetrachloride except

    a. the reactive metabolite is formed by cytochrome P450 3A4

    b. the reactive metabolite is a free radical

     c. chronic ethanol exposure can enhance the injury

     d. the injury involves lipid peroxidation

Q.8 All of the following are true regarding ethanol and the liver except

     a. ethanol inhibits the transfer of triglycerides from liver to adipose tissue

     b. alcohol dehydrogenase is the only inducible enzyme in chronic alcoholism

     c. an inactive form of acetaldehyde dehydrogenase is formed in 50% of Asians

     d. the catalase pathway is a minor route for ethanol metabolism

Q.9 All of the following hepatic sites are matched with the appropriate preferential toxicant except

     a. zone 1 hepatocyte—iron

     b. bile duct cells—ethanol

     c. stellate cells—vitamin A

     d. zone 3 hepatocyte—carbon tetrachloride

Q.10 All of the following cause nonimmune idiosyncratic live toxicity except

     a. tienilic acid

     b. isoniazid

     c. amiodarone

     d. ketoconazole

Answers

1. d; 2. b; 3. c; 4. a; 5. b; 6. c; 7. a; 8. b; 9. b; 10. a.

Exercise 13

Q.1 Which of the following is associated with pathological hypertrophy of the heart?

     a. Hypertension

     b. Exercise

     c. Pregnancy

     d. None of the above

Q.2 Myocardial accumulation of collagen is not associated with

     a. ischemic cardiomyopathy

     b. myocardial infarction

     c. pathological hypertrophy

     d. adaptive hypertrophy

Q.3 Counter-regulatory mechanism in response to compensatory mechanisms to cardiac hypertrophy leads to

     a. decrease in heart size

     b. myocardial remodeling

     c. decrease in cardiac fibrosis

     d. decrease in salt/water retention

Q.4 Inflammatory lesions in the vascular system are termed

     a. vasculitis

     b. embolitis

    c. thrombitis

    d. angio-inflammation

Q.5 The most prevalent vascular structural injury is

    a. capillary hyperplasia

    b. varicose veins

    c. angioma

    d. atherosclerosis

Q.6 Cardiac glycosides-like digoxin

    a. increase the sensitivity of myocytes to calcium

    b. inhibit sodium/potassium ATPase

    c. cause sinus tachycardia

    d. inhibit sympathetic outflow at high doses

Q.7 Which of the following is the most sensitive clinical indicator of myocardial cell damage?

    a. Urine creatine phosphokinase (CPK)

    b. Serum troponin

    c. Serum alanine aminotransferase (ALT)

    d. Serum creatinine

Q.8 Which of the following is an indicator of fluid overload in congestive heart failure?

    a. Urine pH

    b. Serum CPK

    c. Brain natriuretic peptide (BNP)

    d. First-degree atrioventricular (AV) block on ECG

Q.9 Moxifloxacin is associated with

    a. acute congestive heart failure

    b. prolongation of the QT interval

    c. coronary artery thrombotic events

    d. toxic cardiomyopathy

Q.10 COX-2 inhibits presumably increase the risk for cardiovascular events by causing

    a. heart block

    b. systolic dysfunction

    c. toxic cardiomyopathy

    d. coronary artery thrombotic events

Q.11 Which of the following statements is not correct?

    a. Many nephrotoxicants appear to have the primary site of action on (in) the proximal tubule.

    b. The proximal convoluted tubule is the primary site of reabsorption of glucose and amino acids.

    c. The pars recta (S3) has a greater capacity to absorb organic compounds than the distal tubule.

    d. The loop of Henle is the site of damage produced by chronic administration of analgesic mixtures.

    e. The collecting duct appears relatively insensitive to most nephrotoxicants.

Q.12 Acetaminophen-induced liver injury is
   a. periportal
   b. midzonal
   c. centrilobular
   d. biliary
   e. diffuse

Q.13 The grayanotoxins found in many species of *Rhododendron* produce effects similar to
   a. cyanogenic glycosides
   b. veratrum alkaloids
   c. lycopenes
   d. disulfiram
   e. taxol
      Choose: a if 1, 2, and 3 are correct; b if 1 and 3 are correct; c if 2 and 4 are correct; d if only 4 is correct; e if all are correct.

Q.14 What is/are the most likely mechanism(s) by which glomerular nephrotoxicants such as antibiotics induce proteinuria?
   a. By increasing the diameter of pores in the glomerular basement membrane
   b. By enhancing the carrier-mediated transport of protein across the glomerular membrane
   c. By inhibiting the lysosomal protease activity
   d. By reducing the number of fixed anionic charges on glomerular structural elements

Answers

1. a; 2. d; 3. b; 4. a; 5. d; 6. b; 7. b; 8. c; 9. b; 10. d; 11. c; 12. c; 13. b; 14. d.

4.12.3 FILL IN THE BLANKS

Exercise 14

Q.1 The major toxic effect of hydrogen cyanide exposure is _____

Q.2 Ionizing radiations have the shortest range _____ (i.e., travels the shortest distance in tissue) for the same initial energy.

Q.3 Chloracne is associated with _____

Q.4 Convulsion in acute poisoning can be treated by _____

Q.5 Vitamin K is recommended in the treatment of poisoning due to _____

Q.6 The main target organ of paraquat poisoning is _____

Q.7 The major organ affected by diquat poisoning is _____

Q.8 Thalidomide giving birth to deformed children with _____.

Q.9 After a lot a R&D potential drug candidates fail because of
_____.

Q.10 Drug toxicity, also called _____ or
_____.

Answers

1. INHIBITION OF MITOCHONDRIAL RESPIRATION; 2. α-PARTICLE;
3. PROMINENT HYPERKERATOSIS OF THE FOLLICULAR CANAL;
4. BARBITURATES; 5. SWEET CLOVER; 6. LUNG; 7. KIDNEY;
8. SHORTENED LIMBS AND NO EXTERNAL EARS; 9. TOXICITY;
10. ADVERSE DRUG REACTION (ADR) OR ADVERSE DRUG EVENT
(ADE).

4.12.4 MATCH THE STATEMENTS

Exercise 15

Q. Match the following statements in Columns A and B.

Column A	Column B
1. Indomethacin	a. Spinal bifida
2. Cocaine	b. Staining of teeth
3. Phenytoin	c. Virilization of female fetus
4. Ampicillin	d. Neonatal hypothyroidism
5. Amiodarone	e. Relatively safe
6. Progestins	f. Premature closure of ductus arteriosis
7. Valproic acid	g. Fetal hydantoin syndrome
8. Tetracycline	h. Decreased urine blood flow

Answers

Column A	Column B
1. Indomethacin	f. Premature closure of ductus arteriosis
2. Cocaine	h. Decreased urine blood flow
3. Phenytoin	g. Fetal hydantoin syndrome
4. Ampicillin	e. Relatively safe
5. Amiodarone	d. Neonatal hypothyroidism
6. Progestins	c. Virilization of female fetus
7. Valproic acid	a. Spinal bifida
8. Tetracycline	b. Staining of teeth

Exercise 16

Column A	Column B
1. Oral contraceptives	a. Metal associated with essential hypertension
2. Homocysteine	b. Cardiac hemangiosarcoma in laboratory animals
3. β-Amyloid	c. Abortion and abruption placentae
4. Carbon disulfide	d. Noncirrhotic portal hypertension in humans
5. Mercury	e. Increased risk of thrombotic events in users who smoke
6. Particulate matter	f. Preglomerular vasoconstriction and disruption of blood–brain barrier
7. Arsenic	g. Elevated serum levels are associated with increased risk of atherosclerosis and venous thrombosis
8. Cocaine	h. Associated with increased cardiovascular and respiratory morbidity and mortality
9. Lead	i. May contribute to Alzheimer's disease
10. 1,3-butadiene	j. Endothelial damage and hypothyroidism
11. Hydrazine benzoic acid	k. Smooth muscle tumors in mice

Answers

Column A	Column B
1. Oral contraceptives	e. Increased risk of thrombotic events in users who smoke
2. Homocysteine	g. Elevated serum levels are associated with increased risk of atherosclerosis and venous thrombosis
3. β-Amyloid	i. May contribute to Alzheimer's disease
4. Carbon disulfide	j. Endothelial damage and hypothyroidism
5. Mercury	f. Preglomerular vasoconstriction and disruption of blood–brain barrier
6. Particulate matter	h. Associated with increased cardiovascular and respiratory morbidity and mortality
7. Arsenic	d. Noncirrhotic portal hypertension in humans
8. Cocaine	c. Abortion and abruption placentae
9. Lead	a. Metal associated with essential hypertension
10. 1,3-butadiene	b. Cardiac hemangiosarcoma in laboratory animals
11. Hydrazine benzoic acid	k. Smooth muscle tumors in mice

FURTHER READING

Bloom, J.C., Schade, A.E., Brandt, J.T., 2013. Toxic responses of the blood. In: Klaassen, C.D. (Ed.), Casarett and Doull's Toxicology: The Basic Science of Poisons, eighth ed. McGraw-Hill, New York, NY, pp. 527–558.

Capen, C.C., Hoyer, P.B., Flaws, J.A., 2013. Toxic responses of the endocrine system. In: Klaassen, C.D. (Ed.), Casarett and Doull's Toxicology: The Basic Science of Poisons, eighth ed. McGraw-Hill, New York, NY, pp. 907–932.

Faubert Kaplan, B.L., Solantic, C.E.W., Holsapple, M.P., Kaminski, N.E., 2013. Toxic responses of the immune system. In: Klaassen, C.D. (Ed.), Casarett and Doull's Toxicology: The Basic Science of Poisons, eighth ed. McGraw-Hill, New York, NY, pp. 559–638.

Foster, P.M.D., Gray Jr., L.E., 2013. Toxic responses of the reproductive system. In: Klaassen, C.D. (Ed.), Casarett and Doull's Toxicology: The Basic Science of Poisons, eighth ed. McGraw-Hill, New York, NY, pp. 861–906.

Fox, D.A., Boyes, W.K., 2013. Toxic responses of the ocular and visual system. In: Klaassen, C.D. (Ed.), Casarett and Doull's Toxicology: The Basic Science of Poisons, eighth ed. McGraw-Hill, New York, NY, pp. 767–798.

GoldsTein, B.D., Henifin, M.S., 2011. Reference guide on toxicology, Reference Manual on Scientific Evidence, third ed. National Research Council; Federal Judicial Center; Policy and Global Affairs; Committee on Science, Technology, and Law; Committee on the Development, pp. 633–685. <https://www.nap.edu/read/13163/chapter/13#653>

Gupta, P.K., 1988. Veterinary Toxicology. Cosmo Publications, New Delhi, India (Chapter 7).

Jaeschke, H., 2013. Toxic responses of the liver. In: Klaassen, C.D. (Ed.), Casarett and Doull's Toxicology: The Basic Science of Poisons, eighth ed. McGraw-Hill, New York, NY, pp. 639–664.

James Kang, Y., 2013. Toxic responses of the heart and vascular system. In: Klaassen, C.D. (Ed.), Casarett and Doull's Toxicology: The Basic Science of Poisons, eighth ed. McGraw-Hill, New York, NY, pp. 799–838.

Julian Preston, R., Hoffmann, G.R., 2013. Genetic toxicology. In: Klaassen, C.D. (Ed.), Casarett and Doull's Toxicology: The Basic Science of Poisons, eighth ed. McGraw-Hill, New York, NY, pp. 445–480.

Klaunig, J.E., 2013. Chemical carcinogenesis. In: Klaassen, C.D. (Ed.), Casarett and Doull's Toxicology: The Basic Science of Poisons, eighth ed. McGraw-Hill, New York, NY, pp. 394–444.

Leikauf, G.D., 2013. Toxic responses of the respiratory system. In: Klaassen, C.D. (Ed.), Casarett and Doull's Toxicology: The Basic Science of Poisons, eighth ed. McGraw-Hill, New York, NY, pp. 691–732.

Mehendale, H.N., 2010. Hepatic toxicity. In: second reprint Gupta, P.K. (Ed.), Modern Toxicology: Basis of Organ and Reproduction Toxicity, vol. 1. PharmaMed Press, Hyderabad, India, pp. 226–276.

Moser, V.C., Aschner, M., Richardson, R.J., Philbert, M.A., 2013. Toxic responses of the nervous system. In: Klaassen, C.D. (Ed.), Casarett and Doull's Toxicology: The Basic Science of Poisons, eighth ed. McGraw-Hill, New York, NY, pp. 733–766.

Mukherjee, K.C., Dhawan, B.N., 2010. Behavioral and neurotoxicity. In: second reprint Gupta, P.K. (Ed.), Modern Toxicology: Basis of Organ and Reproduction Toxicity, vol. 1. PharmaMed Press, Hyderabad, India, pp. 159–224.

Rice, R.H., Mauro, T.M., 2013. Toxic responses of the skin. In: Klaassen, C.D. (Ed.), Casarett and Doull's Toxicology: The Basic Science of Poisons, eighth ed. McGraw-Hill, New York, NY, pp. 839–860.

Rogers, J.M., 2013. Developmental toxicology. In: Klaassen, C.D. (Ed.), Casarett and Doull's Toxicology: The Basic Science of Poisons, (eighth ed. McGraw-Hill, New York, NY, pp. 481–524.

Schnellmann, R.G., 2013. Toxic responses of the kidney. In: Klaassen, C.D. (Ed.), Casarett and Doull's Toxicology: The Basic Science of Poisons, eighth ed. McGraw-Hill, New York, NY, pp. 665–690.

Vettorazzi, G., 2010. Reproduction toxicity and teratogenicity. In: second reprint Gupta, P.K. (Ed.), Modern Toxicology: Basis of Organ and Reproduction Toxicity, vol. 1. PharmaMed Press, Hyderabad, India, pp. 340–393.

Witschi, H., 2010. Pulmonary toxicology. In: Gupta, P.K. (Ed.), Modern Toxicology: Basis of Organ and Reproduction Toxicity, second reprint, vol. 1. PharmaMed Press, Hyderabad, India, pp. 277–339.

Pesticides (agrochemicals)

5

CHAPTER OUTLINE

5.1 DEFINITIONS

Q. Define pesticides.

Pesticides are defined that are used to control, kill, or repel pests. They are also known as economic poisons, regulated by federal and state laws.

Q. What is acetylcholine (ACh)?

ACh is a chemical neurotransmitter found widely in the body. It triggers the stimulation of postsynaptic nerves, muscles, and exocrine glands.

Q. What is acetylcholinesterase (AChE)?

AChE (generally referred to as cholinesterase) is an enzyme that rapidly breaks down the neurotransmitter, ACh, so that it does not overstimulate postsynaptic nerves, muscles, and exocrine glands.

Q. What is AChE inhibitor?

AChE inhibitor (generally referred to as cholinesterase inhibitor) is a chemical that binds to the enzyme, cholinesterase, and prevents it from

Illustrated Toxicology. DOI: http://dx.doi.org/10.1016/B978-0-12-813213-5.00005-5

breaking down the neurotransmitter, ACh. With toxic doses, the result is that excessive levels of the ACh build up in the synapses and neuromuscular junctions and glands.

5.2 CLASSIFICATION OF PESTICIDES

Q. Classify pesticides.

Depending on what a compound is designed to do, pesticides have been subclassified into a number of categories.

1. Insecticides

2. Herbicides

3. Fungicides

4. Rodenticides

5. Fumigants.

In addition there are other groups of pesticides such as nematicide, acaricide, algicides, bird repellents, and mammal repellents.

Q. How animals are exposed to pesticides?

The most common exposure scenarios for pesticide-poisoning cases are:

1. Accidental;

2. suicidal poisonings;

3. occupational exposure;

4. by exposure to off-target drift;

5. through environmental contamination, e.g., aerial spray.

Q. Which pesticides are commonly used for malicious poisoning in animals?

The most common pesticides used for malicious poisoning in animals (Fig. 5.1) are:

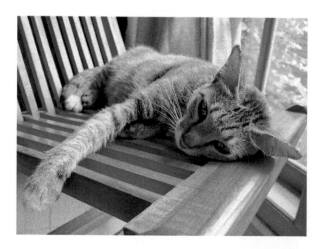

FIGURE 5.1

Insecticide intoxication in cats.

http://www.petmd.com/sites/default/files/insecticide-toxicity-cat.jpg.

1. organophosphorus (OP) insecticides;
2. carbamates (CM);
3. rodenticides;
4. fumigants such as aluminum phosphide and zinc phosphide;
5. pyrethroid insecticides.

5.3 INSECTICIDES

Q. Define insecticides.

An insecticide is a substance used to kill insects. They include ovicides and larvicides used against insect eggs and larvae, respectively. Insecticides are used in agriculture, medicine, industry, and by consumers.

Q. Classify insecticides.

1. Organochlorine (OC)
2. Organophosphorus (OP)
3. Carbamate (CM)
4. Pyrethrins and pyrethroids
5. Formamidines, nicotinoids
6. Natural products (rotenone and nicotine).

5.3.1 ORGANOCHLORINE

Q. What are organochlorine (OC) insecticides? Give examples.

An organochloride, OC compound, chlorocarbon, or chlorinated hydrocarbon is an organic compound containing at least one covalently bonded atom of chlorine that has an effect on the chemical behavior of the molecule, e.g., aldrin, chlordecone, dichlorodiphenyltrichloroethane (DDT), dieldrin, endosulfan, endrin, heptachlor, hexachlorobenzene, lindane (γ-hexachlorocyclohexane), dicofol, mirex, kepone, and pentachlorophenol.

Q. What is the mode of action of OC insecticides?

The chlorinated hydrocarbons are neurotoxicants and cause acute effects by interfering with the transmission of nerve impulses. There are two main groups of OC insecticides. Their mechanism of action differs slightly. The two groups are:

1. DDT-like compounds
2. Chlorinated alicyclics or cyclodienes.

The DDT-like compounds work on the peripheral nervous system. At the axon's sodium channel, they prevent gate closure after activation and membrane depolarization. Sodium ions leak through the nerve membrane and create a destabilizing negative "after potential" with hyperexcitability of the nerve. This leakage causes repeated discharges in the neuron either spontaneously or after a single stimulus.

Chlorinated cyclodienes include aldrin, dieldrin, endrin, heptachlor, chlordane, and endosulfan. Two- to eight-hour exposure leads to depressed central nervous system (CNS) activity, followed by hyperexcitability, tremors, and then seizures. The mechanism of action is the insecticide binding at the $GABA_A$ site in the γ-aminobutyric acid (GABA) chloride ionophore complex, which inhibits chloride flow into the nerve.

Q. What makes these compounds toxic?

OC insecticides are persistent organic pollutants (POPs) because they are:

1. highly lipophilic (soluble in oils and fats);
2. stable;
3. mobile;
4. resistant to break down in the environment.

Insecticides such as the DDT are POPs and accumulate in food chains (Fig. 5.2) and causes reproductive problems (e.g., egg shell thinning) in

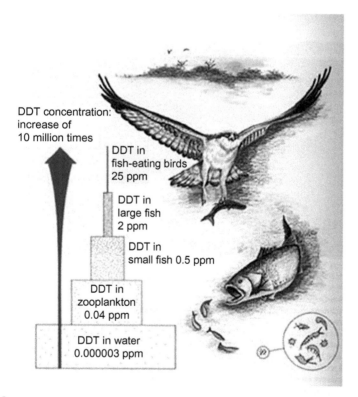

DDT concentration: increase of 10 million times

DDT in fish-eating birds 25 ppm

DDT in large fish 2 ppm

DDT in small fish 0.5 ppm

DDT in zooplankton 0.04 ppm

DDT in water 0.000003 ppm

FIGURE 5.2

Accumulation in food chains.

Image courtesy of US Fish and Wildlife Service.
http://mollykellyddt.weebly.com/uploads/1/7/8/2/17828633/8235025_orig.jpeg.

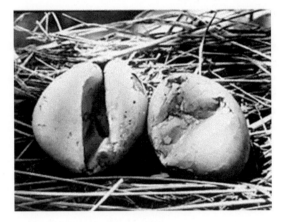

FIGURE 5.3

Thinning of egg shells.

Reproduced with permission from St David's Poultry Team.

certain bird species (Fig. 5.3). Due to their cumulative effects, the use of some of them has been banned. Some OC compounds, such as sulfur mustards, nitrogen mustards, and Lewisite, are even used as chemical weapons due to their toxicity.

5.3.2 OP AND CM COMPOUNDS

Q. What are organophosphate (OP) insecticides? Give examples.

An organophosphate (sometimes abbreviated OP) or phosphate ester is the general name for esters of phosphoric acid. They are used as insecticides, acaricides, soil nematicides, fungicides, herbicides, defoliants, rodenticides, insecticides synergists, insect repellents, chemosterilants, and warfare agents. Examples of OP compounds include acephate, chlorpyrifos, chlorpyrifos-methyl, diazinon, malathion, and parathion. They are known to inhibit esterases (cholinesterase, ChE).

Q. Define CM insecticides? Give examples.

CMs are often used as insecticides. Unlike OPs, CM compounds are not structurally complex and are not considered to be persistent, because these are readily hydrolyzed, e.g., carbaryl and bendiocarb.

Q. Why OPs and CMs are preferred over OC insecticides?

As compared to OC, OPs and CMs are:

1. much less environmentally persistent;
2. much more biodegradable;
3. less subject to biomagnifications;
4. usually unstable in the presence of sunlight;
5. much more acutely toxic to nontarget species.

Q. Out of OC, OP, and CM insecticides, which of them have more acute toxic effects?

Both OP and CM insecticides are often involved in serious fatal human, animal, and wildlife poisoning incidences. Victims are usually children, farmers, and unskilled labor and are considered most dangerous orally or through the skin.

Q. Describe in brief OP nerve agents/gases.

OP nerve agents include tabun (GA), sarin (GB), soman (GD), cyclosarin (GF), venom toxin (VX), and Russian VX (VR). These compounds are highly toxic and pose continuous threats for the lives of humans as well as animals, because they can be used as chemical weapons of mass destruction (WMD). So far these agents have been used by dictators and terrorists. In some incidents, animals have been victims of military operations. These compounds produce toxicity by directly inhibiting AChE, and much more potent than OP insecticides, as they cause lethality to animals in the micrograms range.

Q. What is OP-induced intermediate syndrome (IMS)?

OP-induced IMS was first reported in human patients in Sri Lanka in 1987. After exposure to methamidophos, fenthion, dimethoate, and monocrotophos, 10 patients within 24—96 hours reported symptoms of acute cholinergic poisoning. To date, OPs that are known to cause IMS include bromophos, chlorpyrifos, diazinon, dicrotophos, dimethoate, disulfoton, fenthion, malathion, methamidophos, methyl parathion, monocrotophos, omethoate, parathion, phosmet, and trichlorfon. IMS is usually observed in individuals who have ingested a massive dose of an OP insecticide either accidentally or in a suicide attempt.

Explanation: Clinically, this disease is characterized by acute paralysis and weakness in the areas of several cranial motor nerves, neck flexors, and facial, extraocular, palatal, proximal limb, and respiratory muscles. Generalized weakness, depressed deep tendon reflexes, ptosis, and diplopia are also evident. These symptoms may last for several days or weeks depending on the OP involved. A similar syndrome has also been observed in dogs and cats poisoned maliciously or accidentally with massive doses of certain OPs. It may be pertinent to mention that despite severe AChE inhibition, muscle fasciculations and muscarinic receptor-associated with accumulation of Ach are absent. Although the exact mechanism involved in pathogenesis of IMS is unclear, studies in rats suggest that decrease of AChE and nicotinic ACh receptor mRNA expression occur after oral poisoning with disulfoton. Currently, very little is known about the type of damage at the motor endplate or about risk factors contributing to its development.

Q. Draw a schematic diagram representing mechanism of action of OP and CM insecticides.

Both these groups of insecticides inhibit the AChE enzyme from breaking down ACh, thereby increasing both the level and duration of action of the neurotransmitter ACh. Schematic diagram representing mechanism of action is shown in Fig. 5.4.

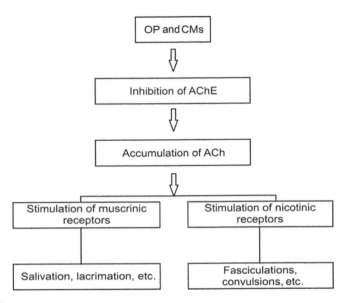

FIGURE 5.4

Schematic representation of mechanism of action of OP and CM insecticides.

In brief OPs and CMs bind ChE and inhibit its functions. This results in excess of Ach in synapses and neuromuscular junction leading to muscarinic and nicotinic symptoms and signs.

Q. How normally ACh is broken down by cholinesterase enzyme?

The positively charged nitrogen in the ACh molecule is attracted to the ionic site on AChE, and hydrolysis is catalyzed at the *esteratic* site to form choline and acetic. The breakdown of ACh by cholinesterase is shown in Fig. 5.5.

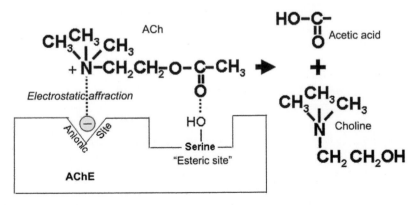

FIGURE 5.5

Breakdown of ACh (normal process).

https://www.atsdr.cdc.gov/csem/cholinesterase/images/acetylcholinesterase.png.

Q. How do cholinesterase inhibitors attach with AChE?

Fig. 5.6 shows how a cholinesterase inhibitor (in this case, a nerve agent) attaches to the serine hydroxyl group on AChE. This prevents ACh from interacting with the cholinesterase enzyme and being broken down.

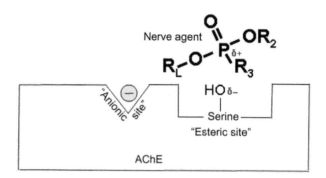

FIGURE 5.6

Partially electropositive phosphorus is attracted to partially electronegative serine. $\delta+$ indicates that phosphorus is partially electropositive and $\delta-$ indicates that oxygen is partially electronegative.

Diagrams modified from Wiener, S.W., Hoffman, R.S., 2004. Nerve agents: a comprehensive review. J. Intens. Care Med. 19 (1), 22–37, https://www.atsdr.cdc.gov/csem/cholinesterase/images/agent_binding.png.

Q. How do cholinesterase inhibitors work?

Fig. 5.7 shows transition state indicating which bonds break and which ones form and Fig. 5.8 shows cholinesterase inhibitor attached to AChE preventing the attachment of ACh.

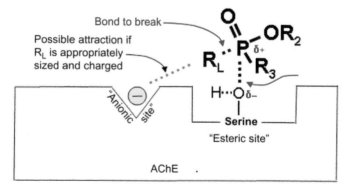

FIGURE 5.7

Transition state showing which bonds break and which ones form.

http://www.atsdr.cdc.gov/csem/cholinesterase/images/transition_state.png.

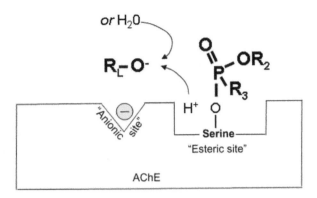

FIGURE 5.8

Cholinesterase inhibitor attached to AChE preventing the attachment of ACh.

http://www.atsdr.cdc.gov/csem/cholinesterase/images/esteric_binding.png.

Q. What are the adverse effects of blocked ACh breakdown?

The adverse effects of blocked ACh breakdown lead to the buildup of excessive levels of the neurotransmitter, ACh, at the skeletal neuromuscular junction and those synapses where ACh receptors are located. Thus, the primary manifestations of acute cholinesterase inhibitor toxicity are those of cholinergic (neurotransmitter) hyperactivity.

Q. What is aging due to cholinesterase inhibitors?

After some time, some inhibitors can develop a permanent bond with cholinesterase, known as aging, where "-doximes" such as pralidoxime (2-PAM) cannot reverse the bond. 2-PAM is often used with atropine (a muscarinic antagonist) to help reduce the parasympathetic effects of organophosphate poisoning.

Q. How do cholinesterase inhibitors can lead to aging?

Phosphorylated cholinesterases may undergo a dealkylation reaction of the OP moiety leading to "aged" enzyme, i.e., conversion of the inhibited enzyme into a nonreactivable form. Aging occurs rapidly when the inhibitor is soman, a powerful nerve agent (Figs. 5.9 and 5.10).

Q. What are the two important classes of cholinesterase inhibitors? How they differ from each other?

Cholinesterase inhibitors fall into two classes, OP and CM compounds. The former has generally higher toxicity, longer duration of action, and usually cause CNS toxicity. The key differences are listed in Table 5.1.

Q. What are toxic symptoms of OP and CM insecticides?

Signs and symptoms of cholinesterase inhibitor poisoning include CNS effects that are due to the presence of both nicotinic and muscarinic receptors and death is usually due to respiratory failure caused by bronchoconstriction,

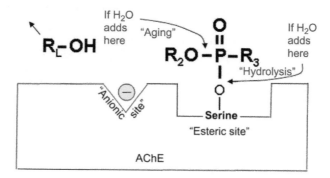

FIGURE 5.9

Cholinesterase is blocked, but it can hydrolyze to original state (slow); regenerate with an oxime (fast); "age" (cannot regenerate).

http://www.atsdr.cdc.gov/csem/cholinesterase/images/cholinesterase_aging.png.

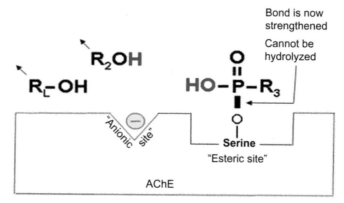

FIGURE 5.10

The "aged" bond (after addition of H_2O to the P—R$_3$ bond. Prior to aging, R_2 was pulling the electrons away from "P." Upon its being removed during the aging process, these electrons are shared with "O"-serine, strengthening its bond, so that it can no longer be hydrolyzed).

Table 5.1 The Key Differences of Cholinesterase Inhibitors (OP and CM Insecticides)

	Organophosphorus Compounds	Carbamates
Toxicity	Higher	Lower
Duration of action	Longer	Shorter
CNS toxicity	More common	Less common

bronchorrhea, central respiratory depression, weakness, and paralysis of respiratory muscles (Table 5.2).

Q. What is the treatment for OP and CM poisoning?

In OP insecticide poisoning, atropine sulfate can be used as an antidote in conjunction with 2-PAM or other pyridinium oximes (such as trimedoxime or obidoxime). Atropine sulfate acts a muscarinic antagonist and thus blocks the action of ACh peripherally. 2-PAM or other pyridinium oximes act as anticholinergic drugs and counteract the effects of excess ACh and reactivate AChE. The use of morphine, aminophylline, phenothiazine, reserpine, etc. is to be avoided.

CM insecticides have similar cholinesterase inhibiting toxicity as OP insecticides and nerve agents. However, the CM—cholinesterase bond spontaneously hydrolyzes, therefore, in the past, 2-PAM was contraindicated in CM poisoning. However, its use in CM toxicity can reduce the clinical severity.

Q. Why fever is observed in atropine poisoning?

Atropine poisoning causes decreased secretions in the body and occasionally, therapeutic doses dilate cutaneous blood vessels, particularly in the "blush" area (atropine flush), and may cause atropine "fever" due to suppression of sweat gland activity, especially in infants and small children.

Table 5.2 OP and CM Insecticide-Induced Muscrinic and Nicotinic Signs of Toxicity

	Site of Action	Physiological Effects
Muscrinic (parasympathetic effects)	Sweat glands	Excessive sweating lead to hypothermia and electrolyte balance
	Pupil	Constricted
	Lacrimal glands	Lacrimation (red tears)
	Salivary gland	Excessive salivation
	Bronchial trees	Wheezing
	GI tract	Cramps, vomiting, diarrhea, tenesmus
	Cardiovascular	Bradycardia, fall in BP
	Ciliary body bladdery	Blurred vision
	Bladder	Urinary inconsistence
Nicotinic effects	Striated muscles	Fasciculations, cramps, weakness, twitching, paralysis, respiratory distress, cyanosis/arrest
	Sympathetic ganglia	Tachycardia, BP raised
	CNS effects	Anxiety, restness, ataxia, convulsions

Q. Describe the mechanism of action of 2-PAM.

In organophosphate poisoning, an organophosphate binds to just one end of the AChE enzyme (the esteric site), blocking its activity (Fig. 5.11). 2-PAM is able to attach to the other half (the unblocked, anionic site) of the AChE enzyme (Fig. 5.12). It then binds to the organophosphate, the organophosphate changes conformation, and loses its binding to the AChE enzyme. The conjoined poison/antidote then unbinds from the site and thus regenerates the enzyme, which is now able to function again (Fig. 5.13).

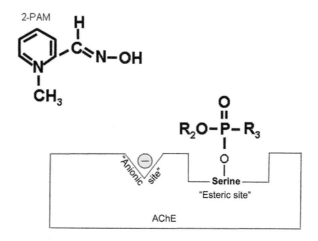

FIGURE 5.11

2-PAM and phosphorylated enzyme.

http://www.atsdr.cdc.gov/csem/cholinesterase/images/2pam_action1.png.

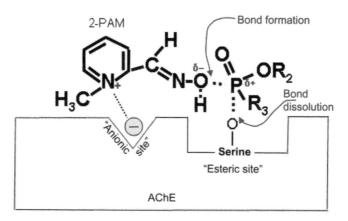

FIGURE 5.12

Partially electropositive nitrogen on 2-PAM is attracted to electronegative anionic site on cholinesterase.

http://www.atsdr.cdc.gov/csem/cholinesterase/images/2pam_action2.png.

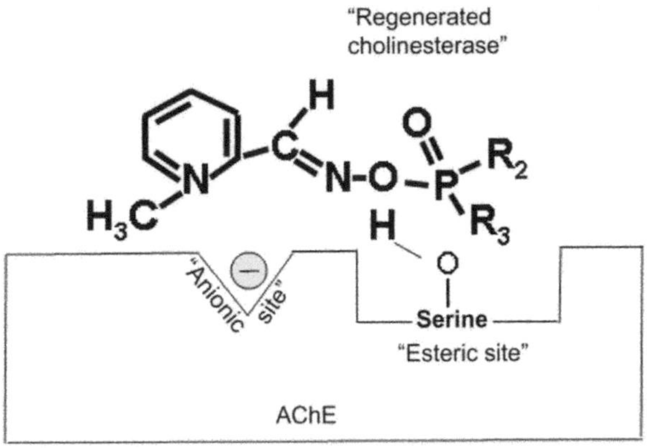

FIGURE 5.13

Regeneration of cholinesterase.

http://www.atsdr.cdc.gov/csem/cholinesterase/images/2pam_action3.png.

Q. What is OP-induced delayed neuropathy (OPIDN)?

Some OP compounds such as tri-*o*-cresyl phosphate (TOCP) was known to produce delayed neurotoxic effects in man and chicken, characterized by ataxia and weakness of the limbs, developing 10−14 days after exposure. This syndrome was called OPIDN. In recent literature, the syndrome has been renamed OP-induced delayed polyneuropathy (OPIDP). OPIDP is characterized by distal degeneration of long- and large-diameter motor and sensory axons of both peripheral nerves and spinal cord. Among all animal species the hen appears to be the most sensitive and therefore used as an animal model. TOCP and certain other compounds have minimal or no anti-AChE property; however, they cause phosphorylation and aging (dealkylation) of a protein in neurons called neuropathy target esterase (NTE), and subsequently lead to OPIDP. Today, many compounds, such as mipafox, tetraethyl pyrophosphate (TEPP), parathion, *o*-cresyl saligenin phosphate, and haloxon, are known to produce this syndrome. Some OP as well as non-OP inhibitors (such as CMs and sulfonyl fluorides) also covalently react with NTE but cannot undergo the aging reaction. As a result, these inhibitors do not cause OPIDP.

5.3.3 PYRETHROIDS

Q. What are pyrethrins and pyrethroids insecticides? Give examples.

A pyrethroid is an organic compound similar to the natural pyrethrins produced by the flowers of pyrethrums (*Chrysanthemum cinerariaefolium* and *Chrysanthemum coccineum*). Pyrethroids now constitute the majority of commercial household insecticides, e.g., allethrin, bifenthrin, cyfluthrin, and cypermethrin.

Q. Describe the important properties of pyrethrins and pyrethroids insecticides.
These compounds are:
1. more persistent,
2. have greater insecticidal activity,
3. photostable,
4. low doses are effective,
5. have low mammalian toxicities.

There are two broad classes of pyrethroids. Type I pyrethroids resemble natural pyrethrins in their structure and activity (e.g., allethrin, pyrethrin, and permethrin) and type II pyrethroids contain a −CYANO group in their structure and are more active and toxic (e.g., deltamethrin, cypermenthrin, and fenvalarate).

Q. Describe mechanism of action of pyrethrins and pyrethroids.
Pyrethrins affect nerve membranes by modifying the sodium and potassium channels, resulting in depolarization of the membranes.
1. The length of tail current is characteristic for each pyrethroid.
2. Both classes have little effect on the activation of channels and current flow, but prolong the inactivation, creating tail currents. Type I pyrethroids produce relatively short tail currents, whereas type II substantially longer ones (Fig. 5.14).

Formulations of these insecticides frequently contain the insecticide synergist piperonyl butoxide [5-{2-(2-butoxyethoxy)ethoxymethyl}-6-propyl-1,3-benzodioxole], which acts to increase the efficacy of the insecticide by inhibiting the cytochrome P450 enzymes responsible for the breakdown of the insecticide.

Q. Describe symptoms of poisoning.
The usual signs of poisoning include restlessness, incoordination, hyperactivity sensory to external stimuli, fine tremors progressing to other parts of body, and hyperthermia.

5.3.4 NATURAL INSECTICIDES

Q. Define natural insecticides. Give examples.
Natural insecticides, such as rotenone, nicotine, pyrethrum, and neem extracts, made by plants as defenses against insects. Natural insecticides are usually nontoxic to humans and pets and safe for the environment.

Q. Name at least three plants having insecticidal properties.
1. Nicotine (Fig. 5.15)
2. Chrysanthemum (Fig. 5.16)
3. *Derris* (Fig. 5.17).

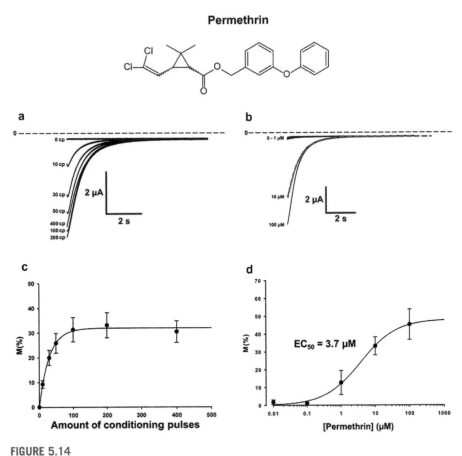

FIGURE 5.14

Characteristic "tail" appearance in type II pyrethroid depolarization.

Reproduced from Springer Nature (https://media.nature.com/lw926/nature-assets/srep/2015/150723/
srep12475/images_hires/srep12475-f6.jpg).

5.3.5 FORMAMIDINE AND NEONICOTINOID

Both formamidine and neonicotinoid are new classes of insecticides that are applied at low dosages and are extremely effective but are relatively nontoxic to humans.

Q. Define neonicotinoids. Give examples.

Neonicotinoids (sometimes shortened to neonics/ˈniːoʊnɪks/) are a class of neuroactive insecticides chemically similar to nicotine. The neonicotinoid family includes acetamiprid, clothianidin, imidacloprid, nitenpyram, nithiazine, thiacloprid, and thiamethoxam. Imidacloprid is the most widely used insecticide in the world.

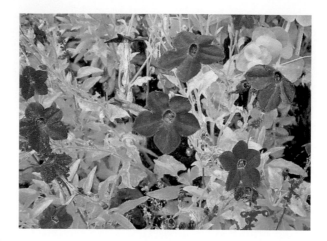

FIGURE 5.15

Nicotine plant.

http://www.thetortoisetable.org.uk/common/files/catalogue/475/large/tobaccoplant_nicotiana%
20spp_solanaceae_lr_oct09%201%206.jpg.

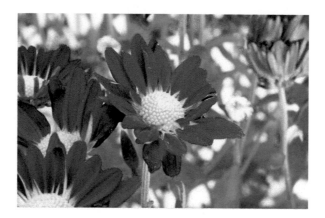

FIGURE 5.16

Chrysanthemum flowers—source of natural pyrethrin.

Reproduced from http://maxpixel.freegreatpicture.com/Chrysanthemum-Flower-Flowers-Red-Chrysanthemum-
1274667.

Q. Define formamidine insecticides. Give examples.

Formamidine insecticides are a relatively new group of acaricides which are particularly useful for the control of Lepidoptera, Hemiptera, phytophagous mites, and cattle ticks. Because of the widespread use for control of cotton insects and cattle ticks, their toxicity is extremely important. This group includes amitraz, chlordimeform, formetanate, formparanate, medimeform, and semiamitraz.

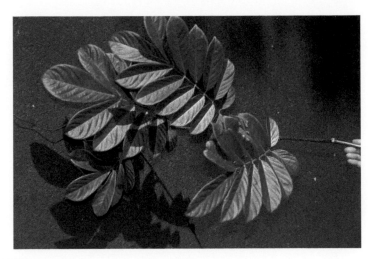

FIGURE 5.17

Derris plant—root is the source of rotenone.

Reproduced from https://commons.wikimedia.org/wiki/File:Starr_990106-3021_Derris_elliptica.jpg.

5.4 HERBICIDES

Q. What are herbicides?

Herbicides control weeds and are the most widely used class of pesticides. This class of pesticide can be applied to crops using many strategies to eliminate or reduce weed populations, e.g., imidazolinones, chlorophenoxy herbicides such as 2,4-D (2,4-dichlorophenoxy acetic acid) and 2,4,5-T (2,4,5-trichlorophenoxy-acetic acid), triazines, bipyridylium family such as paraquat (1,1-dimethyl-4,4-bipyridinium ion as the chloride salt) and diquat.

Q. Classify herbicides.

1. Inorganic (arsenicals, chlorates)
2. Organic (chlorophenoxy and its derivatives, dinitrophenols, bipyridyls, ureas, and other herbicides).

Q. What are the main signs and symptoms of herbicide toxicity?

1. Ingestion: burning pain in mouth, throat, chest, upper abdomen, pulmonary edema, pancreatitis, renal and CNS effects such as nervousness, irritability, combativeness, disorientation, diminished reflexes.
2. Dermal: dry and fissured hands, horizontal ridging or loss of fingernails, ulceration, abrasion. Direct spilling may lead to severe skin injury (Fig. 5.18).

Q. Describe mode of action of paraquat herbicide.

Paraquat is one of bipyridinium compounds. It is caustic and irritant agent which causes ulceration and necrosis of the skin and mucous membranes. Paraquat is actively taken up by the alveolar cells via a diamine or polyamine transport system where it undergoes NADPH-dependent reduction. These are easily reduced to the radical ions, which generates superoxide radical that reacts

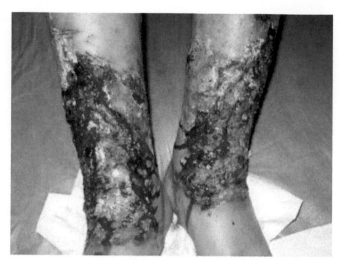

FIGURE 5.18

Skin injury caused by paraquat poisoning.

https://www.spandidos-publications.com/article_images/etm/6/6/ETM-06-06-1504-g00.jpg.

with unsaturated membrane lipids. The excess of superoxide anion radical O_2^- and H_2O_2 causes damage to the cellular membrane in lungs, which reduces the functional integrity of lung cells, affects efficient gas transport and exchange, and results in respiratory impairment including pulmonary fibrosis.

5.5 FUNGICIDES

Q. What are fungicides? Give examples.

Fungicides are chemicals that destroy fungus. Important fungicides include: Chlorothalonil (tetrachloroisophthalonitrile), captan, captafol, folpet, dithiocarbamates, sulfur derivatives of dithiocarbamic acid, metallic dimethyldithiocarbamates, mancozeb, maneb, zineb (zinc ethylenebisdithiocarbamate), and ethylthiourea compounds.

5.6 RODENTICIDES

Q. What are rodenticides? Give examples.

Rodenticides are used to control rodents. The list of rodenticides includes anticoagulants (warfarin, coumatetralyl, chlorophacinone, flocoumafen, difenacoum, bromadiolone, brodifacoum), hypercalcemia (calciferol), metal phosphides aluminum phosphide (fumigant only), calcium phosphide (fumigant only), magnesium phosphide (fumigant only), zinc phosphide (bait only), ANTU (α-naphthylthiourea; specific against brown rat, *Rattus norvegicus*), arsenic trioxide, barium carbonate, chloralose (a narcotic prodrug), etc.

5.7 FUMIGANTS

Toxicity of fumigants has also been discussed in Chapter 15, Veterinary Toxicology.

Q. What are fumigants?

Fumigants are extremely toxic gases used to protect stored products, especially grains, and to kill soil nematodes.

Q. Classify fumigants.

1. Inorganic (aluminum phosphide, hydrogen cyanide, carbon disulfide, sulfur dioxide)

2. Organic (methyl bromide, ethylene dibromide, dibromochloropropane).

Q. Describe in brief aluminum phosphide.

Aluminum phosphide is a solid fumigant pesticide, widely used as a grain preservative. It is used as suicidal and homicidal poisoning. On exposure to air or moisture, it liberates phosphine and can produce multiorgan damage.

5.8 QUESTION AND ANSWER EXERCISES

5.8.1 SHORT QUESTIONS AND ANSWERS

Exercise 1

Q.1 Why OC insecticides are being discouraged/banned?

OC insecticides are not degradable and are persistent in the environment. And due to high lipid solubility, they accumulate in the food chain and enter human and animal bodies. Hence, OC compounds are being discouraged.

Q.2 Why OP compounds are preferred as insecticides for the crops?

OP compounds are biodegradable and hence are not persistent in environment. Further, they are easily destroyed by sunlight, water, microbes, alkalis, metals, etc. Hence, within 2—4 weeks of application, OP compounds are destroyed. However, they have considerable toxicity for mammals if consumed directly.

Q.3 Can we use phenothiazine derivatives as treatment in pyrethroid insecticide poisoning?

No. Use of phenothiazine derivatives is contraindicated.

Q.4 Why lung tissue is primarily affected by paraquat?

1. Paraquat accumulates up to 10 times in lungs.

2. Lung tissue is deficient in superoxide dismutase enzyme, which destroys superoxide radical. Hence, lungs are primarily affected.

Q.5 Despite being highly toxic, why bipyridyl herbicides do not produce toxicity after being sprayed on plants?

  1. Bipyridyl herbicides are used in very low doses, which are not toxic.

  2. They are inactivated immediately upon contact with soil.

Q.6 How do paraquat and diquat differ in their toxicity?

During paraquat exposure, toxicity results from lung injury resulting from both the preferential uptake of paraquat by the lungs and the redox cycling mechanism. Pulmonary fibrosis is the usual cause of death in paraquat poisoning.

During diquat poisoning, renal damage results from both the preferential uptake of diquat by the kidney and the redox cycling mechanism. No progressive pulmonary fibrosis has been noted in diquat poisoning. However, diquat has severe toxic effects on the CNS that are not typical of paraquat poisoning.

Q.7 Does use of oxygen is beneficial in paraquat poisoning?

Use of supplemental oxygen is contraindicated until the patient develops severe hypoxemia.

High concentrations of oxygen in the lung increase the injury induced by paraquat and possibly by diquat as well.

Q.8 Despite being very specific to rats, why ANTU is banned?

Due to carcinogenic potential of α-naphthylamine impurities.

Q.9 What is the difference between pulmonary toxicity caused by ANTU (rodenticide) and paraquat (herbicide)?

ANTU causes pulmonary edema and is fatal, whereas paraquat causes pulmonary fibrosis which is not fatal.

Q.10 How the binding of CM and OP compounds to AChE differs?

  1. CM compounds bind with both anionic and esteratic sites, whereas OP compounds bind only with esteratic site.

  2. CM compounds cause carbomylation, whereas OP compounds cause phosphorylation.

  3. Binding of CMs is reversible, whereas that of OP compounds is irreversible (aging).

Exercise 2

Q.1 Name two main types of cholinergic receptors. Why they are so named?

The two main types of cholinergic receptors are:

  1. nicotinic,

  2. muscarinic.

They are so named because their effects are similar to those of nicotine and muscarine.

Q.2 What is location and function of *nicotinic and muscarinic* receptors?

  1. Are present in different anatomical locations.

  2. Have different functions.

  3. Have different mechanisms by which they trigger signal transmission.

Q.3 What is the key function of nicotinic receptors?

A key function of nicotinic receptors is to trigger *rapid* neural and neuromuscular transmission.

Q.4 Where nicotinic receptors are found in the body?

1. The somatic nervous system (neuromuscular junctions in skeletal muscles)
2. The sympathetic and parasympathetic nervous system (autonomic ganglia)
3. The central nervous system.

Q.5 What are peripheral nervous system clinical findings of nicotinic signs of cholinesterase inhibitor toxicity?

Peripheral nervous system clinical findings of nicotinic signs of cholinesterase inhibitor toxicity include:

1. Fasciculations and myoclonic jerks (CNS effects are discussed later)
2. Weakness and paralysis
3. Sweating
4. Mydriasis (pupillary dilation) (in up to 13% of the cases)
5. Tachycardia, tachydysrhythmias
6. Hypertension
7. Hyperglycemia, glycosuria, ketosis
8. Leukocytosis with a left shift.

The following table provides a mnemonic for remembering the nicotinic signs of cholinesterase inhibitor toxicity.

Nicotinic Mnemonic	Signs of Cholinesterase Inhibitor Toxicity
Monday	Mydriasis (pupillary dilation)
Tuesday	Tachycardia
Wednesday	Weakness
Thursday	Hypertension
Friday	Fasciculations

Q.6 What are the key response differences between muscarinic and nicotinic receptors?

The key response differences between muscarinic and nicotinic receptors are that the response of muscarinic receptors:

1. is slower;
2. may be excitatory or inhibitory;
3. do not affect skeletal muscles, but do influence the activity of smooth muscle, exocrine glands, and the cardiac conduction system. In contrast to skeletal muscle and neurons, smooth muscle and the cardiac conduction system normally exhibit intrinsic electrical and mechanical rhythmic activity. This activity is modulated, rather than initiated, by the muscarinic receptors.

Q.7 Where muscarinic receptors are located?

Muscarinic receptors are located in the:

1. Parasympathetic nervous system
   a. Cardiac conduction system
   b. Exocrine glands
   c. Smooth muscles
2. Sympathetic nervous system
   a. Sweat glands
3. Central nervous system.

Q.8 What are the clinical effects on the peripheral nervous system due to excessive stimulation of muscarinic receptors by cholinesterase inhibitor toxicity?

Excessive stimulation of muscarinic receptors due to cholinesterase inhibitor poisoning results in:

1. Increased parasympathetic cardiac effects
   a. AV blocks, with escape rhythms
   b. Bradycardia
   c. Ventricular dysrhythmias
2. Exocrine gland activity
   a. Bronchorrhea
   b. Hyperamylasemia
   c. Lacrimation
   d. Rhinorrhea
   e. Salivation
3. Smooth muscle activity
   a. Bladder stimulation, sphincter relaxation
   b. Bronchospasm
   c. Miosis (pupillary constriction), eye pain due to ciliary spasm
   d. Nausea, vomiting, cramps, diarrhea.

Exercise 3

Q.1 Why the binding of CMs with AChE is reversible?

CMs causes carbomylation of AChE, which is weaker than phosphorylation caused by OP compounds. Hence, the binding is reversible.

Q.2 Why CMs cannot cause delayed neuropathy?

CMs cannot bind with neurotoxic esterase. Hence delayed neuropathy is not caused.

Q.3 What is bait shyness?

A rodent surviving the exposure to a particular rodenticide will avoid the same rodenticide in the future. This phenomenon is called bait shyness.

Q.4 What is secondary poisoning?

The poisoning that is seen in dogs and cats as a result of consumption of rodenticide poisoned rodents.

Q.5 Why the use of fluoroacetate is restricted?

Fluoroacetate is highly toxic and nonspecific, affecting other species.

Q.6 What are the metabolic active forms of malathion and parathion?

Malaoxon and paraoxon.

Q.7 Why CMs are the most preferred insecticides in veterinary use?

CMs have broad spectrum of activity, low in mammalian toxicity, and undergo rapid degradation in environment. Hence, CMs are preferred for veterinary use (e.g., carbaryl and propoxur).

Q.8 Why sodium fluoroacetate does not produce bait shyness?

Sodium fluoroacetate needs lag period for developing toxicity. Hence, the rodents do not remember the exposure.

Q.9 Why zinc phosphide preparations contain antimony potassium tartrate?

Antimony potassium tartrate is an emetic, which can prevent accidental zinc phosphide toxicity in nontarget species through vomition.

Q.10 Why zinc phosphide is more toxic on full stomach than empty?

On full stomach, the acid production in stomach is increased. As zinc phosphide releases phosphine gas in acidic medium, full stomach increases the toxicity.

Exercise 4

Q.1 How does 2-PAM reactivate the enzyme ChE?

2-PAM attaches to cholinesterase inhibitors that have blocked cholinesterase and removes them from the enzyme, thereby reactivating it.

Q.2 How does aging takes place?

Some cholinesterase inhibitors after a time will form a permanent bond with cholinesterase in a process called aging, after which 2-PAM is no longer effective.

Q.3 Can we give 2-PAM in conjunction with atropine in OP poisoning?

Yes. 2-PAM should be given in conjunction with atropine, with which it has a notable synergistic effect. Although it has been suggested that 2-PAM was absolutely contraindicated in CM poisoning, data are lacking to support this recommendation.

Q.4 When does 2-PAM treatment failure occur?

1. With an inadequate dose
2. When aging has already occurred
3. When active cholinesterase inhibitor absorption or redistribution (e.g., from fat tissue) is continuing to occur.

Q.5 Does aging takes place in CM poisoning?

No. The CM–cholinesterase bond does not age.

Q.6 What is atropine fever?

It is caused due to decreased secretions in the body. Occasionally, therapeutic doses of atropine dilate cutaneous blood vessels, particularly in the "blush" area (atropine flush), and may cause atropine "fever" due to suppression of sweat gland activity, especially in infants and small children.

Q.7 What are signs and symptoms of aluminum phosphide?

Aluminum phosphide has a metallic taste. Symptoms include garlicky odor, nausea, pain in gullet, stomach, abdomen, vomiting, diarrhea, cough dyspnea, respiratory failure, headache, anxiety, hypotension tachy/bradycardia, myocarditis, hepatosplenomegaly, renal failure, and coma.

Q.8 What is the mode of action of warfarin?

Warfarin interferes with normal function of vitamin K and causes coagulation defects characterized by decreased blood concentrations of coagulation protein factors. The decreased coagulation factors lead to massive internal hemorrhages and the affected individuals die due to tissue hypoxia.

Q.9 Describe mode of action of diquat herbicide.

Diquat is a very reactive compound and exerts its action in a similar manner to paraquat but affects liver and kidney but does not cause pulmonary edema or alter lung functions. Signs of CNS excitement and renal impairment occur in severely affected patients.

Q.10 Name the plant from which pyrethrin is obtained.

Chrysanthemum.

Q.11 Jack Daniels is a 50-year-old business manager with a past history of rheumatic fever and a mechanical mitral valve replacement. He takes warfarin to prevent clots forming from the valve replacement. While showering one day, he notices extensive bruising on his abdomen and thighs. He visits his general practitioner who determines the warfarin dose is too high. What drug could be administered to rectify this problem?

Vitamin K is the antidote for warfarin overdose.

5.8.2 MULTIPLE CHOICE QUESTIONS (CHOOSE THE BEST STATEMENT, IT CAN BE ONE, TWO OR MORE OR NONE OR ALL)

Exercise 5

Q.1 Zinc phosphide releases phosphine gas in the following pH:
   a. Acidic
   b. Basic
   c. Neutral
   d. All

Q.2 The following rodenticides require multiple administration to cause death:
   a. Zinc phosphide
   b. Anticoagulants
   c. Vitamin
   d. Strychnine

Q.3 OP compounds can inhibit the following enzyme(s):
   a. AChE
   b. BuChE
   c. NTE
   d. All

Q.4 The following type of toxicity caused by OP compounds is irreversible even with treatment:
   a. Acute

    b. Subacute
    c. Chronic
    d. OPIDN

Q.5 Which of the following insecticides are more specific to arthropods?
    a. OC compounds
    b. OP compounds
    c. CMs
    d. Pyrethroids

Q.6 Paraquat and diquat differ substantially in their
    a. metabolism to a free radical
    b. ability to initiate lipid peroxidation in vivo
    c. uptake by the lung
    d. generation of superoxide anion in vivo
    e. mechanism of cytotoxicity

Q.7 Toxic injury to the cell body, axon, and surrounding Schwann cells of peripheral nerves are referred to, respectively, as
    a. neuropathy, axonopathy, and myelopathy
    b. neuronopathy, axonopathy, and myelinopathy
    c. neuropathy, axonopathy, and gliosis
    d. neuronopathy, dying-back neuropathy, and myelopathy
    e. chromatolysis, axonopathy, and gliosis

Q.8 The following OC insecticides is not persistent in environment:
    a. DDT
    b. Aldrin
    c. Methoxychlor
    d. Endosulfan

Q.9 The most commonly used pyrethroid synergist is
    a. silica
    b. piperonyl butoxide
    c. methyl butyl ether
    d. n-octyl bicycloheptene dicarboximide
    e. toluene

Q.10 The chloronicotinyl compound imidacloprid demonstrates a high insecticidal potency and exceptionally a low mammalian toxicity due to
    a. its high affinity for insect nicotinic ACh receptors and low affinity for mammalian nicotinic ACh receptors
    b. the blood−brain barrier in mammals
    c. the first-pass effect in the liver in mammals
    d. the low pH in the stomach of monogastric mammals
    e. the presence of true AChE in mammals

Answers

1.a; 2.b and c; 3.d; 4.d; 5.d (the LD_{50} of pyrethroids for insects and mammals is 1:4500, which means highly specific action toward insects); 6.a; 7. b; 5.c and d; 9. b; 10.a.

5.8.3 FILL IN THE BLANKS

Exercise 6

Q.1 OP compounds which inhibit AChE without requiring metabolic activation are called _____.

Q.2 Indirect acting OP compounds require metabolic activation and convert to _____ form before producing toxicity.

Q.3 The toxicity of OP compounds_____ during storage in body tissue.

Q.4 The species of animal that is highly sensitive for OP poisoning is _____.

Q.5 The species of animal that is highly sensitive for delayed neuropathy caused by OP compounds (OPIDN) is _____.

Q.6 The site on AChE with which OP compounds bind and cause irreversible inhibition is _____ site.

Q.7 The phosphorylation of AChE by OP compounds resulting in the loss of alkyl group and forming irreversible bond is called _____.

Q.8 The agents which are used to reactivate OP insecticide−inhibited AChE are called _____.

Q.9 Oxime reactivators are ineffective in reactivating AChE after _____ stage.

Q.10 BuChE (pseudocholinesterase) is present in _____.

Answers

1. DIRECT ACTING OP COMPOUNDS (direct acting compounds have $P = O$ (oxon) group, hence act without metabolic activation, e.g., TEPP, dichlorvos, sarin, tabun); 2. OXON (indirect acting agents have $P = S$ (thionate bond) which should be converted to $P = O$ (oxon) form before inhibiting AChE, e.g., malathion, parathion, chlorpyrifos). 3. INCREASES (due to development of toxic isomers in storage); 4. CAT; 5. CHICKEN (chicken brain has higher specific activity of NTE, hence is more susceptible); 6. ESTERATIC; 7. AGING; 5. OXIME REACTIVATORS (e.g., 2-PAM); 9. AGING; 10. PLASMA (inhibition of BuChE is more important in birds than that of AChE inhibition).

Exercise 7

Q.1 OC compound insecticides act by inhibiting _____ receptors.

Q.2 Hyperthermia in OC insecticide poisoning is due to changes in metabolism of _____ and _____ neurotransmitters.

Q.3 The metabolite of DDT is _____.

Q.4 DDT acts as agonist for _____ receptors and DDE acts as antagonist for _____ receptors.

Q.5 DDE, the metabolite of DDT, causes thinning of egg shells due to the inhibition of _____ enzyme.

Q.6 The predominate symptoms in OC insecticide poisoning are
_____ and _____ .

Q.7 The sedatives of choice used in OC insecticide–induced CNS excitation
are _____ .

Q.8 Death in OC compound poisoning is due to _____ failure.

Q.9 Organic insecticides which are esters of phosphorus are _____
compounds.

Q.10 OP insecticides act as irreversible inhibitors of _____ enzyme.

Exercise 8

1. GABA (since GABA are inhibitory receptors, inhibition of GABA receptors
leads to CNS excitation. Cyclodiene OC compounds like aldrin, endrin, and endosulfan follow this mechanism). 2. SEROTONIN and NORADRENALINE. 3. DDE
(dichlorodiphenyldichloroethylene). 4. ESTROGEN, ANDROGEN. 5. CALCIUM
ATPase (DDE is known to cause thinning of egg shells causing decline of birds of
prey (bald eagle, pelican, falcon) chicken, song birds). 6. BEHAVIORAL (nervous), HYPERTHERMIA (OP compounds do not produce behavioral symptoms
and hyperthermia). 7. BENZODIAZEPINES (e.g., diazepam; benzodiazepines also
increase affinity for GABA for its receptors, which is inhibited by OC insecticides); 8. RESPIRATORY (OC causes initial CNS stimulation followed by depression and coma. Hence, ultimately death is due to respiratory failure);
9. ORGANOPHOSPHATE (OP); 10. ACETYLCHOLINESTERASE (AChE)
(AChE inhibition causes excess ACh accumulation producing cholinergic
symptoms).

Exercise 9

Q.1 The use of oxime reactivators is contraindicated in _____
insecticide poisoning.

Q.2 Voltage-gated sodium channels are more sensitive for _____
type of pyrethroids.

Q.3 The metabolite of zinc phosphide that is produced in the body is
_____. (hypophosphite is excreted in urine).

Q.4 Phosphine gas acts as _____ poison.

Q.5 Bait shyness is not observed with _____ rodenticides.

Q.6 Warfarin inhibits clotting factors which are dependent on
_____ for synthesis.

Q.7 Anticoagulant rodenticides decrease vitamin K synthesis through inhibition
of _____ enzyme.

Q.8 Capillary damage seen in warfarin rodenticides is due to the presence of
_____ chemical moiety.

Q.9 The hematological tests used to confirm poisoning from anticoagulants are
_____.

Q.10 The specific treatment for anticoagulant poisoning is _____.

Answers

1. CARBAMATE (as no binding site is available for oxime reactivators, they themselves will cause toxicity); 2. TWO; 3. HYPOPHOSPHITE (hypophosphite is excreted in urine); 4. PROTOPLASMIC (it is also highly irritant to gastrointestinal tract); 5. ANTICOAGULANT (anticoagulants act after a lag time. Further, due to absence of odor and taste, they do not produce bait shyness); 6. VITAMIN K (vitamin K−dependent clotting factors are II (prothrombin), VII, IX, and X); 7. VITAMIN K EPOXIDE REDUCTASE; 8. BENZALACTONE (mere decrease of clotting factors is not enough to cause death, hence, induction of capillary damage is necessary to cause fatal hemorrhage); 9. CLOTTING TIME and PROTHROMBIN TIME (an increase of two to six times in clotting and prothrombin times are noted); 10. PHYTOMENADIONE (vitamin K1) (menadione is a precursor of vitamin K. Menadione from synthetic sources is K3; menaquinone—K2 I from bacteria; phytomenadione—K1 is from plants).

Exercise 10

Q.1 In type II pyrethroid toxicity, characteristic _____ is seen in depolarization phase of action potential.

Q.2 Type II pyrethroids act as inhibitors for ----------------- neurotransmitter receptors.

Q.3 The symptoms in type I pyrethroid toxicity are referred to as _____.

Q.4 Type II pyrethroids produce characteristic syndrome known as _____.

Q.5 A group of tranquilizers contraindicated in pyrethroid poisoning is _____.

Q.6 The roots of *Derris* genus of plants are the sources for the natural insecticide _____.

Q.7 Rotenone is highly toxic for _____ species.

Q.8 The agents which are used to control rodents are known as _____.

Q.9 The toxicity of zinc phosphide (Zn3P2) is due to the release of _____ gas.

Q.10 The characteristic smell of phosphine gas, which can be used for diagnosis of zinc phosphide toxicity, is _____ odor.

Answers

1. TAIL; 2. GABA; 3. T-SYNDROME (tremors); 4. CS SYNDROME (choreoathetosis and salivation); 5. PHENOTHIAZINE; 6. ROTENONE; 7. FISH (hence *Derris* is used to control not only insects but also fish (piscicide)); 8. RODENTICIDES; 9. PHOSPHINE (PH3); 10. FISH LIKE or ACETYLENE.

Exercise 11

Q.1 The breed of rat, which is very sensitive for ANTU, is _____ or _____ rats.

Q.2 The risk of secondary poisoning is very high in _____ rodenticides.

Q.3 Fluoroacetate acts by inhibiting _____ or _____ and lowers energy production in the body.

Q.4 The prominent symptom in fluoroacetate poisoning is _____.

Q.5 The competitive antagonist, which is used in the treatment of fluoroacetate poisoning is, _____.

Q.6 The effective rodenticides in warfarin-resistant rats is _____ compounds.

Q.7 The mechanism of rodenticide action of vitamin D compounds (cholecalciferol) is by producing _____.

Q.8 The treatment for vitamin D rodenticides is administration of _____and _____.

Q.9 The phrase "drowning in one's own fluids" is associated with _____ rodenticide poisoning.

Q.10 Metaldehyde inhibits ------------ neurotransmitter in CNS, which causes excitation.

Answers

1. BROWN or NORWAY; 2. SECOND GENERATION (hence are also called super-warfarins, e.g., bromadiolone and brodifacoum); 3. TCA or KREBS CYCLE; 4. NEUROLOGICAL (brain is severely affected in the event of depletion of energy in the body); 5. GLYCEROL MONOACETATE (however, glyceryl monoacetate is not a specific antidote of fluoroacetate); 6. VITAMIN D (cholecalciferol); 7. HYPERCALCEMIA (hypercalcemia causes calcification of visceral organs like kidney, blood vessels, heart, and lungs); 8. CORTICOSTEROIDS and CALCITONIN (both corticosteroids and calcitonin reduce hypercalcemia); 9. ANTU (α-napthylthiourea) (ANTU causes leakage of fluid into lungs leading to froth formation and death); 10. GABA.

Exercise 12

Q.1 Paraquat selectively accumulates in _____ organ of the body.

Q.2 The mechanism of toxicity of paraquat is through generation of _____ free radical, which affects unsaturated membrane lipids.

Q.3 The bipyridyl herbicide, which can cause pulmonary fibrosis, is _____ .

Q.4 The agents which are used to prevent fungal infestation of plants or seeds are known as _____.

Q.5 Fungicides which can cause act by uncoupling of oxidative phosphorylation are _____.

Q.6 The mechanism of uncoupling of oxidative phosphorylation of PCP is due to _____ activity.

Q.7 Dithiocarbamates such as ziram and thiram are derivatives of
_____.

Q.8 Agents which are used to control snails and slugs are known as
_____.

Q.9 The most commonly used molluscicide is _____.

Q.10 Metaldehyde is extremely toxic though _____ route of exposure.

Q.11 The active metabolite of metaldehyde formed in the body is
_____.

Answers

1. LUNGS; 2. SUPEROXIDE; 3. PARAQUAT; 4. FUNGICIDES; 5. PENTACHLOROPHENOL (PCP); 6. PROTON INOPHORE (PCP being a lipid-soluble weak acid carries protons (H^+) across mitochondrial membrane leading to depletion of proton gradient required for ATP synthesis. Hence, ATP synthesis is inhibited); 7. CARBAMATES; 5. MOLLUSCICIDES; 9. METALDEHYDE; 10. INHALATION; 11. ACETALDEHYDE.

FURTHER READING

ATSDR, 2016. Cholinesterase inhibitors: including insecticides and chemical warfare nerve agents, part 2: What are cholinesterase inhibitors? Case Studies in Environmental Medicine Page (last updated December 19, 2016). Agency for Toxic Substances and Disease Registry, USA. <https://www.atsdr.cdc.gov/csem/csem.asp?csem=11&po=5>.

Costa, L.G., 2013. Toxic effects of pesticides. In: Klaassen, C.D. (Ed.), Casarett and Doull's Toxicology: The Basic Science of Poisons, eighth ed. McGraw-Hill, New York, NY, pp. 933–980.

Gupta, P.K., 1986. Pesticides in the Indian Environment. Interprint, New Delhi, India.

Gupta, P.K., 1988a. Veterinary Toxicology. 1988, Cosmo Publications, New Delhi, India (Chapters 6 and 9).

Gupta, P.K., 2010a. Epidemiology of anticholinesterase pesticides: India. In: Satoh, T., Gupta, R.C. (Eds.), Anticholinesterase Pesticides: Metabolism, Neurotoxicity, and Epidemiology. John Wiley & Sons, USA, pp. 417–431.

Gupta, P.K., 2010b. Pesticides. In: second reprint Gupta, P.K. (Ed.), Modern Toxicology: The Adverse Effects of Xenobiotics, vol. 2. PharmaMed Press, Hyderabad, India, pp. 1–60.

Gupta, P.K., 2017. Herbicides and fungicides. In: Gupta, R.C. (Ed.), Reproductive and Developmental Toxicology, second ed. Academic Press/Elsevier, Amsterdam, pp. 655–677.

Gupta, P.K., 2018a. Toxicity of herbicides. In: Gupta, R.C. (Ed.), Veterinary Toxicology: Basic and Clinical Principles, third ed. Academic Press/Elsevier, San Diego, USA, pp. 553–568.

Gupta, P.K., 2018b. Toxicity of fungicides. In: Gupta, R.C. (Ed.), Veterinary Toxicology: Basic and Clinical Principles, second ed. Academic Press/Elsevier, San Diego, USA, pp. 569–582.

Metals and micronutrients

CHAPTER OUTLINE

6.1 METALS AND MICRONUTRIENTS

Toxicity of metals and micronutrients has also been discussed in Chapter 15, Veterinary Toxicology.

Q. Define metals.

Metals are elements that form cations when compounds of them are in solution and oxides of the elements form hydroxides rather than acids in water. Most metals are conductors of electricity, have crystalline solids with a metallic luster (except mercury, which is liquid), and have a high chemical reactivity.

Illustrated Toxicology. DOI: http://dx.doi.org/10.1016/B978-0-12-813213-5.00006-7

Q. Define micronutrients.

Micronutrient is a chemical element or substance required in trace amounts for the normal growth and the development of living organisms.

6.2 METALS

Q. What is the difference between a metal and a nonmetal?

Metals tend to be malleable and ductile, which means that they can be hammered and drawn into wires, whereas solid nonmetals tend to be hard and brittle. Metals lose electrons easily, and they often corrode easily. The oxides of metals tend to be basic, but the oxides of nonmetals tend to be acidic.

Q. Describe in brief general mechanism of *enzyme inhibition/activation by metals.*

A major site of toxic action for metals is interaction with enzymes, resulting in either enzyme inhibition or activation. Two mechanisms are of particular importance: inhibition may occur as a result of interaction between the metal and sulfhydryl (SH) groups on the enzyme, and the metal may displace an essential metal cofactor of the enzyme. For example, lead may displace zinc in the zinc-dependent enzyme δ-aminolevulinic acid dehydratase, thereby inhibiting the synthesis of heme, an important component of hemoglobin and heme-containing enzymes, such as cytochromes.

Q. How do toxic metals affect subcellular organelles of the tissues?

Toxic metals may disrupt the structure and function of a number of organelles. For example, enzymes associated with the endoplasmic reticulum may be inhibited, metals may be accumulated in the lysosomes, respiratory enzymes in the mitochondria may be inhibited, and metal inclusion bodies may be formed in the nucleus.

Q. Which metals have carcinogenic potential in human beings or animals?

A number of metals have been shown to be carcinogenic in humans or animals. Arsenic, certain chromium compounds, and nickel are known human carcinogens; beryllium, cadmium, and cisplatin are probable human carcinogens. The carcinogenic action, in some cases, is thought to result from the interaction of the metallic ions with DNA.

Q. Which metal(s) has/have kidney as the target organ?

The kidney is a common target organ for metal toxicity.

1. Cadmium
2. Inorganic mercury compounds, which are more water soluble
3. Organic lead compounds.

Q. Which metal(s) has/have nervous system as the target organ?

The nervous system is the target organ for organic metal compounds. For example, methylmercury, because it is lipid soluble, readily crosses the blood—brain barrier (BBB), and enters the nervous system.

Q. Name two metals which are known to have endocrine and reproductive effects.

1. Cadmium is known to produce testicular injury after acute exposure.

2. Lead accumulation in the testes is associated with testicular degeneration, inhibition of spermatogenesis, and Leydig-cell atrophy.

Q. Describe in brief how metal-binding proteins regulate the intracellular bioavailability of metals in the body.

The toxicity of many metals such as cadmium, lead, and mercury depends on their transport and intracellular bioavailability. This availability is regulated to a degree by high-affinity binding to certain cytosolic proteins.

Such ligands usually possess numerous SH-binding sites that can outcompete other intracellular proteins and thus mediate intracellular metal bioavailability and toxicity. These intracellular "sinks" are capable of partially sequestering toxic metals away from sensitive organelles or proteins until their binding capacity is exceeded by the dose of the metal. Metallothionein (MT) is a low molecular weight metal-binding protein (approximately 7000 Da) that is particularly important in regulating the intracellular bioavailability of cadmium, copper, mercury, silver, and zinc. For example, in vivo exposure to cadmium results in the transport of cadmium in the blood by various high molecular weight proteins and uptake by the liver, followed by hepatic induction of MT. Subsequently cadmium can be found in the circulatory system bound to MT as the cadmium—metallothionein complex (CdMT).

Q. How one is exposed to metals?

The exposure to metals is given in Table 6.1.

Table 6.1 Exposure to metals by inhalation

Exposures : Metals
***Exposure* primarily by Inhalation:**

Particulates
- Processes: grinding, cutting, sanding, mixing
- Examples: copper, nickel, zinc

Fumes
- Processes: welding, smelting
- Examples: lead, manganese, hexavalent chromium zinc

Mists (soluble metal compounds)
- Processes: spraying anticorrosives, metal plating
- Examples: hexavalent chromium, nickel chloride

6.2.1 LEAD

Toxic effects of lead are also discussed in Chapter 15, Veterinary Toxicology.

Q. What is the main source of lead poisoning?

Poisoning is more common from chronic occupational exposure among lead smelters, battery manufacturers, painters, decorators, etc. Chronic exposure may also occur at home from paint, pottery, and contaminated drinking water by lead pipes used for city water supply.

Q. What are the common toxic compounds of lead?

The common toxic compounds are lead acetate, lead carbonate, lead chromates, lead oleate, lead oxide, lead sulfide, lead tetroxide, and tetraethyl lead.

Q. What is the fatal dose lead?

Fatal dose depends on toxic compound (20 g of lead acetate). The fatal period is 1−2 days.

Q. What is the health problems associated with acute lead toxicity?

Acute poisoning usually occurs with high dosage of lead acetate, starts with burning and dryness in the throat, salivation and intense thirst, vomiting, colicky pain, and tender abdomen. Constipation is a common feature. Urine is scanty. Finally, there may be peripheral circulatory collapse, headache, insomnia, paresthesia, depression, convulsions, exhaustion, and coma leading to death.

Q. What are the health problems associated with subacute lead poisoning?

Repeated small doses of lead acetate can lead to blue line on the gums (Fig. 6.1) as well as gastrointestinal (GI) symptoms. Urine is scanty and in deep red color. In the later stages, nervous symptoms become prominent with

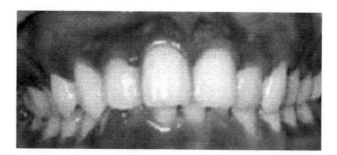

FIGURE 6.1

Gingival lead line on gums.

Reproduced with permission from Springer Nature (http://www.atarasdentalclinic.com/wp-content/uploads/2014/05/s19.jpg).

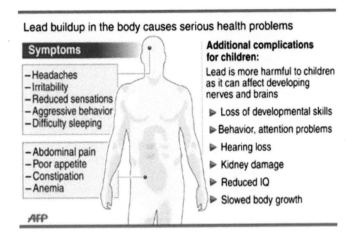

Lead buildup in the body causes serious health problems

Symptoms

- Headaches
- Irritability
- Reduced sensations
- Aggressive behavior
- Difficulty sleeping

- Abdominal pain
- Poor appetite
- Constipation
- Anemia

AFP

Additional complications for children:

Lead is more harmful to children as it can affect developing nerves and brains

▷ Loss of developmental skills

▷ Behavior, attention problems

▷ Hearing loss

▷ Kidney damage

▷ Reduced IQ

▷ Slowed body growth

FIGURE 6.2

Symptoms of lead poisoning.

MedlinePlus/Mayo Clinic. http://metalpedia.asianmetal.com/img/pb/heal1.jpg.

numbness, cramps, and flaccid paralysis of lower limbs. Death is rare but may be followed by convulsions and coma.

Q. What are the health problems associated with chronic lead poisoning (plumbism, saturnism)?

Symptoms of chronic lead poisoning are summarized in Fig. 6.2. In general, chronic poisoning with lead can destroy nerve cells, myelin sheaths in central nervous system (CNS) and also produce cerebral edema. It also exerts toxic effects on kidneys (nephritis) and reproductive system (infertility). Other symptoms include:

Facial pallor: Pallor seen especially around the mouth, also known as circumoral pallor, is due to the vasospasm of the capillaries and arterioles, around the mouth.

Lead colic and constipation: The victim will complain of severe colicky pain abdomen relieved by pressure and bowel irregularities. Abdominal muscles become tense and retracted.

Lead palsy: There is a typical paralysis affecting the extensor muscles of the fingers and wrist causing "wrist drop" and "claw-shaped hand." Similarly, paralysis may extend to the extensor muscles of the foot leading to foot drop.

Lead encephalopathy: Mostly seen in infants presenting with severe ataxia, vomiting, lethargy, stupor, convulsion and coma; cerebral psychic effect may be present.

Cardiorenal manifestations: Elevated blood pressure and arteriosclerotic changes are observed. Urine contains albumin and abnormal quantity of lead, co-protoporphyrin III and δ-aminolevulinic acid. Interstitial nephritis may occur.

Sterility/infertility may be observed.

General manifestations such as weakness, anorexia, metallic taste in the mouth, dyspepsia, and foul breath.

Q. What is Burtonian line?

The Burton line or Burtonian line is a clinical sign found in patients with chronic lead poisoning. It is a stippled blue line seen at the junction of the gums usually nearer to tooth caries, especially in the upper jaw. This is due to the deposition of lead sulfide formed by the action of the combination of lead with hydrogen sulfide which had evolved from the decomposed food debris in the caries tooth.

Q. Define the effect of lead on blood.

Lead causes hypochromic, microcytic anemia with reticulocytosis, and punctate basophilia. Lead can combine with sulfhydryl enzymes and can decrease the synthesis of heme leading to anemia and can bring about hemolysis as well as release immature red blood cells (RBCs) into circulation (reticulocytosis and basophilic stippling (BS) of RBCs) (Fig. 6.3). Platelet count decreases. Anemia is probably due to decreased survival time of RBCs and inhibition of heme synthesis by interference with the incorporation of iron into protoporphyrin.

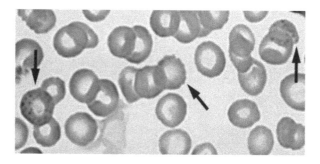

FIGURE 6.3

BS (arrows) of RBCs in a 53-year-old who had elevated blood lead levels due to drinking repeatedly from glasses decorated with lead paint.

https://upload.wikimedia.org/wikipedia/commons/3/3b/Lead_poisoning_-_blood_film.jpg.

Q. What is the effect of lead on bone?

Accumulation of lead in bone is very common. The detection of opaque lines in metaphysis of bones in an X-ray suggests lead poisoning (Fig. 6.4).

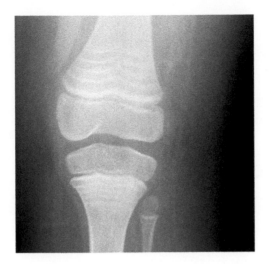

FIGURE 6.4

X-ray revealing opaque lead lines in metaphyses of bone.

http://images.radiopaedia.org/images/14071470/2074a1b10ccd27c37914e434156100_gallery.jpg.

6.2.2 MERCURY

Q. Define important properties of mercury (quick silver, liquid metal, para, padarasa).

Mercury is a liquid metal and is a metallic inorganic irritant poison. It is available in inorganic, organic, and metallic forms. Metallic mercury is a heavy, silvery liquid and is not poisonous. But it volatilizes at room temperature and inhalation of vapors is toxic.

Q. What are the potential sources of mercury poisoning?

Potential source of elemental mercury is at home, which includes mercury switches, mercury-containing devices such as thermometers, thermostats, and barometers. Other sources include laboratories, dental amalgam filling, cosmetics, calomel teething powder, and industrial sources. Absorption is possible through all routes. Pure metallic form is nontoxic. However, the mercurial compounds can act by inactivating sulfhydryl enzymes, which in turn interfere with cellular metabolism. A classic example of environmental contamination due to mercury and its health implications is the outbreak of Minamata disease, an outbreak of children born with Bay disaster in Japan in 1950s, that witnessed a devastating epidemic of mercury poisoning.

Q. What is Minamata disease?

Minamata disease was identified in Japan. This disease is caused due to the consumption of fish contaminated with methylmercury. Observing cats are affected, which led to the identification of fish as the common source of food.

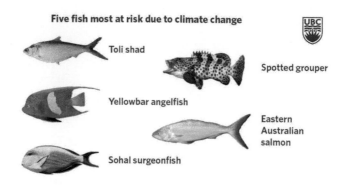

Five fish most at risk due to climate change

Toli shad

Spotted grouper

Yellowbar angelfish

Eastern
Australian
salmon

Sohal surgeonfish

FIGURE 6.5

Mercury poisoning (fish containing mercury is poisonous for cats).

Reproduced from the University of British Columbia (http://oceans.ubc.ca/files/2017/09/Climate-change-fish-risk.jpg).

Later, analysis of fish led to the detection of organic Hg as the root of the problem (Fig. 6.5).

Q. What were the symptoms of methylmercury poisoning outbreak?

Symptoms of methylmercury poisoning outbreak include primitive oral and grasping reflexes, poor coordination, character disorders (unfriendly, nervous, shy, and restless), seizures and epilepsy, deformed limbs, and slow growth.

Q. What was the effect on children born during an outbreak of Minamata disease?

Children were born with severe mental retardation (approximately 6% of children born were affected).

Q. What was the outcome of studies done in 1974 on methylmercury poisoning?

The studies indicated that women who gave birth to congenitally poisoned children had exhibited none of the early symptoms of methylmercury poisoning. This was because the methylmercury easily crosses the placenta and concentrates in the developing fetus. Concentrations in fetal brains were up to four times those in the mother, and fetal blood levels were 28% greater than the mothers.

Q. Draw a schematic diagram of environmental cycling of mercury.

The less toxic inorganic mercury gets converted through biomethylation to more toxic form of mercury. The schematic representation of mercury's environmental cycling, biomethylation, and food chain transfer is under is shown in Fig. 6.6.

Q. Where does mercury in fish come from?

Anthropogenic sources, such as coal burning and mining of iron, can contaminate water sources with methylmercury. Methylmercury is absorbed in

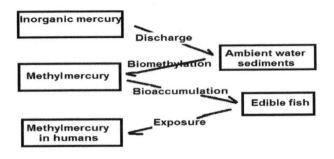

FIGURE 6.6

Environmental cycling and conversion of inorganic mercury to methyl-mercury.

the bodies of fish through the process of biomagnification; mercury levels in each successive predatory stage increase (Fig. 6.7).

Q. What are the major target organs of three forms of mercury?

1. Elemental mercury: the vapors target the respiratory system.
2. Inorganic mercury: mainly affects kidneys and GI tract.
3. Organic mercury: mainly affects the CNS.

Q. Describe in brief toxic potential of different forms of mercury.

Both inorganic and organic forms of mercury are associated with genotoxicity, teratogenicity, and embryotoxicity. Major organs affected along with their manifestation in mercury poisoning are summarized in Table 6.2.

6.2.3 ARSENIC

Q. Which form of arsenic is nonpoisonous?

Arsenic is a heavy metallic inorganic irritant poison. Metallic arsenic is not poisonous as it is insoluble in water and cannot be absorbed from the GI tract.

Q. How arsenic gets into the body?

Arsenic may be inhaled in particulate form, ingested, or absorbed through skin and mucous membranes. The minimum lethal dose is 100–200 mg of arsenic trioxide. Workers in the metallurgy industry or arsenic-containing dust emitted from smelters are the major sources of arsenic poisoning. The action of acid on metal ore contaminated with arsenic causes release of arsine gas.

Q. What is the mode of action of arsenic?

Arsenic compounds act by inactivating the sulfhydryl enzymes, which in turn interfere with the cellular metabolism, in the liver, lungs, intestinal wall, and spleen. Arsenic can replace phosphorus in the bones where it may remain for years. It also gets deposited in the hairs.

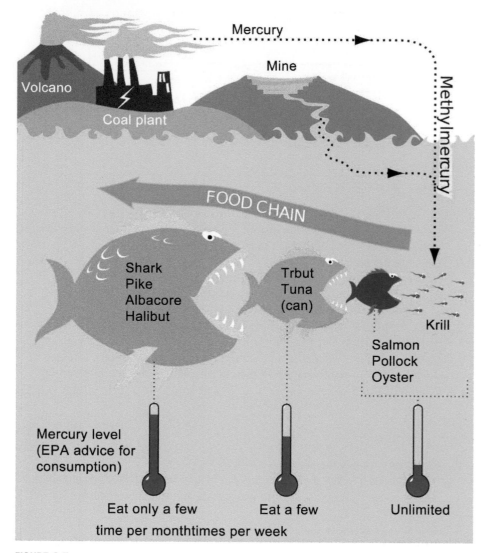

FIGURE 6.7

Through the process of biomagnifications, mercury levels in each successive predatory stage increase in fish.

https://upload.wikimedia.org/wikipedia/commons/thumb/0/07/MercuryFoodChain.svg/1200px-MercuryFoodChain.svg.png.

Q. Describe the symptoms of acute exposure to arsenic.

Acute exposure to a toxic dose initially produces a dry burning sensation in the mouth and throat and a constricted feeling in the throat. This is followed by severe abdominal pain, cramping, diarrhea, and

Table 6.2 Major organs affected along with their manifestation in mercury poisoning

Organ or system affected	Manifestations
Brain	Memory loss, attention deficit, ataxia, impairment of hearing & vision, sensory disturbances, fatigue, autism in children
Motor system	Disruption of motor function, decreased muscular strength, late walking in children
Kidney	Increased plasma creatinine level
Heart	Alteration of normal cardiovascular homeostasis
Immune	system Decreased immunity, multiple sclerosis, autoimmune thyroiditis
Reproductive system	Decreased fertility rate, abnormal offspring

vomiting. The diarrhea begins with "rice water" stools progressing to a bloody discharge. Stools and breath may have a garlicky odor. Vertigo develops, followed by delirium, coma, and often convulsions. Circulatory collapse with hepatic and renal failure ensues. In exposure to the gaseous form, inhalation of toxic amounts of arsine gas results in headache, malaise, weakness, dizziness, and dyspnea accompanied by GI distress.

Usually, hemolysis occurs 4–6 hours after the onset of symptoms and dark red urine is noticed. Jaundice develops 24–48 hours later. The patient may have fever, tachycardia, and tachypnea. Acute oliguric renal failure occurs because concentration of arsenic in the proximal tubules and binding to proteins of tubular epithelium damages the tubules.

Q. Describe the symptoms of subacute and chronic exposure to arsenic.

Environmental exposure to well water containing inorganic arsenic can result in skin hyperpigmentation or an eczematous dermatitis. Peripheral vascular involvement may occur, with acrocyanosis and the appearance of a Raynaud-like picture. In addition, a sensorimotor distal neuropathy may occur (Fig. 6.8) that presents like Guillain–Barré syndrome, and sideroblastic anemia—a state of ineffective erythropoiesis characterized by the presence of erythroid precursors containing mitochondria with stainable iron granules. Although a similar hematopoietic picture is seen in lead toxicity, the mechanism producing the anemia is not believed to be the same. Leukopenia is a common finding.

Q. What is raindrop pigmentation in arsenic poisoning?

Raindrop pigmentation is known to produce milk and roses complexion followed by patchy brown pigmentation of the skin (especially face), which resembles the raindrops (Fig. 6.9). It might also show hyperkeratosis of the skin of the palm and soles (Fig. 6.10), which is prone to change into

The most common neurologic effect of chronic arsenic intoxication is a sensory-predominant peripheral neuropathy in a "stocking-glove" pattern, as shown in the diagram to the right.

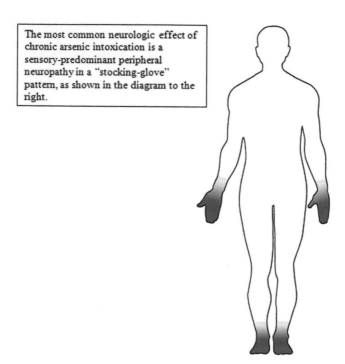

FIGURE 6.8

Major signs of arsenic poisoning in human beings.

Reproduced from Agency for Toxic Substances and Disease Registry (ATSDR).

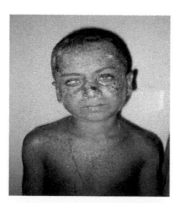

FIGURE 6.9

Arsenicosis—patchy brown pigmentation of the skin (especially face), which resembles the raindrops.

https://encrypted-tbn0.gstatic.com/images?q=tbn: ANd9GcTXZHiDyFQbiUQOHwkB2agAUil2iLNXzLYGzIwFcuGxBg_2mwDm.

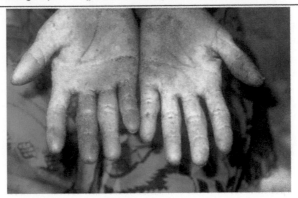

Arsenic keratoses (below) on the palms of a patient who ingested arsenic from a contaminated well over a prolonged period (photo courtesy Dr. Joseph Graziano).

FIGURE 6.10

Arsenicosis—hyperkeratosis of the skin of the palm.

Reproduced from Agency for Toxic Substances and Disease Registry (ATSDR) (https://www.atsdr.cdc.gov/ csem/arsenic/images/arsenic_pic7.jpg).

basal cell carcinoma at a later stage. The scalp may also show alopecia (baldness).

Q. What are Meese's lines?

Meese's lines are lines of discoloration across the nails of the fingers and toes (whitish lines 1—2 mm breadth) across the nail of the finger and toes representing the deposition of the poison as a result of high sulfhydryl content of the keratin. The lines are seen after chronic arsenic poisoning.

6.2.4 CADMIUM

Q. What is the source of toxicity of cadmium?

Cadmium occurs in nature primarily in association with lead and zinc ores and is released near mines and smelters processing these ores.

Q. How one is exposed to cadmium?

1. Industrially cadmium is used as a pigment in paints and plastics, in electroplating, and in making alloys and alkali storage batteries (e.g., nickel—cadmium batteries).

2. Environmental exposure to cadmium is mainly from contamination of groundwater from smelting and industrial uses as well as the use of sewage sludge as a food-crop fertilizer.

3. Grains, cereal products, and leafy vegetables usually constitute the main source of cadmium in food.

Q. Which is a metal-binding protein for cadmium?

Cadmium readily binds to and induces the production of MT; binding to MT does not have a major effect on the uptake of cadmium, but is, in part, responsible for the retention of cadmium within the cells. MT does this by decreasing the cadmium elimination, especially in bile.

Q. What is itai-itai disease?

Itai-itai disease was the name given to the mass cadmium poisoning of Toyama Prefecture, Japan, starting around 1912. The term "itai-itai disease" was coined by locals for the *severe* pains felt in the spine and joints of victims (Fig. 6.11). The disease resulted from the consumption of cadmium-contaminated rice.

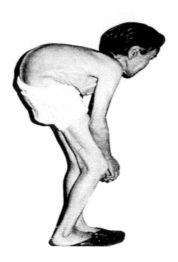

FIGURE 6.11

Symptoms of "itai-itai disease," *severe* pains felt in the spine and joints of victims.

http://parts.igem.org/wiki/images/2/2c/2015SCUT-0-1.jpg.

Q. What are the common symptoms of cadmium toxicity?

Acute effects of exposure to cadmium result primarily from local irritation. After ingestion, the main effects are nausea, vomiting, and abdominal pain. Inhalation exposure may result in pulmonary edema and chemical pneumonitis.

Chronic effects are of particular concern because cadmium is very slowly excreted from the body. Thus low levels of exposure can result in considerable accumulation of cadmium. The main organ of damage following long-term exposure is the kidney, with the proximal tubules being the primary site of action.

Q. What is the mechanism of toxicity of cadmium?

Cadmium is present in the circulatory system bound primarily to the metal-binding protein, metallothionein (CdMT), produced in the liver. Following glomerular filtration in the kidney, CdMT is reabsorbed efficiently by the proximal tubule cells, where it accumulates within the lysosomes.

Subsequent degradation of the CdMT complex releases Cd^{+2}, which inhibits lysosomal function, resulting in cell injury. The mechanism of chromium (Cr^{+6}) carcinogenicity in the lung is believed to be its reduction to Cr^{+3} and generation of reactive intermediates, leading to bronchogenic carcinoma.

Q. What are the long-term effects of cadmium?

Low levels of exposure can result in considerable accumulation of cadmium. The main organ of damage following long-term exposure is the kidney, with the proximal tubules being the primary site of action. In humans, occupational exposure to cadmium has been associated with renal dysfunction and osteomalacia with osteoporosis. One of the earliest effects of chronic cadmium exposure is renal tubular damage with proteinuria. Other chronic effects can include liver damage, emphysema (through inhalation), osteomalacia, neurological impairment, testicular, pancreatic and adrenal damage, and anemia.

6.2.5 ALUMINUM

Q. Which form of aluminum is toxic?

Aluminum (Al) is the third most abundant element that occurs naturally in the earth's crust. Poisoning in human beings and animals by Al is rare. Among all Al compounds, Al phosphide is of major concern to animals, because at a low stomach pH, phosphide converts to toxic phosphine (PH_3) gas.

Q. Define in brief toxicity of aluminum.

Toxicity of Al depends on its chemical form, route of exposure, and animal species. The CNS and skeletal system appear to be the two major target organs for Al toxicity. It has been known for a while that Al is involved in neurodegenerative diseases like Alzheimer's, encephalopathy, and amyotrophic sclerosis. Problems associated with chronic exposure to Al are summarized in Table 6.3.

Table 6.3 Problems Asssociated with Aluminum toxicity

Alzheimer's disease	Hypoparathyroidism
Amyotropic lateral sclerosis	Kidney dysfunction
Anemia	Liver dysfunction
Hemolusis	Neuromuscular disorders
Leucocytosis	Osteomalacia
Porphyria	Parkinson's disease
Colitis	Ulcers
Dental cavities	

6.3 MICRONUTRIENTS

6.3.1 COPPER

Toxic effects of copper are also discussed in Chapter 15, Veterinary Toxicology.

Q. Which salts of copper are poisonous?

Copper, an inorganic metallic irritant, is not poisonous in metallic state, but some of its salts are poisonous, e.g., copper sulfate (blue vitriol) and copper subacetate (verdigris). Copper toxicity, also called copperiedus, refers to the consequences of an excess of overuse of copper sulfate as an algicide has been speculated to have caused a copper poisoning epidemic on Great Palm Island in 1979.

Q. Define in brief symptoms of acute copper poisoning.

Acute symptoms of copper poisoning by ingestion include vomiting, hematemesis (vomiting of blood), hypotension (low blood pressure), melena (black "tarry" feces), coma, jaundice (yellowish pigmentation of the skin), and GI distress. Individuals with glucose-6-phosphate deficiency may be at an increased risk of hematologic effects of copper. Hemolytic anemia resulting from the treatment of burns with copper compounds is infrequent.

Q. Define in brief long-term effects of copper poisoning.

Chronic (long-term) effects of copper exposure can damage the liver and kidneys. Mammals have efficient mechanisms to regulate copper stores such that they are generally protected from excess dietary copper levels. Gums appear unhealthy with bluish lining. There is mucosal atrophy. Liver and kidneys show varying degrees of degeneration (Fig. 6.12). Gunmetal kidneys are characteristics in copper poisoning, because hemoglobin released during hemolysis clogs the renal tubules and leads to darkening and necrosis of kidneys. Hence, gunmetal-like kidneys are seen.

Vomitus is blue or green in color. Stool is brownish or bloody. Oliguria, hematuria, and uremia may develop in some. There may also be low urinary output with casts and albumin in urine. Jaundice occurs in severe cases due to centrilobular necrosis and biliary stasis. Later muscular spasms cramps, coma, and circulatory collapse precede death.

6.3.2 IRON

Q. What are the sources of iron toxicity?

Iron is an inorganic metallic irritant. Most exposures involve children less than 6 years of age who have ingested pediatric multivitamin preparations. Concentrated iron supplement overdoses more often result in serious poisoning.

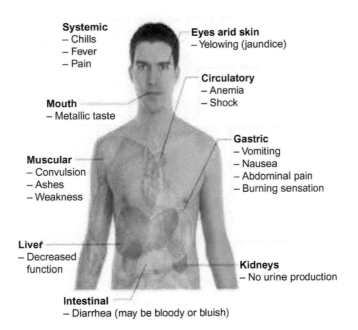

Systemic
– Chills
– Fever
– Pain

Eyes arid skin
– Yelowing (jaundice)

Circulatory
– Anemia
– Shock

Mouth
– Metallic taste

Gastric
– Vomiting
– Nausea
– Abdominal pain
– Burning sensation

Muscular
– Convulsion
– Ashes
– Weakness

Liver
– Decreased
  function

Kidneys
– No urine production

Intestinal
– Diarrhea (may be bloody or bluish)

FIGURE 6.12

Main symptoms of copper poisoning.Copper poisoning is not uncommon among people working with tanning solutions in the leather industry. However, the more common cause of copper toxicity might be with the use of unlined, poor quality copper pots and pans used as cookware. Copper is a good conductor of heat and has been used for many years for making pots and pans.

https://encrypted-tbn3.gstatic.com/images?q=tbn:
ANd9GcRX3ONWFOkFrwYvlA7NJUNfNGsRutlThz1GzA4x1iN9BirMP7.

Q. What are the complications of iron overload in human beings?
  Iron overload and complications of iron toxicity are summarized in Table 6.4.

Q. Numerate various steps involved in the catabolism of heme.
  Various steps involved in the catabolism of heme include:
  • Generation of bilirubin
  • Transport to liver
  • Conjugation in liver
  • Excretion of bilirubin in intestine
  • Fate of conjugated bilirubin in intestine
  • Enterohepatic circulation
  • Final excretion.

Q. Name the specific antidote of iron toxicity.
  Deferoxamine (desferrioxamine) is the specific antidote. A solution of 2 g in 1 L of water can be used for gastric lavage; followed by 2 g in 10 mL

Table 6.4 Iron toxicity and overload

- Iron is essential for cellular metabolism, but too much can be toxic
- Upper limit has been set at 45mg/day from all sources
- Iron poisoning can be life threatening. It can damage the intestine lining and cause abnormalities in body pH, shock and liver failure
- Iron overload can happen over time and accumulates in tissues such as the heart and the liver
- The most common form of iron overload is hemochromatosis.

sterile water should be left in stomach. 2 g of this is then given IM or by a slow IV infusion at the rate of 15 mg/kg body weight per hour to a maximum of 80 mg/kg in 24 hours.

6.3.3 COBALT DEFICIENCY

See Chapter 15, Veterinary Toxicology.

6.3.4 CHROMIUM

Q. What is the source of chromium poisoning?
1. Chromium occurs in ores; environmental levels are increased by mining, smelting, and industrial uses.
2. Chromium is used in making stainless steel, various alloys, and pigments. The levels of this metal are generally very low in air, water, and food, and the major source of human exposure is occupational.

Q. In which form chromium is available?

Chromium occurs in a number of oxidation states from Cr^{+2} to Cr^{+6}, but only the trivalent (Cr^{+3}) and hexavalent (Cr^{+6}) forms are of biological significance.

Q. Describe in brief toxicity of chromium.

The trivalent compound is the most common form found in nature. The hexavalent form is of greater industrial importance. In addition, hexavalent chromium, which is not water soluble, is more readily absorbed across cell membranes than is trivalent chromium. In vivo the hexavalent form is reduced to the trivalent form, which can complex with intracellular macromolecules, resulting in toxicity. Chromium is a known human carcinogen and induces lung cancers among exposed workers.

6.3.5 NICKEL

Q. Describe some properties of nickel.

Nickel is used in various metal alloys, including stainless steels and in electroplating. Major properties of nickel alloys include strength, corrosion resistance, and good thermal and electrical conductivity.

Q. Describe in brief toxicity of nickel.

Nickel-induced contact dermatitis is the most common adverse health effect from nickel exposure and is found in 10%—20% of the general population (Fig. 6.13). Nickel sensitization usually arises from prolonged contact with nickel or exposure to a large dose of nickel. The resulting dermatitis is an inflammatory reaction mediated by type IV delayed hypersensitivity. Metallic nickel combines with carbon monoxide to form nickel carbonyl ($Ni[CO]_4$), which decomposes to nickel and carbon monoxide on heating to 200°C (the Mond process). This reaction provides a convenient and efficient method for nickel refining. However, nickel carbonyl is extremely toxic, and many cases of acute toxicity have been reported. Intoxication begins with headache, nausea, vomiting, and epigastric or chest pain, followed by cough, hyperpnea, cyanosis, GI symptoms, and weakness. The symptoms may be accompanied by fever and leukocytosis. The more severe cases can progress to pneumonia, respiratory failure, and eventually to cerebral edema and death. Nickel compounds are responsible for lung and nasal cancers.

Q. What is the line of treatment for nickel toxicity?

Sodium diethylcarbodithioate is the preferred drug. Disulfiram, another nickel-chelating agent, has been used in nickel dermatitis and in nickel carbonyl poisoning. Other chelating agents, such as D-penicillamine and 2,3-dimercapto-1-propanesulfonic acid (DMPS), provide some degree of protection from clinical effects.

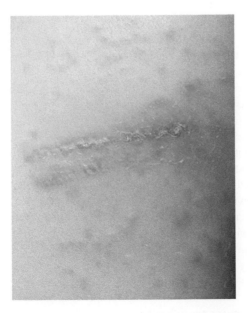

FIGURE 6.13

Nickel allergy.

Reproduced from Wikipedia(https://upload.wikimedia.org/wikipedia/commons/thumb/a/a8/ Contact_dermatitis_around_wound.jpg/300px-Contact_dermatitis_around_wound.jpg).

6.3.6 MOLYBDENUM

Q. Define in brief properties of molybdenum.

Molybdenum (Mo) was first separated from lead and graphite in 1778. Molybdenum was derived from Greek molybdos meaning "lead-like." As an essential element, molybdenum acts as a cofactor for at least three enzymes in humans: sulfite oxidase, xanthine oxidase, and aldehyde oxidase. Molybdenum exists in five oxidation states but the predominant species are Mo^{4+} and Mo^{6+}. Molybdenum concentration in food varies considerably depending on the local environment. Molybdenum is added in trace amounts to fertilizers to stimulate plant growth. The human requirement for molybdenum is low and easily provided by a common US diet.

Q. Describe toxicity of molybdenum.

Molybdenum is of low toxicity. Chronic exposure to excess molybdenum in humans is characterized by high uric acid levels in serum and urine. A gout-like syndrome has been observed in inhabitants exposed to high levels of environmental molybdenum or among workers exposed to molybdenum in a copper—molybdenum plant. When inhaled, both metallic molybdenum and sparingly soluble molybdenum trioxide have been reported to cause pneumoconiosis.

6.3.7 ZINC DEFICIENCY

Q. What is zinc deficiency?

Zinc deficiency or hypozincemia is caused by a lack of zinc in the diet. It can also be caused by other diseases such as liver disease, cystic fibrosis, and even congenital abnormalities.

According to WHO, about 31% of the entire population is at risk of zinc deficiency. In fact, zinc deficiency is one of the leading risk factors for disease in developing countries.

Q. Describe in brief importance of zinc.

Zinc is widely distributed in the body—in bones, teeth, hair, skin, liver, muscle, white blood cells, and testes. It is a component of more than 100 enzymes, including those involved in the formation of RNA (ribonucleic acid) and DNA (deoxyribonucleic acid). The level of zinc in the body depends on the amount of zinc consumed in the diet. Zinc is necessary for healthy skin, healing of wounds, and growth.

Q. What are the main causes of zinc deficiency?

The primary causes of zinc deficiency or hypozincemia are the following:
- Inadequate zinc in the diet.
- Diseases or conditions that disrupt proper digestion. Diarrhea and malabsorption is one of them.
- Physiological states such as during pregnancy, or during the early stage of growth of infants and young children, which require increased intake of zinc.

- Disease in kidney or liver.
- After undergoing bariatric surgery (removal of parts of the stomach or intestines to induce weight loss).
- Heavy metal exposure to zinc, e.g., people living near zinc smelters.
- Tartrazine (artificial orange-yellow dye used commonly as food coloring) can disrupt the body's ability to absorb zinc.
- Vitamin A and D deficiency. Studies have shown that the body's ability to maintain zinc levels is dependent on A and D vitamins.

Q. What are the symptoms of zinc deficiency?
- Eczema, skin rashes, and many other skin conditions.
- Diarrhea and pneumonia.
- Acne.
- Vision loss and poor sense of smell and taste—zinc is vital for the development of our five senses.
- Anorexia (prolonged loss of appetite)—zinc is an appetite stimulator.
- Low testosterone production in men.
- Dysmenorrhea.

Q. What are the foods rich in zinc?

Animal foods are actually richer in zinc than plant foods. A few of food items include oysters, wheat germ, calf liver, roast beef, pumpkin seeds, dried watermelon seeds, cocoa or dark chocolate, lamb (mutton), crab, cabbage, sea vegetables, baked beans, soy foods, peanuts, sesame or pumpkin seeds, and peas.

Q. What are the problems associated with zinc deficiency?

The problems associated with zinc deficiency include:
- loss of appetite and hair.
- sluggishness,
- loss of sense of taste.
- white spot on the nails, skin acrodermatitis enteropathica, erosive dermatitis. and erythema are the well-recognized entities caused by an inherited defect in zinc absorption leading to hypozincemia. Common symptoms of zinc deficiency and toxicity due to zinc are summarized in Figs. 6.14 and 6.15.

6.4 QUESTION AND ANSWER EXERCISES

6.4.1 SHORT QUESTIONS AND ANSWERS

Exercise 1

Q.1 Which form of arsenic is more toxic?

Arsenites (As^{3+} or trivalent) are 5—10 times more toxic than arsenates (As^{5+} or pentavalent) due to higher solubility.

Q.2 Malicious poisoning is very common with which arsenic compound?

Arsenic trioxide.

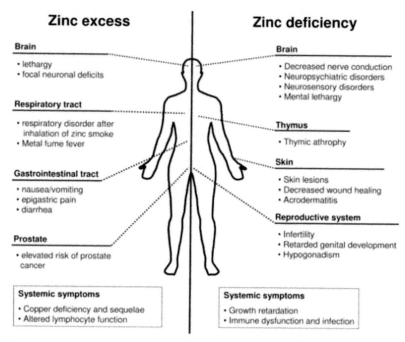

FIGURE 6.14

Symptoms associated with zinc deficiency and toxicity in human beings deficiency or toxicity in human beings.

Reproduced from U.S. National Library of Medicine.

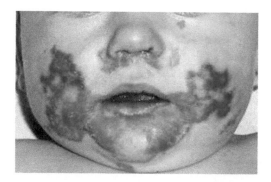

FIGURE 6.15

Congenital zinc deficiency.

http://www.pyroenergen.com/articles13/images/congenital-zinc-deficiency.jpg.

Q.3 Why arsenic tends to accumulate in keratin-rich tissues such as hair and nails?

Arsenic has high affinity for sulfhydryl groups (−SH). Since hair and nails contain −SH-rich keratin, arsenic accumulates in them.

Q.4 Is arsenic cumulative in animals?

No. Arsenic is rapidly detoxified and is completely eliminated in few days.

Q.5 Why arsenic can cause abortions but not nervous symptoms?

Arsenic can cross placental barrier (PB). Hence can cause abortions but in most of the species it cannot cross BBB, hence, is unable to cause nervous symptoms.

Q.6 In which species of animals, organic arsenicals cause nervous symptoms?

Swine. Nervous symptoms include ataxia and incoordination.

Q.7 What are the prominent postmortem findings in arsenic poisoning?

Severe gastroenteritis.

Q.8 How is arsenic differentiated from lead poisoning?

In arsenic poisoning, severe gastroenteritis and absence of nervous symptoms is observed, whereas in lead poisoning, the symptoms are just the reverse.

Q.9 How zinc administration decreases development of copper toxicity?

Zinc induces the synthesis of mucosal metallothioneins in GI tract, which bind to copper and prevent Cu absorption. Hence, zinc supplementation decreases the development of copper toxicity.

Q.10 List some common metals used in industrial processes which can give rise to toxicity. Indicate what element forms are involved and what kind of toxicity is produced.

1. Lead (II) ions
   a. These ions possibly reduce fertility—possible effects on baby in the womb—anemia; brain and kidney damage—death.
2. Mercury
   a. Common symptoms of mercury poisoning include peripheral neuropathy, presenting as paresthesia or itching, burning, pain, or even a sensation that resembles small insects crawling on or under the skin (formication); skin discoloration (pink cheeks, fingertips, and toes); swelling; and desquamation (shedding or peeling of skin). Affected children may show red cheeks, nose, and lips, loss of hair, teeth, and nails, transient rashes, hypotonia (muscle weakness), and increased sensitivity to light. Other symptoms may include kidney dysfunction (e.g., Fanconi syndrome) or neuropsychiatric symptoms such as emotional lability, memory impairment, or insomnia.

Exercise 2

Q.1 Which form of arsenic is more toxic? Why?

Arsenites (As^{3+} or trivalent, arsenic trioxide) are 5−10 times more toxic than arsenates (As^{5+} or pentavalent) due to their higher solubility.

Q.2 Why arsenic tends to accumulate in keratin-rich tissues such as hair and nails?

Arsenic has high affinity for sulfhydryl groups (−SH). Since hair and nails contain −SH-rich keratin, arsenic accumulates in them.

Q.3 What are the prominent postmortem findings in arsenic poisoning?

Severe gastroenteritis.

Q.4 Why arsenic can cause abortions but not nervous symptoms?

Arsenic can cross PB, hence can cause abortions. It cannot cross BBB, hence is unable to cause nervous symptoms.

Q.5 How zinc deficiency is caused?

Much of the zinc consumed in the diet is not absorbed and leads to zinc deficiency. A diet high in fiber and phytate (present in whole-grain bread, bran, beans, soybeans, other legumes, and nuts), various disorders, alcoholism, and use of diuretics reduce zinc absorption.

Q.6 How do you treat zinc deficiency?

Zinc deficiency can be treated by taking dietary zinc supplements, or by eating foods that are rich and fortified with zinc.

Q.7 What is the cure for zinc deficiency?

Zinc deficiency can be treated by taking dietary zinc supplements, or by eating foods that are rich and fortified with zinc.

Q.8 What is half-life of cadmium?

Half-life of cadmium is about 30 years.

Q.9 What is arsenical neuritis?

The victim presents with polyneuritis, optic neuritis, anesthesias, paresthesias, atrophy of extensors resulting in wrist drop, etc.

Q.10 Which form of arsenic is poisonous?

Arsenious oxide or arsenic trioxide (sankhyal or somalker) is poisonous. They are found in shell fish, cod fish, and haddock. Sources of poisoning include soil, well water, shellfish, and arsenic compounds. Inorganic arsenicals, a by-product of smelting of ore containing copper, lead, and zinc, are more toxic than the organic.

6.4.2 MULTIPLE CHOICE QUESTIONS (CHOOSE THE BEST STATEMENT, IT CAN BE ONE, TWO OR ALL OR NONE)

Exercise 3

Q.1 Exposure to fumes of which of the following metals is most likely to cause acute chemical pneumonitis and pulmonary edema?
  a. Lead
  b. Zinc
  c. Cadmium
  d. Copper
  e. Magnesium

Q.2 Which of the following is NOT true about arsine?
    a. It is a gas at room temperature.
    b. It produces acute intravascular hemolysis.
    c. It has a garlic-like odor.
    d. Acute renal failure is a common man infestation of arsine poisoning.
    e. Significant hepatotoxicity often occurs as part of arsine poisoning.

Q.3 Which of the following is NOT commonly associated with mercury vapor poisoning?
    a. Acute, corrosive bronchitis
    b. Interstitial pneumonitis
    c. Tremor
    d. Increased excitability
    e. Vomiting and bloody diarrhea

Q.4 Which form of mercury was the predominant cause of Minamata Bay disease?
    a. Metallic mercury
    b. Mercuric salts
    c. Mercurous salts
    d. Organic mercury compounds
    e. Mercury was not the causative agent

Q.5 Which is the only arsenical that can cause blindness?
    a. Arsenic trioxide
    b. Arsenic pentoxide
    c. Arsine
    d. Arsanilic acid

Q.6 Copper has inverse interrelationship with the following element(s):
    a. Iron
    b. Molybdenum
    c. Sulfur
    d. Both b and c

Q.7 In lead poisoning, BS are commonly seen in this species:
    a. Cattle
    b. Sheep
    c. Dog
    d. Horse

Q.8 The following chelating agent(s) that is/are used for treating mercury poisoning:
    a. Dimercaprol (BAL)
    b. D-penicillamine
    c. DMSA (dimercaptosuccinic acid) (succimer)
    d. Na-thiosulfate.
    e. All the above

Q.9 Which of the following nutrient(s) can counteract toxicity of organic mercurial?
- **a.** Vitamin A
- **b.** Vitamin D
- **c.** Vitamin E
- **d.** Selenium

Q.10 Which of the following forms of Hg is more toxic?
- **a.** Elemental
- **b.** Monovalent
- **c.** Divalent
- **d.** Organic

Q.11 Mercury can cross the following barriers in the body:
- **a.** Blood—brain barrier (BBB)
- **b.** Placental barrier (PB)
- **c.** Both
- **d.** No barrier

Q.12 The following properties can be attributed to methylmercury (organic Hg):
- **a.** Mutagenic
- **b.** Carcinogenic
- **c.** Embryotoxic
- **d.** Teratogenic
- **e.** All of the above

Answers

1. c; 2. e; 3. e; 4. d; 5. d; 6. d (both b and c); 7. c (dog; BS are remnants of RNA seen in RBC which take up basophilic stain, but BS are not pathognomonic for lead); 8. e (all of the above. It should be noted that all these chelating agents are rich in −SH groups. As Hg has high affinity for −SH groups, it is easily removed by chelation); 9. c and d (mercury produces free radicals which are counteracted by vitamin E, which is a free radical scavenger. Selenium and vitamin E have interrelationship); 10. d (organic form of Hg is more toxic); 11. c (both; as Hg can cross BBB causing neurological symptoms and crossing PB leads to accumulation in fetus and abortions); 12. e (all of the above).

6.4.3 FILL IN THE BLANKS

Exercise 4

Q.1 The detection of opaque lines in metaphyses of bones in an X-ray suggests _____.

Q.2 In lead poisoning, the estimation of _____ enzyme in blood is of diagnostic value.

Q.3 The lead content in liver and kidney indicative of lead poisoning is more than _____.

Q.4 The specific antidote for lead toxicosis is _____.

Q.5 Meat from food animals recovered from lead poisoning is _____ for human consumption.

Q.6 The species of animals that are most susceptible to lead poisoning are _____, _____ and _____.

Q.7 The species of animal that is considered as indicator for lead in the environment is _____.

Q.8 The species of animal that is very resistant to lead poisoning is _____.

Q.9 The most common route of lead exposure is ----------------.

Q.10 Roaring in horses due to lead poisoning is caused due to _____ nerve paralysis.

Answers

1. LEAD; 2. ALA-D SYNTHASE; 3. >4 ppm; 4. CALCIUM DISODIUM EDTA; 5. FIT (however, bones should not be consumed as they store lead); 6. DOG, CATTLE, and HORSES (dogs live close to soil have the habit of frequent digging of soil; cattle and horses tend to lick walls and chew on paints); 7. DOG; 8. SWINE; 9. ORAL ROUTE; 10. RECURRENT LARYNGEAL.

Exercise 5

Q.1 Elemental mercury is toxic when exposed through _____ route.

Q.2 The common source of mercury poisoning in animals is through _____.

Q.3 Arsenic tends to accumulate in _____ and _____ (name the organ of the body).

Q.4 Minamata disease in Japan is caused due to the consumption of fish contaminated with _____.

Q.5 The species of animal which is more sensitive to Hg poisoning is _____.

Q.6 In body, lead tends to accumulate in tissues such as _____ and _____.

Q.7 The process of accumulation of Hg in marine animals to a very high concentration over a period of time is known as _____.

Q.8 In body, heavy metals such as mercury and cadmium tend to accumulate in _____ (name the organ of body).

Q.9 The mechanism of toxicity of mercury involves binding with _____, _____ groups of proteins and enzymes.

Q.10 The predominant symptoms of organic mercury poisoning are _____.

Answers

1. INHALATION (ingested mercury is not likely to cause toxicity, but is toxic through inhalation route. Guess, which of the following situations is more dangerous: a child biting on a thermometer and ingesting mercury or a thermometer falling on to the floor leading to evaporation of mercury?); 2. FOOD; 3. HAIR

and SKIN; 4. METHYLMERCURY (observing cats being affected led to the identification of fish as the common source of food. Later, analysis of fish led to the detection of organic Hg as the root of the problem); 5. CATTLE (cow and calves); 6. BONE AND TEETH; 7. BIOACCUMULATION or BIOMAGNIFICATION; 8. KIDNEY; 9. −SH, THIOL; 10. NEUROLOGICAL (ataxia, incoordination, convulsions, abnormal behavior, etc.).

Exercise 6

Q.1 The predominant symptom in inorganic mercury poisoning is

_____.

Q.2 The predominant symptom in elemental mercury poisoning is

_____.

Q.3 Elemental mercury (Hg) is toxic only through _____ route of exposure.

Q.4 The most frequently encountered heavy metal poisoning in veterinary cases is _____.

Q.5 The sample of choice for detection of inorganic mercury intoxication is

_____.

Q.6 The sample of choice for detection of organic mercury intoxication is

_____.

Q.7 Neurological and renal damage caused in mercury poisoning are

_____.

Q.8 The lead compound which is added to petrol and gasoline as anti-knocking is _____.

Q.9 The lead compound that was used for sweetening of wine is

_____.

Q.10 The carcass of animal affected with mercury poisoning is _____ for human consumption.

Q.11 Acute zinc deficiency causes _____ in children.

Q.12 The common source of mercury poisoning in animals is through

_____.

Answers

1. GASTROENTERITIS; 2. PULMONARY SYMPTOMS; 3. INHALATION ROUTE; 4. LEAD POISONING or PLUMBISM; 5. URINE (urinary concentration is a reliable indicator of inorganic Hg poisoning); 6. KIDNEY (organic Hg tends to accumulate in visceral organs including brain. A concentration of 10 mg/kg in kidney is indicative of Hg poisoning); 7. IRREVERSIBLE (even with treatment); 8. TETRAETHYL LEAD (TEL) (the tendency for fuels to auto-ignite and damage the engine is knows as knocking. Addition of TEL to petrol is banned in India since 1996); 9. LEAD ACETATE (the above process along with usage of lead pipes for water supply leads to the downfall of Roman empire due to lead toxicosis, which caused cognitive disorders and dementia); 10. UNFIT (as Hg

accumulates in body); 11. EROSIVE DERMATITIS; 12. FOOD (predatory animals at the end of food chain are more likely to accumulate Hg, which causes poisoning).

FURTHER READING

Garland, T., 2018. Arsenic. In: Gupta, R.C. (Ed.), Veterinary Toxicology: Basic and Clinical Principles, third ed. Academic Press/Elsevier, San Diego, USA, pp. 411−416.

Gupta, P.K., 1988. Veterinary Toxicology. Cosmo Publications, New Delhi, India (Chapter 7).

Gupta, R.C., Milatovic, D., Lall, R., Srivastava, A., 2018. Mercury. In: Gupta, R.C. (Ed.), Veterinary Toxicology: Basic and Clinical Principles, third ed. Academic Press/Elsevier, San Diego, USA, pp. 455−462.

Hooser, S.B., 2018. Cadmium. In: Gupta, R.C. (Ed.), Veterinary Toxicology: Basic and Clinical Principles, third ed. Academic Press/Elsevier, San Diego, USA, pp. 417–422.

Liu, J., Goyer, R.A., Waalkes, M.P., 2013. Toxic effects of metals. In: Klaassen, C.D. (Ed.), Casarett and Doull's Toxicology: The Basic Science of Poisons, eighth ed McGraw-Hill, New York, NY, pp. 931−980.

Pillay, V.V., 2008. Comprehensive Medical Toxicology, second ed. Paras Medical Publisher, Hyderabad, India.

Squibb, K.S., Kardish, R.M., Carmichael, N.G., Fowler, B.A., 2010. Metal toxicity. In: second reprint Gupta, P.K. (Ed.), Modern Toxicology: The Adverse Effects of Xenobiotics, vol. 2. PharmaMed Press, Hyderabad, India, pp. 61−130.

Thompson, L.J., 2017. Copper. In: Gupta, R.C. (Ed.), Veterinary Toxicology: Basic and Clinical Principles, third ed. Academic Press/Elsevier, Amsterdam (in press).

Toker, E.J., Boyd, W.A., Freedman, J.R., Waalkes, M.P., 2013. Toxic effects of metals. In: Klaassen, C.D. (Ed.), Casarett and Doull's Toxicology: The Basic Science of Poisons, eighth ed. McGraw-Hill, New York, NY, pp. 981−1030.

Nonmetals and micronutrients

CHAPTER OUTLINE

7.1 DEFINITIONS

Q. Define nonmetals.

There is no rigorous definition of a nonmetal. They show more variability in their properties than do metals. In brief one can say nonmetal is an element or a substance that is not a metal.

Q. Define the properties of nonmetals.

Chief characteristics of nonmetals are as follows:

- Unlike metals, which are nearly all solid and closely packed, if solid, they generally have a submetallic or dull appearance and are brittle, as opposed to metals, which are lustrous, ductile, or malleable.
- They usually have lower densities than metals.
- They are poor conductors of heat and electricity when compared to metals.

Illustrated Toxicology. DOI: http://dx.doi.org/10.1016/B978-0-12-813213-5.00007-9

- They have significantly lower melting points and boiling points than those of metals (with the exception of carbon).
- They usually exist as anions or oxyanions in aqueous solution.
- Generally nonmetals form ionic or interstitial compounds when mixed with metals.
- Unlike metals, which form alloys, they have acidic oxides, whereas the common oxides of the metals are basic.

Q. Classify nonmetals.

The distinction between nonmetals and metals is by no means clear. The result is that a few borderline elements lacking a preponderance of either nonmetallic or metallic properties are classified as metalloids, and some elements classified as nonmetals are instead sometimes classified as metalloids, or vice versa. For example, selenium (Se), a nonmetal, is sometimes classified instead as a metalloid.

Q. Describe in brief actions of nonmetal chemicals.

Nonmetal chemicals such as phosphorus, chlorine, bromine, iodine, formaldehyde, methyl aldehyde, methylene oxide act as irritant poisons and produce inflammation on the site of contact, especially in the gastrointestinal (GI) tract, respiratory tract, and the skin. When a poison has a systemic effect and death occurs, then it is classified as a cerebral poison or a spinal poison. (Irritant poisons should be differentiated from certain natural disease of GI tract such as cholera, acute gastritis, acute gastroenteritis, perforated gastric ulcer, peritonitis, and colic.) In general, after ingestion, irritant poisons will manifest action within 30–60 minutes.

Q. Describe in general gastric symptoms of nonmetal toxicity.

GI symptoms of *nonmetals* include burning pain in mouth, throat, esophagus, and stomach, which radiates all over the abdomen, and intense thirst, but dysphasic due to painful deglutition. So not taking water or food leads to dehydration and starvation with continuous painful vomiting. Initially vomitus shows normal contents, but later turns bilious or contains altered blood. The patient will show continuous severe diarrhea and tenesmus. Stools initially will be soft, loose, but later mixed with mucus and blood.

Collapse due to shock with rapid, feeble pulse, pale anxious face, cold clammy skin, sighing respiration, cramps in leg muscles, etc.; convulsions, loss of consciousness, extreme exhaustion, and death when not treated properly (if survives may develop stricture esophagus later, which can contribute to dysphagia leading to starvation).

Q. Describe in general respiratory symptoms due to nonmetal toxicity.

Respiratory symptoms include cough, feeling of constriction of chest, breathlessness, suffocation, pulmonary edema, and hemoptysis.

Q. Describe in general dermal symptoms due to nonmetal toxicity

Dermal symptoms are (as in the case of radioactive substances, insect and snake bites, marking nut, etc.) pain, irritation, itching, redness and, vesication, and blisters.

7.2 PHOSPHORUS

Q. Describe the major action of phosphorus on our body.

Phosphorus acts as a protoplasmic poison due to which normal metabolism is disturbed and cellular oxidation is severely affected. This results in specific changes in liver, bone, kidneys (acute renal failure), and lungs.

Q. Describe the major action of phosphorus on liver.

The changes in liver include necrobiosis, which resemble ischemia, and prevent cellular metabolism and inhibit glycogen deposition with excess fat deposition, resulting in extensive fatty degeneration and acute hepatic necrosis. Thus phosphorus is a hepatotoxic substance.

Q. Describe the major action of phosphorus on bone.

The major change observed in bone is called Phossy jaw. Phossy jaw is a type of osteomyelitis of jaws observed in chronic cases of phosphorus poisoning, wherein bone formation under the epiphyseal cartilage, haversian, and marrow canals increases. This results in a decrease in the blood circulation to bone, thereby necrosis and sequestration of bone (Figs. 7.1 and 7.2).

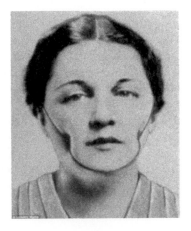

FIGURE 7.1

Phossy jaw—phosphorus poisoning—degeneration of jaw bone.

From https://s-media-cache-ak0.pinimg.com/236x/0d/b5/c9/0db5c909ef102fd79f8c86e57a6a9f71.jpg.

Q. Describe the major action of phosphorus on lung.

Phosphene (PH_3) gas released in the environment reduces oxyhemoglobin in blood and may prove fatal if more than 20 parts of phosphene is present in 100,000 parts of air. It can also bring about respiratory inflammation and develop pulmonary symptoms.

Q. Describe the major action of phosphorus on kidney.

Kidney changes constitute renal damage with acute renal failure.

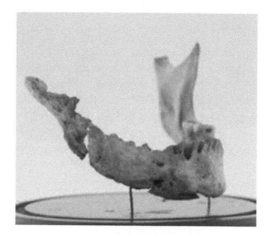

FIGURE 7.2

Mandible showing damage caused by "phossy jaw" at the Hunterian Museum.

From https://encrypted-tbn0.gstatic.com/images?q = tbn:
ANd9GcSyYaG_pKTpxFAng3UpTMdw2TpiJJgRtudGZhF_ipD_JrDMy8qp.

Q. What are the signs and symptoms of phosphorus poisoning?

Massive intake of phosphorus (more than 1 g) results in fulminating poisoning. The chief clinical feature is peripheral vascular collapse and death in 12−48 hours. Acute poisoning is observed in three phases: (1) primary phase, due to local irritant action on the GI tract, (2) dormant or silent secondary phase and, (3) tertiary phase, due to action of absorbed poison.

Primary phase: It occurs within 2−6 hours of ingestion and may last up to 3 days. Occasionally, the onset may be immediate. The initial features include garlicky taste, and severe burning sensation in the mouth, throat, retrosternal area, and epigastrium, followed by nausea, vomiting, and diarrhea. Breath and vomitus has a garlicky odor. The vomitus and stools are luminous in dark. There may be hematemesis. The stools may give rise to faint fumes constituting the smoky stool syndrome.

Secondary phase: It is a symptom free phase and patient feel well enough and may last for 2 to 6 days or even more after the subsidence of primary phase.

Tertiary phase: It is due to systemic effects of the absorbed poison. The original symptoms of primary phase will reappear with increased severity along with manifestations of hepatic damage. There will be tender hepatomegaly, jaundice, pruritus, and bleeding from multiple sites and anemia. Finally, hepatic encephalopathy develops, leading to stupor and coma; and oliguria, hematuria, albuminuria, and acute renal failure leading to death.

Chronic poisoning is usually observed in industrial workers due to long-term (2−5 years) occupational exposure to phosphorus fumes, resulting in a condition known as Phossy jaw.

7.3 CHLORINE

Q. Describe the mode of action of chlorine.

Chlorine is a halogen, which is an inorganic nonmetallic irritant poison. It is a yellowish green gas with irritating pungent odor. Chlorine acts as a direct irritant of the mucous membrane of respiratory tract by locally forming hydrochloric acid as it comes in contact with moisture.

Q. What are the signs and symptoms of exposure to chlorine?

Main symptoms after inhalation are choking, suffocation, and a feeling of tightness in the chest with laryngeal spasm. Headache, nausea, sore throat, lacrimation, rhinorrhoea, and cough are also seen. Breathlessness is due to the collection of secretions inside the respiratory passage. Death occurs due to laryngeal or pulmonary edema.

Fatal dose is greater than 400 ppm for few minutes (inhalation) or 1 part of chlorine in 1000 parts of air exposed for 5 minutes.

7.4 BROMINE

Q. What are the characteristics of bromine?

Bromine is a reddish-brown liquid, volatilizing to red fumes at room temperature and emitting an unpleasant odor. Bromides are more often in use as a medicine, acts as a sedative and cough elixir.

Q. Describe the signs and symptoms of acute bromine toxicity.

If taken in liquid form, bromine acts as a corrosive poison. Intense burning pain throughout the GI tract, dysphagia, vomiting, eructation of offensive vapors, and purging are due to the corrosive action of bromine liquid on the GI tract.

If inhaled in gaseous form, bromine causes violent catarrhal inflammation of the respiratory tract. There is cough, feeling of constriction of the chest, pulmonary edema and hemoptysis, edema of the glottis and larynx, and death from suffocation.

Q. Describe the signs and symptoms of chronic bromine toxicity.

Chronic bromide poisoning is known as "bromism," and occurs due to repeated administration of bromides of ammonium, sodium, and potassium as sedatives in medical doses, over a prolonged period. Clinically, bromism manifests with:

- Skin rashes in the form of red papules (bromine rash), similar to acne vulgaris, which may transform into a pustular lesion/uncerate at the hair roots (bromoderma), on the face, neck, and upper part of chest.
- There may be a problem of memory loss, muscular weakness, and incoordination.

- May suffer from delusion, hallucinations, and personality changes in severe cases.
- Fatal dose and period is uncertain. The maximum permissible level of vapor in air is 0.1 ppm.

7.5 IODINE

Q. What are the characteristics of iodine?

Iodine is a type of halogen, an inorganic nonmetallic irritant poison. It is a volatile crystalline substance with purple glittering color, a characteristic odor, and an acrid taste. It gives violet fumes/vapors at room temperature. It acts as an antiseptic. It is a powerful irritant and vesicant.

Q. Describe the signs and symptoms of acute iodine toxicity.

- Burning pain from mouth to epigastrium, intense thirst, excessive salivation, vomiting, purging, giddiness, cramps, convulsions, and fainting.
- Lips and mouth are stained brownish.
- Vomitus and stool are dark yellow/bluish in color and show the presence of blood and emits iodine odor.
- Urine is suppressed, reddish-brown in color and shows the presence of albumin.
- Pulse—low and weak.
- Skin—cold and clammy, the patient passes into a state of uremia and collapse, but consciousness is retained till death.

Q. Describe the signs and symptoms of chronic iodine toxicity.

Iodine toxicity is also known as "iodism." The problem occurs in patients who take large doses of potassium iodine continuously as medication. The symptoms include erythema, urticaria (Fig. 7.3), acne, inflammation of all mucous membranes, parotitis, lymphadenopathy, anorexia, and insomnia. Fatal dose is 2−4 g of iodine or 30−60 mL (1−2 ounces) of tincture iodine. The fatal period is about 24 hours.

Q. What is iodine deficiency?

Iodine deficiency is a lack of the trace element iodine. It may result in goiter (the so-called endemic goiter) (Fig. 7.4), as well as cretinism, which results in the developmental delays and other health problems. Iodine deficiency is an important public health issue as it is a preventable cause of intellectual disability.

7.6 FORMALDEHYDE (FORMALIN, METHYL ALDEHYDE, METHYLENE OXIDE)

Q. Describe the characteristics of formaldehyde.

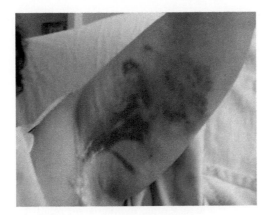

FIGURE 7.3

Erythema, blistering, and necrosis in distribution of axillary skin folds from exposure to povidone—iodine

From http://escholarship.org/uc/item/14h5d8wq/1.jpg.

HYPERTHYROIDISM

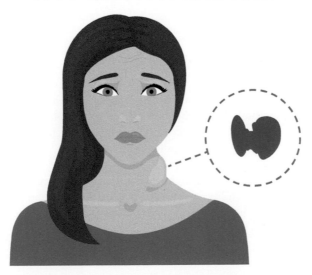

FIGURE 7.4

Iodine deficiency leads to hyperthroidism.

Reproduced from www.shutterstock.com/th/image-vector/woman-enlarged-hyperthyroid-gland-hyperthyroidism-symbol-508392580?src = 1T1IIfRB31_14Sdx7GEoKg-1-6.

Formaldehyde is an irritant poison. It is a colorless gas with pungent odor. However, commercially it is available as formalin, which is a 40% aqueous solution of formaldehyde gas.

Formalin is a disinfectant, antiseptic, deodorant, tissue fixative, and embalming agent. It has an irritant action also and can act by all routes of absorption.

Q. What are the signs and symptoms of acute formaldehyde poisoning?

Inhalation of vapors can bring about irritation of respiratory tract, resulting in headache, rhinitis, dyspnea, lacrimation, cough, etc.

Oral ingestion can result in corrosion of GI tract with painful abdomen, nausea, vomiting, and diarrhea. Pupils will be constricted and the face is flushed. It can cause severe acidosis which results from rapid conversion of formaldehyde to formic acid. Coma, hypotension, renal failure, etc. are usual complications in severe ingestion cases.

Q. What are the main signs and symptoms of chronic formaldehyde poisoning?

It is known to be a carcinogenic in animal experiments, but its relationship to occupational cancer is uncertain. Repeated exposure to formaldehyde may cause some persons to become sensitized to it and may cause asthmatic reaction at levels which is too low to create any symptoms in normal people.

Fatal dose is 30–90 mL and the fatal period ranges from 24 to 48 hours.

7.7 SELENIUM TOXICITY/DEFICIENCY

Toxic effects of selenium are also discussed in Chapter 15, Veterinary Toxicology.

Q. Describe the properties of selenium.

Selenium (Se) was discovered in 1817, and named after the Greek word *selene* meaning moon. Although technically a nonmetal, certain forms have metal-like properties. Selenium is an essential element found in selenoproteins and deficiency is recognized in humans and animals.

Q. What is selenosis?

Selenium is also toxic and high doses cause overt selenium poisoning (*selenosis*). The availability and the toxic potential of selenium compounds are related to their chemical forms and, most importantly, to solubility.

Q. Define acute toxicity of selenium.

Acute selenium toxicity in humans is rare. Intentional or accidental ingestion of a large dose of sodium selenate or sodium selenite can be life-threatening. Symptoms of fatal selenium intoxication include nausea and vomiting, followed by pulmonary edema and rapid cardiovascular collapse.

Q. Define subacute and chronic toxicity of selenium.

Chronic (long-term) exposure to high levels of selenium in food and water results in discoloration of the skin, deformation, and loss of nails, reversible loss of hair (baldness) excessive tooth decay and discoloration, a garlic odor to the breath, weakness, lack of mental alertness, and listlessness.

In humans, effects are mainly dermal and neurological including hair and fingernail loss, tooth discoloration, numbness, paralysis, and occasional hemiplegia.

7.8 FLUORIDE TOXICITY/DEFICIENCY

Toxic effects of fluoride in animals are discussed in Chapter 15, Veterinary Toxicology.

Q. What are the sources of fluoride poisoning?

Fluoride is present at low levels in virtually all feed and water sources, while a small amount of fluoride in the diet has been shown to improve bone and teeth development; a chronic excess of fluoride can have adverse effects on teeth, bone, and other body systems. Sodium fluoride is readily absorbed from the digestive tract and is several times more biologically available than fluoride compounds from feed or environmental sources.

Q. Which countries are mostly affected by fluorosis?

The chronic disease which occurs due to continuous ingestion of small doses of fluoride is known as fluorosis. Fluorosis is endemic in at least 22 countries worldwide (Fig. 7.5).

Q. How fluoride excess affects teeth and bones of animals and human beings?

Chronic excess fluoride ingestion affects the teeth and bones of affected animals and human beings. Fluoride substitutes for hydroxyl groups in the hydroxyapatite of the bone matrix which alters the mineralization and crystal structure of the bone. Bone changes induced by excess fluoride

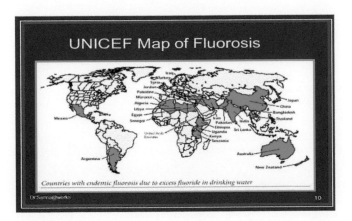

FIGURE 7.5

Worldwide distribution of endemic fluorosis—22 counties are affected.

From http://slideplayer.com/224204/1/images/10/UNICEF+Map+of+Fluorosis.jpg.

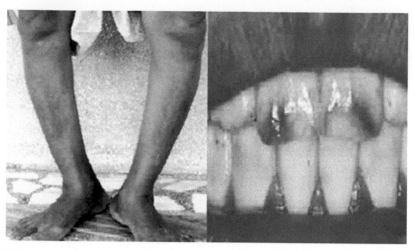

FIGURE 7.6

Severe fluorosis of legs and teeth.

Reproduced from Avicenna Journals (http://www.ajournals.com/wp-content/uploads/2016/03/Figure5.png).

ingestion, termed skeletal fluorosis or osteofluorosis, include the interference of the normal sequences of osteogenesis and bone remodeling with the resulting production of abnormal bone or the resorption of normal bone. The fluoride content of bone can increase over a period of time without other noticeable changes in the bone structure or function of teeth (Figs. 7.6 and 7.7).

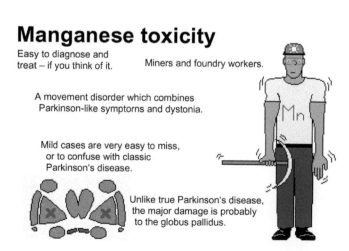

FIGURE 7.7

Mn-induced parkinsonism.

From http://metalpedia.asianmetal.com/img/mn/health2.jpg.

7.9 MANGANESE TOXICITY/DEFICIENCY

Q. What are the sources of manganese (Mn) poisoning?

The uptake of Mn by humans mainly takes place through food.

The following fresh food groups (in descending order) are most important in manganese content: Nuts, whole cereals, dried fruits, roots, tubers and stalks, fruits, nonleafy vegetables, meat, poultry products, fish and seafoods. Leafy vegetables also rank high on the list when expressed in dry-weight terms. Tea also has a very high level of manganese, about 10 times that of cereals.

Q. Describe the role of manganese (Mn) as an essential trace metal.

The human body contains 12−20 mg of manganese, most of which is found in the liver, bones, and kidneys. This trace element is a cofactor for several important enzymes, thus it is essential to ensuring the health and well-being of humans. The functions of manganese are as follows:

- Normal skeletal growth and development
- Essential for glucose utilization
- Lipid synthesis and lipid metabolism
- Cholesterol metabolism
- Pancreatic function and development
- Prevention of sterility
- Important for protein and nucleic acid metabolism
- Activates enzyme functions
- Involved in thyroid hormone synthesis.

Q. Describe the adverse effects of manganese (Mn) deficiency.

Because manganese is an essential element for human health, shortages of manganese can cause adverse health effects. Mn deficiency can result in the following ill effects:

- Ataxia
- Fatness
- Blood clotting
- Skin problems
- Lowered cholesterol levels
- Skeleton disorders
- Birth defects
- Reduced immune function
- Impaired glucose metabolism
- Changes of hair color
- Neurological symptoms.

Q. Describe the toxic potential of manganese (Mn).

Despite its essentiality, Mn overexposure can cause a variety of toxic effects in humans and animals. Mn has been linked to a peculiar extrapyramidal syndrome in occupational workers since 1837 (Mn-induced parkinsonism, Fig. 7.7). Clinical investigations include bradykinesia, rigidity, masked face diminished blinking, impaired dexterity, gait abnormalities, hypophonia, and micrographia (Fig. 7.8). Long-term exposure to excess levels may cause kidney failure, hallucinations, as well as diseases of the central nervous system, and reproductive and developmental effects.

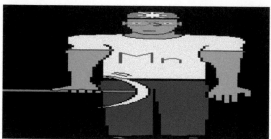

Manganese toxicity can result in a permanent neurological disorder known as manganism with symptoms that include tremors, difficulty walking, and facial muscle spasms. These symptoms are often preceded by other lesser symptoms, including irritability, aggressiveness, and hallucinations.

FIGURE 7.8

Micrographia in a patient with chronic manganese toxicity.

7.10 SULFUR

Toxic effects of sulfur in animals are discussed in Chapter 15, Veterinary Toxicology.

7.11 CYANIDE

Toxic effects of cyanide in animals are discussed in Chapter 15, Veterinary Toxicology.

Q. What is cyanide poisoning?

Cyanide poisoning is a form of histotoxic hypoxia because the cells of an organism are unable to use oxygen, primarily through the inhibition of cytochrome c oxidase enzyme.

Q. How do cyanides are produced in nature?

Cyanides are produced by certain bacteria, fungi, and algae, and are found in a number of plants. Cyanides are found in substantial amounts in certain seeds and fruit stones, e.g., those of apricots, apples, and peaches. In plants, cyanides are usually bound to sugar molecules in the form of cyanogenic glycosides and defend the plant against herbivores. Cassava roots (also called manioc), an important potato-like food grown in tropical countries (and the base from which tapioca is made), also contain cyanogenic glycosides.

Q. What are the common routes of cyanide exposure?

The common routes of exposure include (Fig. 7.9):

ingestion;

inhalation;

skin (dermal).

Q. The consumption of which cassava root is responsible for chronic form of cyanide toxicity in humans?

Chronic form of cyanide toxicity observed in humans due to consumption of cassava root is *konzo* (Fig. 7.10).

Explanation: Cassava is a vitally important crop worldwide, serving as a major source of calories for 200–300 million people. It produces more carbohydrate per acre than any other plant. One of the reasons it is so prolific is that the plant comes with its own insecticide. The glycoside linamarin releases cyanide when it comes into contact with the enzyme linamarase, which is also found in the root. This reaction occurs when the plant is bruised or eaten raw. The elaborate, lengthy preparation of cassava for human consumption involves grating the root and soaking it in warm water for several days—a procedure that releases and dissipates cyanide before the plant is consumed.

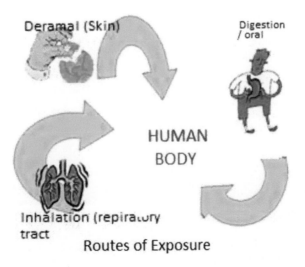

FIGURE 7.9

Common routes of cyanide exposure.

From http://3.bp.blogspot.com/-Osq7OnndSwA/UAGwHoLlpzI/AAAAAAAAADg/oUKd4VHne_g/s1600/routes.jpg.

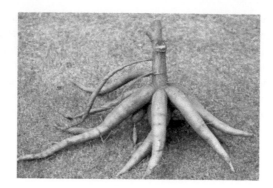

FIGURE 7.10

Cassava root—causes chronic cyanide poisoning.

From http://www.thepoisonreview.com/wp-content/uploads/cassava-ethanol1.jpg.

Q. What are the signs and symptoms of cyanide toxicity?

Signs and symptoms of toxicity include:

Mild to toxicity: nausea, dizziness, drowsiness.

Moderate toxicity: loss of consciousness for a short period, convulsions, vomiting, and cyanosis.

Severe toxicity: deep coma, dilated nonreactive pupils, deteriorating cardiorespiratory function.

The onset of signs and symptoms of cyanide intoxication via inhalation are very fast and can cause death in 6—8 minutes (Fig. 7.11).

Q. What is the mechanism of cyanide toxicity?

The cyanide ion halts cellular respiration by inhibiting the enzyme cytochrome c oxidase found in the mitochondria. It attaches to the iron within this protein. The binding of cyanide to this enzyme prevents transport of electrons from cytochrome c to oxygen. As a result, the electron transport

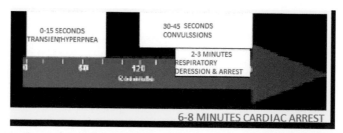

FIGURE 7.11

Schematic representation of onset of signs and symptoms of cyanide intoxication via inhalation. It can cause death in 6—8 min.

chain is disrupted, meaning that the cell can no longer aerobically produce ATP for energy. Tissues that depend highly on aerobic respiration, such as the central nervous system and the heart, are particularly affected. This is an example of histotoxic hypoxia.

Q. Describe the mechanism of action of sodium nitrite in cyanide poisoning.

Mechanism of action of sodium nitrite in cyanide poisoning is depicted in Fig. 7.12. The figure shows that cyan-cytochrome oxidase has more affinity for methemoglobin to form cyan-methemoglobin.

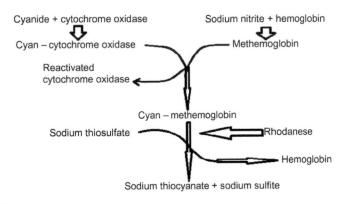

FIGURE 7.12

Mechanism of action of sodium nitrite in cyanide poisoning.

7.12 OXALATE POISONING

Toxicity of oxalates is also discussed in Chapter 15, Veterinary Toxicology.

Q. What are oxalates?

Oxalates belong to a group of substances known as antinutrients. Antinutrients are, as their name would suggest, compounds which prevent the nutritive value of foods from being effective, either by preventing the absorption of nutrients, by being toxic themselves, or by one or more other methods of action.

Q. Name some plants and foods that contain oxalates.

There are several plants and food that contain oxalates. For example, *Dieffenbachia* plant, vegetables and fruits such as spinach, Swiss chard, rhubarb, soy nuts, plantains, almonds, cashews, sesame seeds, and yucca (Fig. 7.13).

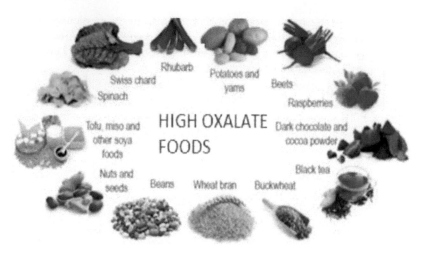

FIGURE 7.13

Foods that contain oxalates.

7.13 QUESTION AND ANSWER EXERCISES

7.13.1 SHORT QUESTIONS AND ANSWERS

Exercise 1

Q.1 Why fluorine is not available in free form?

Fluorine is the most reactive nonmetal (due to its high electron gravity) and hence is not available in free form. It is seen in combination with other elements as fluorides.

Q.2 Name the nonmetal toxicity that could occur during some festivals and in war zones.

Phosphorus, because yellow phosphorus is used in the manufacture of fire crackers and military ammunition.

Q.3 Why burns due to phosphorus causes higher mortality than other agents?

The absorption of phosphorus through raw burnt surface leads to multiorgan failure. Hence, burns due to phosphorus are more dangerous than other burns.

Q.4 Why oily purgatives such as mineral oils are contraindicated in phosphorus poisoning?

Oils increase the absorption of phosphorus. Hence they are contraindicated in phosphorus poisoning.

Q.5 What is Phossy jaw?

Phossy jaw, formally phosphorus necrosis of the jaw, is an occupational disease of those who work with white phosphorus, also known as *yellow phosphorus*, without proper safeguards. It was most commonly seen in workers in the match industry in the 19th and early 20th centuries.

Q.6 What are the different forms of phosphorus and name their common derivatives?

Phosphorus exists in two forms—white or yellow and red phosphorus. Derivatives of phosphorus include aluminum phosphide, zinc phosphide, and phosphine gas.

Q.7 What is the antidote of iodine poisoning?

Sodium thiosulfate solution (1%–5%) orally, in iodism, liberal intake of sodium chloride or sodium bicarbonate is useful.

Q.8 What are the different forms of selenium?

Selenium occurs in nature and in biological systems as selenate (Se^{6+}), selenite (Se^{4+}), selenide (Se^{2+}), and elemental selenium (Se^{0}).

Q.9 What is the toxic principle of cyanogenic plants?

Cyanogenic glycosides or cyanogens (amygdalin, prunasin, dhurrin, linamarin).

Hydrogen cyanide is formed when the glycosides are hydrolyzed by enzymes in plants or by rumen microorganisms.

Q.10 Name the compounds that produce cyanide ions?

Common poisonous cyanide compounds include hydrogen cyanide gas and the crystalline solids, potassium cyanide, and sodium cyanide.

Exercise 2

Q.1 Why cyanide has more affinity for cytochrome oxidase than hemoglobin, which also contains iron?

Cyanide has more affinity for ferric (Fe^{3+}) form of iron. In hemoglobin, iron is present in ferrous (Fe^{3+}) form, whereas cytochrome oxidase has ferric (Fe^{3+}) iron. Hence, cyanide prefers cytochrome oxidase.

Q.2 Why *Halogeton glomeratus* and *Oxalis pes-caprae* commonly cause oxalate poisoning?

The oxalates present in the above plant species are soluble. Hence, these plants cause oxalate poisoning. In *H. glomeratus*, both sodium and potassium oxalates are present, whereas in *O. pes-caprae*, only potassium oxalates are present.

Q.3 Do you recommend use of administration of oil or fat in phosphorus poisoning? Give reasons.

No. Oral administration of oil, fat, egg, etc. is not recommended because phosphorus is soluble in these agents and would enhance its absorption.

Q.4 What are the main postmortem findings in iodine poisoning?

Brownish stains of skin and mucosa, characteristic iodine odor, congestion of all the viscera. Stomach may show blue content if starchy food is present. Heart and liver may show fatty degeneration and kidneys glomerular/tubular necrosis.

Q.5 Name the compounds that produce cyanide ions.

Common poisonous cyanide compounds include hydrogen cyanide gas and the crystalline solids such as potassium cyanide and sodium cyanide.

Q.6 What are the different compounds of sulfur?

Sulfur can react with all metals except gold and platinum, forming sulfide. It also forms compounds with several nonmetallic elements. It forms compounds in oxidation states; -2 (sulfide, S^{2-}), $+4$ (sulfite, SO_3^{2-}), and $+6$ (sulfate, SO_4^{2-}). Millions of tons of sulfur are produced each year, mostly for the manufacture of sulfuric acid, which is widely used in industry.

Q.7 Is sulfur important for our body, if so how?

Yes. The "beauty mineral," *sulfur*, is necessary for healthy skin, hair, and nails. It is also an important element of body detoxification: as a part of detox enzymes and sulfur-containing amino acids cysteine and methionine, it binds to toxic heavy metal contaminants—especially aluminum—making its elimination much easier. Sulfur also helps regeneration of joint cartilage, both by helping it rebuild and by suppressing copper, whose high levels promote joint degeneration. Sulfur is useful in reducing allergic reactions and parasitic infections.

Sulfur is also a component of insulin, thus necessary for proper metabolism of carbohydrates. Thus low sulfur levels can aggravate symptoms of diabetes.

Q.8 What are the symptoms of inorganic sulfur compound toxicity?

Inorganic (not carbon-bonded) sulfur compounds, such as those found in fossil fuels and their emissions, pesticides, industrial compounds, food additives, and drugs, can aggravate allergies, chemical sensitivities, symptoms of diabetes, impair immune system's antibody response, and, possibly, even alter the DNA/RNA function.

Q.9 What are the short-term effects of high sulfur supplementation?

The short-term effects of high sulfur supplementation can cause digestive disturbance, while long-term exposure can result in lowering body levels of potassium and calcium.

Q.10 How do oxalates damage the body?

These chemicals are present in plants (and some animal foods) that bind with minerals in the body, such as magnesium, potassium, calcium, and sodium, creating oxalate salts. Most of these salts are soluble and pass quickly out of the body. However, oxalates that bind with calcium are practically insoluble and these crystals solidify in the kidneys (kidney stones) or the urinary tract, causing pain and irritation. These crystals can then easily settle out as sediments from the urine, causing kidney stones.

Some serious chronic diseases—like Crohn's and Lou-Gehrig—are further aggravated by sulfur intake. On the other hand, extra sulfur intake helps with Alzheimer's, as well as chronic toxicity caused by heavy metals.

7.13.2 MULTIPLE CHOICE QUESTIONS (CHOOSE THE BEST STATEMENT, IT CAN BE ONE, TWO OR ALL OR NONE)

Exercise 3

Q.1 Which of the following form of phosphorus is/are toxic?
    a. White
    b. Red
    c. Yellow
    d. Black

Q.2 Fluoride inhibits pyruvic acid synthesis by inhibiting an enzyme
    a. enolase
    b. transaminase
    c. phosphatase
    d. phosphodiesterase

Q.3 The most serious consequence of crude oil or kerosene ingestion by cattle is
    a. liver damage
    b. kidney damage
    c. aspiration pneumonia
    d. central nervous system stimulation
    e. leukemia

Q.4 After a period of drought or cloudy weather, the cyanide content in the plant
    a. increases
    b. decreases
    c. does not change
    d. becomes zero

Q.5 Cyanide has more affinity for the following:
    a. Hemoglobin
    b. Cytochrome oxidase
    c. Met-hemoglobin
    d. Myoglobin

Q.6 The oxalate salt of the following element(s) is/are soluble:
    a. Sodium
    b. Potassium
    c. Magnesium
    d. Calcium

Q.7 The most appropriate sample to be collected in case of nitrate/nitrite poisoning is
    a. blood
    b. rumen contents
    c. fodder
    d. CSF
    e. aqueous humor
    f. all of above

Q.8 Which of the following leads to the deposition of oxalate crystals in the urinary tract?

a. Dieffenbachia (dumbcane)
b. Propylene glycol
c. Methoxyflurane
d. Philodendron
e. Ethylene glycol

Q.9 Which of the following conditions represents a manifestation of moderate chronic fluoride toxicity?

a. Osteomalacia
b. Osteosclerosis
c. Osteopetrosis
d. Osteopenia
e. Osteolysis

Q.10 Intoxication from consumption of wild cherry or apricot pits would best be treated by

a. hyperbaric oxygen
b. artificial respiration
c. inhalation of amyl nitrite
d. intravenous sodium nitrite and sodium thiosulfate
e. oral sodium nitrate

Answers

1. a and c (white and yellow phosphorus are soluble and readily absorbed, hence cause toxicity, whereas red phosphorus is insoluble, hence is nontoxic); 2. a; 3. c; 4. a; 5. c. (hence, sodium nitrate is used as a therapeutic strategy to convert hemoglobin to methemoglobin, which removes cyanide from cytochrome oxidase); 6. a and b; 7. d; 8. a; 9. b; 10. d.

7.13.3 FILL IN THE BLANKS

Exercise 4

Q.1 In selenium toxicity, depleted glutathione levels can be restored by administering _____ during treatment.

Q.2 Bran disease in horses is caused due to excess feeding of wheat bran, which contains high amount of _____.

Q.3 In selenium poisoning, the level of selenium detected in blood is _____ and in hooves _____.

Q.4 Garlic-like odor of breath or stomach contents luminous in dark is indicative of _____ poisoning.

Q.5 Phosphorus is eliminated from the body through _____ and _____.

Q.6 Dermal exposure to white/yellow phosphorus leads to _____.

Q.7 The use of _____ metal chelator is contraindicated in selenium toxicity.

Q.8 The immediate symptom upon oral ingestion of phosphorus is _____.

Q.9 The organs which are damaged in phosphorus poisoning are _____ and _____.

Q.10 In chronic phosphorus poisoning, the necrosis of jaw which is observed is called as _____.

Q.11 The best material for diagnosis of phosphorus poisoning is _____ or _____.

Q.12 The prognosis in case of phosphorus poisoning is _____ to _____.

Q.13 Cyanide inhibits cellular respiration by binding with _____.

Q.14 The conversion of methemoglobin to hemoglobin by methylene blue depends on the availability of _____.

Answers

1. ACETYL CYSTEINE; 2. PHOSPHORUS; 3. 1–4 ppm, 5–20 ppm; 4. PHOSPHORUS; 5. URINE and BREATH (hence the breath has garlic-like odor); 6. SKIN BURNS; 7. DIMERCAPROL (BAL); 8. EMESIS (hematemesis) (phosphorus is a strong irritant with corrosive properties, hence it causes GI tract irritation leading to vomition); 9. LIVER, KIDNEY; 10. PHOSSY JAW; 11. VOMITUS or STOMACH CONTENTS; 12. GUARDED to GRAVE; 13. CYTOCHROME OXIDASE (cyta3) (cyanide has more affinity toward metalloporphyrin (Fe)-containing enzymes); 14. $NADPH_2$.

FURTHER READING

Barceloux, D.G., Bond, G.R., Krenzelok, E.P., et al., 2002. American Academy of Clinical Toxicology practice guidelines on the treatment of methanol poisoning. J. Toxicol. Clin. Toxicol. 40, 415–446.

Bird, M.G., Greim, H., Snyder, R., Rice, J.M., 2005. International symposium: recent advances in benzene toxicity. Chem. Biol. Interact. 153–154.

Bruckner, J.V., Satheesh Anand, S., Alan Warren, D., 2013. Toxic effects of solvents and vapors. In: Klaassen, C.D. (Ed.), Casarett and Doull's Toxicology: The Basic Science of Poisons, eighth ed. McGraw-Hill, New York, NY, pp. 981–1050.

Gupta, P.K., 2014. Essential Concepts in Toxicology. BSP Pvt Ltd, Hyderabad, India (Chapter 19).

Gupta, P.K., 2016. Fundamental in toxicology: essential concepts and applications in toxicology. Elsevier/BSP, San Diego, USA (Chapter 19).

Sills, R.C., Morgan, D.L., Harry, G.J., 1998. Carbon disulfide neurotoxicity in rats: introduction and study design. Neurotoxicology 19, 83–88.

Sills, R.C., Harry, G.J., Valentine, W.M., Morgan, D.L., 2005. Interdisciplinary neurotoxicity inhalation studies: carbon disulfide and carbonyl sulfide research in F344 rats. Toxicol. Appl. Pharmacol. 207, S245–S250.

Solvents, vapors, and gases

8

CHAPTER OUTLINE

8.1 SOLVENTS

Q. What is a solvent?

A solvent can be defined as "a liquid that has the ability to dissolve, suspend, or extract other materials, without chemical change to the material or solvent."

Q. What are the properties of solvents?

Solvent chemicals have variable lipophilicity and volatility. These properties, coupled with small molecular size and lack of charge, make inhalation the major route of solvent exposure and provide for ready absorption across the lung, gastrointestinal (GI) tract, and skin.

Q. What are the uses of solvents?

Solvents are so widely used in the modern world as to be ubiquitous and are employed in paints, pharmaceuticals, degreasants, adhesives, printing inks,

Illustrated Toxicology. DOI: http://dx.doi.org/10.1016/B978-0-12-813213-5.00008-0

pesticides, cosmetics, and household cleaners. The largest end user is the coatings industry where solvents play an important role in the quality and durability of paints and varnishes.

Q. Classify solvents.

Commercial solvents are frequently complex mixtures and may include nitrogen- or sulfur-containing organics—gasoline and other oil-based products. The common solvents fall into the following groups:

1. *Aliphatic hydrocarbons*, such as hexane. These may be straight or branched-chain compounds and are often present in mixtures.
2. *Halogenated aliphatic hydrocarbons*. The best-known examples are methylene dichloride, chloroform, and carbon tetrachloride, although chlorinated ethylenes are also widely used.
3. *Aliphatic alcohols*. Common examples are methanol and ethanol.
4. *Glycols and glycol ethers*. Ethylene and propylene glycols (PG), for example, in antifreeze give rise to considerable exposure of the general public. Glycol ethers, such as methyl cellosolve, are also widely used.
5. *Aromatic hydrocarbons*. Benzene is probably the one of greatest concern, but others, such as toluene, are also used.

Explanation: Most solvent exposures involve a mixture of chemicals, rather than a single compound. Our knowledge of the toxicity of solvent mixtures is rudimentary relative to the toxicology of individual solvents. While the assumption is frequently made that the toxic effects of multiple solvents are additive, solvents may also interact synergistically or antagonistically.

Q. How solvents are absorbed?

The majority of systemic absorption of inhaled volatile organic compounds (VOCs) occurs in the alveoli, although limited absorption has been demonstrated to occur in the upper respiratory tract. Gases in the alveoli are thought to equilibrate almost instantaneously with blood in the pulmonary capillaries.

Q. What are the commonly used solvents?

The commonly used solvents include isopropanol, toluene, xylene, and solvent mixtures such as white spirits and the chlorinated solvents, methylene chloride, trichloroethylene (TCE), and perchloroethylene.

In the recent past, 1-bromopropane has been introduced, to replace ozone-depleting agents such as 1,1,1-trichloroethane (methylchloroform).

Q. Define factors which govern toxicity from solvent exposure.

1. Solvent exposure is dependent on several factors:
2. Toxicity of the solvent
3. Exposure route
4. Amount or rate of exposure
5. Duration of exposure
6. Individual susceptibility
7. Interactions.

Q. What are the main dangers of solvents?
1. Toxic effects
2. Corrosive effects
3. Flammable effects
4. Reactive nature-incompatible chemicals.

Q. Give some examples of serious but potentially reversible effects of solvents.
- Liver and kidney damage—toluene-containing substances and chlorinated hydrocarbons (correction fluids, dry-cleaning fluids)
- Blood oxygen depletion—organic nitrites (*poppers*, *bold*, and *rush*) and methylene chloride (varnish removers, paint thinners).

Q. What is solvent abuse?

The use of certain volatile organic solvents as intoxicants by inhalation, e.g., glue-sniffing, is known as solvent abuse (inhalant users inhale vapor or aerosol propellant gases using plastic bags held over the mouth or by breathing from a solvent-soaked rag or an open container). The practices are known colloquially as "sniffing," "huffing," or "bagging."

Q. Describe the routes of exposure of solvents.
1. Oral
2. Inhalation (major)
3. Skin.

Q. What are biological properties of solvents?

From a biological perspective the most important properties of solvents are:
1. volatility;
2. high-fat solubility (lipophilicity);
3. small molecule size.

Explanation: Solvents with these characteristics are termed VOCs. Under normal working conditions solvents readily evaporate into the air, from where they enter the lungs. The high lipid solubility and small molecule size means they are quickly absorbed across lung membranes and enter the blood supply. Blood from the lung moves directly to the brain and other body organs before reaching the liver, where metabolism of the solvent occurs. With ongoing exposure, equilibrium is reached between the amount in the body and the concentration of the solvent in the air.

Q. What are the common toxic effects of organic solvents?

General toxic effects of organic solvents are listed in Table 8.1.

Q. What is a painter's syndrome?

The painter's syndrome was first described in Scandinavia in the late 1970s and became a recognized occupational disease in these countries. The cluster of symptoms includes headache, fatigue, sleep disorders, personality changes, and emotional instability, which progress to impaired intellectual function and ultimately, dementia. Early symptoms are often reversible if exposure is stopped.

Table 8.1 General Toxic Effects of Organic Solvents

Respiratory System

- Asphyxiation
- Irritation—asthma, bronchitis, pneumonitis
- Sensitization and allergy bronchoconstriction
- Lung cancer

Skin

- Irritant contact dermatitis
- Allergic contact dermatitis

The Nervous System

- Short-term effects—tiredness, disorientation, a sense of intoxication, drowsiness, euphoria, dizziness, confusion, and eventually, unconsciousness
- Long-term effects—memory impairment, coordination impairment, deterioration of personality and depression

8.1.1 TRICHLOROETHYLENE

Q. How trichloroethylene (TCE) is released into the atmosphere?

TCE is a widely used solvent identified so far. It is released into the atmosphere from vapor degreasing operations; however, direct discharges to surface waters and groundwater from disposal operations have been the frequent occurrences. As a result, TCE can be released to indoor air by vapor intrusion through underground walls and floors and by volatilization from the water supply.

Q. Describe in brief toxicity of tetrachloroethylene.

Tetrachloroethylene (perchloroethylene) is commonly used as a dry cleaner, fabric finisher, degreaser, rug and upholstery cleaner, paint and stain remover, solvent, and chemical intermediate. The highest exposures usually occur in occupational settings via inhalation. Much attention is now focused on adverse health effects that may be experienced by dry cleaners and other persons living in the proximity of such facilities. The chemical is well absorbed from the lungs and GI tract, distributed to tissues according to their lipid content. Dry-cleaning workers exposed to these chemicals show modest changes in a few indices of liver or kidney cell functions. More effects may occur in humans exposed for longer periods. Moderate-to-high doses of TCE, as with other halocarbons, are associated with a number of noncancer toxicities. TCE has been implicated in the development of autoimmune disorders and immune system dysfunction, and has been investigated for its potential as a male reproductive toxicant. Several studies indicate that TCE can cause cancer.

8.1.2 CARBON TETRACHLORIDE

Q. How carbon tetrachloride ($CC1_4$) is released into the atmosphere?

$CC1_4$ has widespread use as a solvent, cleaning agent, fire extinguisher, synthetic intermediate, grain fumigant, and human anthelmintic. Nevertheless, $CC1_4$ appears to be ubiquitous in ambient air in the United States, and it is still found in groundwater from some wells and waste sites.

Q. Describe in brief toxicity of chloroform ($CHCl_3$).

The primary use of $CHCl_3$ (trichloromethane) is in the production of the refrigerant chlorodifluoromethane (Freon 22), but this use is expected to diminish as chlorine-containing fluorocarbons are phased out under the Montreal Protocol. $CHCl_3$ was among the first inhalation anesthetics, but it was replaced by safer compounds after about 1940. The reproductive and developmental toxicities of $CHCl_3$ are unremarkable. Inhalation of 100–300 ppm $CHCl_3$ by pregnant rats caused a high incidence of fetal resorption, retardation of fetal development, and a low incidence of fetal anomalies. Under certain conditions $CHCl_3$ is hepatotoxic and nephrotoxic. These toxicities are potentiated by aliphatic alcohols, ketones, and Dichloroacetate (DCA) and trichloroacetic acid (TCA). The status of $CHCl_3$ as a rodent carcinogen is indisputable. It causes liver and kidney tumors that are species-, strain-, sex-, and route of exposure-dependent.

8.1.3 BENZENE

Q. Describe in brief toxicity of benzene.

Benzene produced commercially in the United States is derived primarily from petroleum. Benzene has been utilized as a general-purpose solvent, but it is now used principally in the synthesis of other chemicals. The percentage by volume of benzene in gasoline is 1%–2%. Benzene plays an important role in unleaded gasoline due to its antiknock properties. Inhalation is the primary route of exposure in industrial and in everyday settings. Cigarette smoke is the major source of benzene in the home. The most important adverse effect of benzene is hematopoietic toxicity. Chronic exposure to benzene can lead to bone marrow damage, which may be manifest initially as anemia, leukopenia, thrombocytopenia, or a combination of these. Bone marrow depression appears to be dose dependent in both laboratory animals and humans. Continued exposure may result in marrow aplasia and pancytopenia, an often fatal outcome. Survivors of aplastic anemia frequently exhibit a preneoplastic state, termed myelodysplasia, which may progress to myelogenous leukemia.

8.1.4 TOLUENE

Q. Describe in brief toxicity of toluene.

Toluene is present in paints, lacquers, thinners, cleaning agents, glues, and many other products. Toluene is also used in the production of other chemicals. Gasoline, which contains 5%−7% toluene by weight, is the largest source of atmospheric emissions and exposure of the general populace. Inhalation is the primary route of exposure, though skin contact occurs frequently. Toluene is a favorite of solvent abusers, who intentionally inhale high concentrations to achieve a euphoric effect. Large amounts of toluene enter the environment each year by volatilization. Relatively small amounts are released into industrial wastewater. Toluene is frequently found in water, soil, and air at hazardous waste. The central nervous system (CNS) is the primary target organ of toluene and other alkylbenzenes. Manifestations of acute exposure range from slight dizziness and headache to unconsciousness, respiratory depression, and death. Occupational inhalation exposure guidelines are established to prevent significant decrements in psychomotor functions. Acute encephalopathic effects are rapidly reversible upon cessation of exposure. Subtle neurological effects have been described in some groups of occupationally exposed individuals. Exposure to approximately 100 ppm toluene for years may result in subclinical effects.

8.1.5 XYLENES AND ETHYLBENZENE

Q. Describe in brief toxicity of xylenes and ethylbenzene.

Large numbers of people are exposed to xylenes and ethylbenzene occupationally and environmentally. Xylenes and ethylbenzene, like benzene and toluene, are the major components of gasoline and fuel oil. The primary uses of xylenes industrially are as solvents and synthetic intermediates. Most of these aromatics that are released into the environment evaporate into the atmosphere. They may also enter groundwater from oil and gasoline spills, leakage of storage tanks, and migration from waste sites. The toxicokinetics and acute toxicity of toluene, xylenes, and other aromatic solvents are quite similar. They are well absorbed from the lungs and GI tract, distributed to tissues according to tissue blood flow and lipid content, exhaled unchanged to some extent. Xylenes and ethylbenzene appear to have very limited capacity to adversely affect organs other than the CNS. Mild, transient liver and/or kidney toxicity have occasionally been reported in humans exposed to high vapor concentrations of xylenes.

8.2 ALCOHOLS

Q. Describe in brief toxicity of alcohols.

Alcohols comprise a class of organic compounds composed of a hydrocarbon chain and a hydroxyl group. Alcohols that have one hydroxyl group are called monohydric, which include methanol, ethanol, and isopropanol. These three alcohols are most commonly responsible for alcohol toxicosis. Alcohols are also classified as primary, secondary, or tertiary, according to the number of carbon atoms bonded to the carbon atom to which the hydroxyl group is bonded. Ethanol and methanol are primary alcohols, and isopropanol is a secondary alcohol.

Q. Describe in brief toxicity of ethanol.

Many humans experience greater exposure to ethanol (ethyl alcohol and alcohol) than to any other solvent. Not only is ethyl alcohol used as an additive in gasoline, as a solvent in industry, in many household products, and in pharmaceuticals, but it is also heavily consumed in intoxicating beverages. Frank toxic effects are less important occupationally than injuries resulting from psychomotor impairment. Driving under the influence of alcohol is, of course, the major cause of fatal auto accidents. In many states in the United States, a blood alcohol level of 80 mg/100 mL blood (80 mg%) is prima facie evidence of "driving while intoxicated." Gender differences in responses to ethanol are well recognized. Women are more sensitive to alcohol and exhibit higher mortality at lower levels of consumption than men. Alcohol-induced hepatotoxicity is postulated to be caused by elevation of endotoxin in the bloodstream. Endotoxin, released by the action of ethanol on gram-negative bacteria in the gut, is believed to be taken up by Kupffer cells, causing the release of inflammatory mediators that are cytotoxic to hepatocytes and chemoattractants for neutrophils. These mediators include interleukins, prostaglandins, free radicals, and tumor necrosis factor-α (TNF-α). Proinflammatory cytokines and oxidative stress stimulate collagen synthesis by hepatic stellate cells, leading to alcoholic fibrosis. There is a concern about the role of ethyl alcohol in carcinogenesis, due to the frequent consumption of alcoholic beverages by millions of people.

Q. Describe in brief toxicity of methanol.

Methanol (methyl alcohol, wood alcohol, and CH_3OH) is primarily used as a starting material for the synthesis of chemicals such as formaldehyde, acetic acid, methacrylates, ethylene glycol (EG), and methyl tertiary-butyl ether. CH_3OH is found in windshield washer fluid, carburetor cleaners, antifreeze, and copy machine toner, and serves as fuel for Sterno heaters, model airplanes, and Indianapolis 500 racecars. It also functions as a denaturant for some ethyl and isopropyl alcohols, rendering them unfit for consumption. Ingested methanol is absorbed quickly from the GI tract, and peak methanol concentrations occur within 30−60 minutes following ingestion. Toxicosis has also been reported following inhalation or dermal absorption. Methanol is much more toxic to human beings and nonhuman primates than it is to other mammals. Methanol is metabolized by alcohol dehydrogenase (ADH) to formaldehyde, which is oxidized to formic acid by formaldehyde dehydrogenase. Formic acid is responsible for ocular and CNS lesions in primates as a result of inhibition of cytochrome oxidase. Blindness and permanent neurological abnormalities are common sequel in primates.

Q. Describe in brief toxicity of isopropanol.

Isopropanol (isopropyl alcohol) has the structural formula $CH_3CH(OH)CH_3$; a molecular weight of 60 Da; and is found in rubbing alcohol (70%), antifreeze, detergents, window cleaning products, and disinfectants. Ingestion is the usual cause of poisoning in humans, although toxicity from inhalation and topical absorption has been reported. Isopropanol toxicosis is rare in domestic animals, possibly due to its bitter taste. Isopropanol is approximately twofold more toxic than ethanol. It is rapidly absorbed from the GI tract, and approximately 80% is metabolized to acetone, which is also a CNS depressant, but acetone has a much longer half-life (16−20 hours) than does alcohol.

8.3 GLYCOLS

Q. Describe in brief toxicity of ethylene glycol (EG).

EG (1,2-dihydroxyethane) is a constituent of antifreeze, deicers, hydraulic fluids, drying agents, and inks, and is used to make plastics and polyester fibers. Workers may be exposed dermally or by inhalation when solutions containing EG are heated or sprayed. The most important exposure route is ingestion, as EG may be accidentally swallowed, taken deliberately in suicide attempts, or used as a cheap substitute for ethanol. "Antifreeze" poisoning occurs frequently in cats and dogs that find its taste appealing.

Acute poisoning entails three clinical stages after an asymptomatic period, during which EG is metabolized:

1. A period of inebriation, the duration, and degree depending on dose.

2. The cardiopulmonary stage 12−24 hours after exposure, characterized by tachycardia and tachypnea, which may progress to cardiac failure and pulmonary edema.

3. The renal toxicity stage 24−72 hours post exposure.

Metabolic acidosis, due largely to glycoxylic acid (GA) accumulation, can develop and become progressively more severe during stages 2 and 3. Hypocalcemia can result from Ca^{2+} chelation by oxalic acid (OA) to form Ca^{2+} oxalate monohydrate crystals. Deposition of these crystals in kidney tubules is associated with organ damage and potentially acute renal failure. Nephrotoxicity appears to be an acute, high-dose phenomenon, as no demonstrable kidney damage has been reported in occupational studies of groups.

Q. Describe in brief toxicity of diethylene glycol (DEG).

DEGs use as an excipient in a liquid sulfanilamide preparation resulted in 105 deaths in the United States in 1937. This incident prompted the passage of the Food, Drug, and Cosmetic Act of 1938. Use of DEG-contaminated PG or glycerin in various pharmaceuticals has caused multiple fatalities from renal failure in Nigeria, Bangladesh, India, and Haiti. In the Haitian incident,

109 cases of acute renal failure (with 88 deaths) were identified in children who received locally manufactured acetaminophen syrup containing DEG-contaminated glycerin. Renal failure was the "hallmark" finding in these cases, but hepatitis, pancreatitis, and severe neurological manifestations (e.g., encephalopathy, optic neuritis with retinal edema, and unilateral facial paralysis) were frequently seen.

Q. Describe in brief toxicity of propylene glycol (PG).

PG is used as an intermediate in the synthesis of polyester fibers and resins, as a component of automotive antifreeze/coolants, and as a deicing fluid for aircraft. As PG is "generally recognized as safe" by the Food and Drug Administration (FDA), it is a constituent of many cosmetics, processed foods, and tobacco products, and serves as a diluent for oral, dermal, and IV drug preparations. The most important routes of exposure in the general population are ingestion and dermal contact with products containing the compound. PG has a very low order of acute and chronic toxicity. No organ system has been identified as a target for acute or chronic injury by PG, and there have been no accounts of human fatalities.

8.4 PETROLEUM PRODUCTS

Q. Describe in brief toxicity of petroleum.

Health effects from exposure to petroleum products vary depending on the concentration of the substance and the length of time that one is exposed. Breathing petroleum vapors can cause nervous system effects (such as headache, nausea, and dizziness) and respiratory irritation. Very high exposure can cause coma and death. Liquid petroleum products which come in contact with the skin can cause irritation and some can be absorbed through the skin. Chronic exposure to petroleum products may affect the nervous system, blood, and kidneys. Gasoline contains small amounts of benzene, a known human carcinogen. Animals exposed to high levels of some petroleum products have developed liver and kidney tumors. Whether specific petroleum products can cause cancer in humans is not known; however, there is evidence that occupationally exposed people in the petroleum refining industry have an increased risk of skin cancer and leukemia.

Petroleum toxicity is more common in domestic and wild animals. Crude petroleum can be released into the environment during well blowouts, leaks at wellheads, pipeline leaks, land and sea shipping disasters, and other events and activities. Emissions can be from venting storage tanks, blowouts of gas wells, burning petroleum that has been spilled, or burning unwanted gaseous material. In general, chemicals associated with petroleum intoxication in cattle are the gaseous, liquid, and solid crude petroleum that contain natural gas, crude oil, and bitumen. Natural gas contains H_2S, other sulfur compounds, methane, and other petroleum hydrocarbons, and is known as sour gas. Sour gas is extremely irritating to the eyes and respiratory tract. Many of the chemicals used have limited toxicological information, and the toxicology of chemical mixtures is unknown.

8.5 GASES

Q. Define gases.

Gas is defined as a state of matter consisting of particles that have neither a defined volume nor a defined shape at standard temperatures and pressures.

8.6 VAPORS

Q. Define vapor.

A vapor represents the gas phase of components from substances that are either solid or liquid at standard temperatures and pressures.

8.7 INHALANTS

Q. What are inhalants?

Inhalants are a broad range of intoxicative drugs whose gases or volatile vapors are breathed in via the nose or mouth. They are taken by room temperature volatilization or from a pressurized container (e.g., nitrous oxide), and do not include drugs that are sniffed after burning or heating. For example, amyl nitrite and toluene—the solvent used in contact cement and model airplane glue—are considered inhalants, but tobacco, cannabis, and crack are not, even though the latter are also inhaled (as smoke).

Q. What are short-term effects of solvent abuse that are inhaled by kids?

Within seconds of inhalation, the user experiences intoxication along with other effects similar to those produced by alcohol. Alcohol-like effects may include slurred speech, an inability to coordinate movements, dizziness, confusion, and delirium. Nausea and vomiting are other common side effects.

Q. What physical damages inhalants cause in the short term?

The physical damages inhalants cause in the short term include the following:
- Drowsiness
- Lack of energy
- Risk-taking behavior

- Light-headedness
- Agitation
- Belligerence (hostility)
- Lack of concern about surroundings or life
- Poor judgment
- Inability to function in school, work, or social situations
- Slurred speech
- Poor reflexes
- Muscle weakness
- Headache
- Poor coordination
- Loss of sensations
- Confusion and delirium
- Nausea and vomiting
- Unconsciousness
- Sudden death.

Q. What physical damages inhalants cause in the long term?

The physical damages inhalants cause in the long term include the following:

- Compulsive use
- Withdrawal
- Unwanted weight loss
- Muscle weakness
- Disorientation
- Inability to concentrate
- Poor coordination
- Irregular or rapid heart rate
- Irritability
- Depression
- Impaired thinking ability
- Dementia (lost contact with reality)
- Lost sense of touch
- Deafness
- Blindness
- Reproductive complications
- Bone marrow injury
- Heart damage
- Lung damage
- Liver damage, including cirrhosis
- Kidney damage
- Damaged nerve cells
- Brain shrinkage.

After heavy use of inhalants, abusers may feel drowsy for several hours and experience a lingering headache. Because intoxication lasts only a few minutes, abusers frequently seek to prolong their high by continuing to inhale repeatedly over the course of several hours. By doing this, abusers can suffer loss of consciousness and death.

Q. Give some examples of the irreversible effects caused by inhaling specific solvents.
- Hearing loss—toluene (paint sprays, glues, dewaxers) and TCE (cleaning fluids, correction fluids)
- Peripheral neuropathies or limb spasms—hexane (glues, gasoline) and nitrous oxide (whipping cream, gas cylinders)
- CNS or brain damage—toluene (paint sprays, glues, dewaxers)
- Bone marrow damage—benzene (gasoline).

Q. What is sudden sniffing death syndrome (SSDS)?

SSDS is the most common killer of inhalant abusers. An especially exciting or frightening hallucination could also trigger SSDS. When the abuser is surprised or startled, he has a sudden surge of the hormone *epinephrine*.

Explanation: Epinephrine is also called adrenaline. Epinephrine aids in regulating the functions of the body that are beyond a person's conscious control, like heart rate. When a person is highly stimulated (by fear or challenge, for example) extra amounts of epinephrine are released into the bloodstream to prepare the body for energetic action. Epinephrine increases blood pressure, heart rate, and cardiac output. The presence of the chemical inhalants in the body makes the heart muscle more sensitive to epinephrine. When the surge of epinephrine reaches the heart, the heart suffers an arrhythmia (irregular heart beat). This massive arrhythmia kills the user in seconds.

Q. What adverse effects inhalants have on the CNS and how?

Many of the chemicals found in commonly abused inhalants cause severe and permanent brain and nerve cell damage. Brain scans of inhalant abusers show dramatic shrinkage in the overall size of the brain. Abusers also lose "white matter" in the brain, which is responsible for conducting nerve impulses throughout the body. The white matter is destroyed because each cell is encased in *myelin*, a *lipid* or fat, and many commonly used inhalants are lipid-solvents, i.e., their purpose is to break down lipids. Chronic inhalant abusers suffer massive CNS damage, which results in dementia (lost contact with reality) and loss of cerebellum function. The cerebellum is the portion of the brain that coordinates movements of the voluntary muscles. Abusers lose the ability to think, reason, learn, and remember. Their gait (way of walking) becomes abnormal and they lose coordination.

Q. How one can know a person has an inhalant abuse?

Here are some signs to look for:
- Paint or stains on body or clothing
- Spots or sores around the mouth

- Red or runny nose
- Watery, red eyes
- Chemical breath odor
- Drunk, dazed, or dizzy appearance
- Drowsiness or unconsciousness
- Nausea, loss of appetite
- Anxiety, excitability, irritability
- Inability to concentrate
- Substance odor on breath and clothes
- Poor muscle control
- Change in sleep patterns
- Prefers group activity to being alone
- Reduced attendance in school
- Lower grades
- Bags or rags containing dried solvents at home or in locker at school
- Discarded containers of various sprays or gases
- Small bottles labeled "incense" (users of butyl nitrite).

8.8 QUESTION AND ANSWER EXERCISES

8.8.1 SHORT QUESTIONS AND ANSWERS

Exercise 1

Q.1 List three organic solvents that can cause hazards and risks.
1. Chloroform
2. Carbon tetrachloride
3. Ethanol.

Q.2 What are the hazards and risks of chloroform?
1. Effective fat solvent, easily ingested, attacks the liver and the brain and nervous system, causing loss of control and anesthesia.
2. Removes natural oils from skin, causing blistering.
3. Dissolves sealants in plumbing systems.
4. Vapors are poisonous, affects the nervous system: not flammable.

Q.3 What are hazards and risks of carbon tetrachloride?
1. Effective fat solvent, easily ingested, attacks the liver and the brain and nervous system, causing loss of control and anesthesia.
2. Removes natural oils from skin, causing blistering.
3. Dissolves sealants in plumbing systems.
4. Liver damage may lead to liver cancer.
5. Not flammable.

Q.4 What are hazards and risks of ethanol?
1. Effective fat solvent, after ingestion attacks the liver and the brain and nervous system, causing loss of control and anesthesia.

2. Dissolves natural oils from the skin.

3. Vapors are poisonous, affects the nervous system.

4. Flammable.

Q.5 List the possible ways global warming could change the climate and ecology of our planet and alter toxic effects of chemicals.

1. Global warming melts the polar ice caps and reduces the size of ice fields; this increases sea levels, affecting the world's coastline.

2. Local changes: Marshlands will become flooded; lakes and rivers increase in size; human settlements become flooded—increased evaporation in dry areas increases desert.

Q.6 What information should appear on a chemical safety card for ethanol?

Ethanol

1. Highly flammable

2. Intoxication if inhaled or ingested

3. Causes drying of the skin or mucous tissues

4. Causes damage to the eyes

5. Is miscible with water.

Q.7 What information should appear on a chemical safety card for ethanoic acid (acetic acid)?

Ethanoic acid

1. Flammable

2. Causes severe burns

3. Causes severe irritation if ingested

4. Irritating odor

5. Miscible with water.

Q.8 Give examples of products containing solvents that are abused by kids.

Examples of products kids abuse to get high include:

Model airplane glue, nail polish remover, cleaning fluids, hair spray, gasoline, the propellant in aerosol whipped cream, spray paint, fabric protector, air conditioner fluid (freon), cooking spray, and correction fluid.

Q.9 How solvents are misused to get high?

These products are sniffed, snorted, bagged (fumes inhaled from a plastic bag), or "huffed" (inhalant-soaked rag, sock, or roll of toilet paper in the mouth) to achieve a high. Inhalants are also sniffed directly from the container.

Q.10 What is Kaposi's sarcoma (KS)?

Amyl and butyl nitrites have been associated with Kaposi's sarcoma (KS), the most common cancer reported among AIDS patients. Early studies of KS showed that many people with KS had used volatile nitrites. Researchers are continuing to explore the hypothesis of nitrites as a factor contributing to the development of KS in HIV-infected people.

8.8.2 MULTIPLE CHOICE QUESTIONS (CHOOSE THE BEST STATEMENT, IT CAN BE ONE, TWO OR ALL OR NONE)

Exercise 2

Q.1 The major toxic effect of hydrogen cyanide exposure is
  a. lung damage
  b. hemoglobin alteration
  c. hemolysis of red blood cells (RBCs)
  d. inhibition of mitochondrial respiration
  e. lipid peroxidation

Q.2 In regard to chemically induced adverse effects on the eye,
  a. no chemical has been shown to cause glaucoma
  b. nonionic detergents damage the eye more than cationic detergents
  c. 2,4-dinitrophenol, corticosteroids, and naphthalene are known to cause cataracts in humans
  d. methanol produces blindness by rendering the cornea and lens opaque
  e. acids usually produce late-appearing ocular toxicity as contrasted to alkalis which produce immediate damage

Q.3 Which of the following agents would NOT likely produce reactive airways dysfunction syndrome?
  a. Carbon monoxide
  b. Chlorine
  c. Ammonia
  d. Toluene diisocyanate
  e. Acetic acid

Q.4 The most serious consequence of crude oil or kerosene ingestion by cattle is
  a. liver damage
  b. kidney damage
  c. aspiration pneumonia
  d. CNS stimulation
  e. leukemia

Q.5 Benzene is similar to toluene
  a. in its metabolism to redox-active metabolites
  b. regarding covalent binding of its metabolites to proteins
  c. in its ability to produce CNS depression
  d. in its ability to produce acute myelogenous leukemia
  e. in its ability to be metabolized to benzoquinone

Q.6 Sorbitol and other sugar alcohols have been associated with
  a. respiratory distress syndrome
  b. osmotic diarrhea
  c. hepatotoxicity
  d. immediate hypersensitivity reaction
  e. CNS depression

Q.7 Chloroform is NOT
   a. CNS depressant
   b. hepatotoxic
   c. metabolized to phosgene
   d. peroxisome proliferator
   e. contaminant of chlorinated water

Q.8 Each of the following solvents is paired with a correct target organ of toxicity EXCEPT
   a. methanol:retina
   b. EG:kidney
   c. EG monomethyl ether:kidney
   d. dichloromethane: CNS
   e. carbon tetrachloride:liver

Q.9 Which of the following is NOT associated with spermatotoxicity in rats?
   a. EG monomethyl ether
   b. EG monoethyl ether
   c. Ethoxy acetic acid
   d. Methoxy acetic acid
   e. PG monomethyl ether

Q.10 Methyl bromide (CH3Br)
   a. is a liquid used primarily as a fumigant
   b. has essentially no warning properties, even at physiologically hazardous concentrations
   c. is extremely flammable
   d. is of greater concern from its oral toxicity than from its inhalation toxicity
   e. would not be expected to be readily absorbed through the lungs

Answers

1. d; 2. c; 3. a; 4. c; 5. c; 6. b; 7. d; 8. c; 9. e; 10. b.

8.8.3 MATCH THE STATEMENTS

Exercise 3

Q. Match the statements in Columns A and B.

Column A	Column B
1. Ethylene glycol	a. Hematopoietic toxicity
2. Benzene	b. Hepatotoxicity
3. Alkylbenzene	c. Reproductive toxicity
4. Methanol	d. Pulmonary toxicity
5. Ethanol	e. CNS toxicity
6. Chlorinated hydrocarbons	f. Ocular toxicity

Answers

Column A	Column B
1. Ethylene glycol	c. Reproductive toxicity
2. Benzene	a. Hematopoietic toxicity
3. Alkylbenzene	e. CNS toxicity
4. Methanol	f. Ocular toxicity
5. Ethanol	b. hepatotoxicity
6. Chlorinated hydrocarbons	d. Pulmonary toxicity

FURTHER READING

ATSDR, 2000. Agency for Toxic Substances and Disease Registry: Toxicological Profile for Toluene. Public Health Service, Atlanta, GA.

ATSDR, 2005. Agency for Toxic Substances and Disease Registry: Toxicological Profile for Carbon Tetrachloride. Public Health Service, Atlanta, GA.

ATSDR, 2006a. Agency for Toxic Substances and Disease Registry: Tox FAQs for Trichloroethylene (TCE). Public Health Service, Atlanta, GA.

ATSDR, 2006b. Agency for Toxic Substances and Disease Registry: Toxicological Profile for 1,1,1-Trichloroethane (Update). Public Health Service, Atlanta, GA.

ATSDR, 2006c. Agency for Toxic Substances and Disease Registry: Toxicological Profile Benzene. Public Health Service, Atlanta, GA.

ATSDR, 2006d. Agency for Toxic Substances and Disease Registry: Toxicological Profile for Xylenes. Public Health Service, Atlanta, GA.

Bruckner, J.V., Satheesh Anand, S., Warren, D.A., 2013. Toxic effects of solvents and vapors. In: Klaassen, C.D. (Ed.), Casarett and Doull's Toxicology: The Basic Science of Poisons, eighth ed. McGraw-Hill, New York, NY, pp. 1031−1112.

Coppock, R.W., Christian, R.G., 2018. Petroleum. In: Gupta, R.C. (Ed.), Veterinary Toxicology: Basic and Clinical Principles, third ed. Academic Press/Elsevier, Amsterdam, pp. 659−674.

Gupta, P.K., 2016. Fundamental in Toxicology: Essential Concepts and Applications in Toxicology. Elsevier/BSP, San Diego, USA (Chapter 20).

Slice, S., Thrall, M.A., Hamar, D.W., 2018. Alcohols and glycols. In: Gupta, R.C. (Ed.), Veterinary Toxicology: Basic and Clinical Principles, third ed. Academic Press/Elsevier, San Diego, USA, pp. 647−658.

Witschi, H., 2010. Pulmonary toxicology. In: second reprint Gupta, P.K. (Ed.), Modern Toxicology: Basis of Organ and Reproduction Toxicity, vol. 2. PharmaMed Press, Hyderabad, India, pp. 277−339.

Poisonous and venomous organisms

CHAPTER OUTLINE

9.1 DEFINITIONS

Q. Define venomous animal.

A venomous animal can produce venom in specialized glands or cells and deliver it either by biting or stinging or in some cases by acquiring or spitting.

Q. Define poisonous animal.

A poisonous animal possesses a toxin(s) within its tissue that can have deleterious effects when ingested.

Q. How one can differentiate toxin, poison, and venom?

- Toxins are proteins that lead to immune reaction.
- Poisons are chemical substances (not injected by biological vector), i.e., if poison is injected by snake it becomes venom.
- Venoms are biological poisons.

Q. What is neurotoxin? Give examples.

Neurotoxins are toxins that are poisonous or destructive to nerve tissue (causing neurotoxicity). *Neurotoxins* are an extensive class of exogenous chemical neurological insults that can adversely affect the function in both developing and mature nervous tissues. For example, king cobra (*Ophiophagus hannah*) (known as hannahtoxin containing α-neurotoxins), sea snakes (Hydrophiinae) (known as erabutoxin), many-banded krait (*Bungarus multicinctus*) (known as α-bungarotoxin), and cobras (*Naja* spp.) (known as cobratoxin).

Illustrated Toxicology. DOI: http://dx.doi.org/10.1016/B978-0-12-813213-5.00009-2

Q. What is the difference between poison and venom?

Poison is contained in the tissues and is delivered through eating, e.g., puffer fish—tetrodotoxin (poison) and must be inhaled, ingested, or delivered via touch, while venom is produced by a specialized gland and is delivered either injected into a wound or through biting or stinging (generally venom will not hurt if delivered in other than this mode, even if you swallow it), e.g., snake venom.

9.2 SNAKES

Q. What is the difference between poisonous and nonpoisonous snakes?

The shape of the head, pupil, fangs, and tail is the biggest and the most easily recognizable feature that can be used to determine the difference between venomous and nonvenomous snakes (Figs. 9.1 and 9.2 A,B).

Q. Classify poisonous snakes.

There are about 3200 species of snakes. Approximately 1300 species are venomous. Venomous snakes are usually defined as those which possess venom glands and specialized venom-conducting fangs, which enable then to

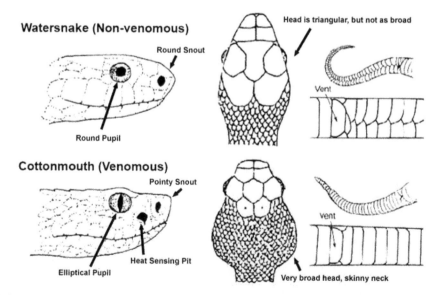

FIGURE 9.1

Difference between poisonous and nonpoisonous snakes.

Reproduced from 247wildlife (http://www.247wildlife.com/images/identify3.jpg).

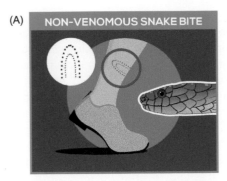
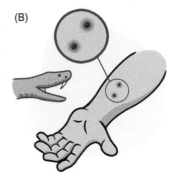

FIGURE 9.2

Bite marks of nonvenomous snakebites (A) and venomous snake bite (B).

(A) Reproduced from Shutterstock https://thumb7.shutterstock.com/display_pic_with_logo/1163873/
540753625/stock-vector-non-venomous-snake-bite-in-the-leg-snakebite-beware-of-snakes-flat-vector-
illustrations-540753625.jpg (B) https://thumb1.shutterstock.com/display_pic_with_logo/2179469/
191494484/stock-vector-first-aid-and-snake-bite-on-arm-191494484.jpg.

inflict serious bites upon their victims. In general, there are five families of venomous snakes recognized:

1. The Colubridae, which possess small rear fangs
2. The Elapidae and Hydrophidae, which possess small front-fanged
3. The viper group, which consists of the Viperidae and Crotalidae.

Venomous snakes are widespread throughout the world. However, they do not occur in several islands such as New Zealand, Ireland, Iceland, the Azores and Canaries.

Q. What is the general nature of snake venom?

Snake venom is highly modified saliva containing zootoxins. It contains more than 20 different compounds, mostly proteins and polypeptides. A complex mixture of proteins, enzymes, and various other substances with toxic and lethal properties serves to immobilize the prey animal. Enzymes play an important role in the digestion of prey, and various other substances are responsible for important but nonlethal biological effects.

Q. Describe the mode of action of neurotoxic venomous snakes.

The venoms of different types of venomous snakes are different in composition. Elapidae and Hydrophidae venoms are rich in neurotoxic polypeptides. These venoms are typically fast acting on nerve tissue and neurotransmitters, often degrading neurotransmitters or depolarizing the axonal membrane for long periods of time, thereby preventing nervous impulses from being conducted.

Q. Describe the mode of action of cardiotoxic venomous snakes.

Cobra cardiotoxins depolarize cardiac cell membranes, which leads to systolic arrest. Cardiotoxic venoms have an affinity for cardiac tissue. These venoms are typically fast acting on nerve tissue and neurotransmitters, often degrading neurotransmitters or depolarizing the axonal membrane for long periods of time, thereby preventing nervous impulses from being conducted.

Q. Describe the mode of action of viper and crotalid neurotoxic venomous snakes.

The venoms of these snakes are neurotoxins that are not membrane depolarizing, but rather are antagonistic to acetylcholine and act as a blocking agent at the neuromuscular junction. Phospholipases, proteases, and lytic factors contained in venom tend to cause hemolytic effects and are largely responsible for the necrosis that follows viper and crotalid bites. Cell metabolism is interrupted by the inhibition of oxidative phosphorylation, which leads to an insufficient supply of ATP for the cell. Mitochondrial electron transport is also interrupted as Q-cytochrome c, an electron acceptor protein in the electron transport chain, is denatured.

Q. Describe the general symptoms of snakebite.

The general symptoms include bloody wound discharge, fang marks or swelling at wound, extreme localized pain, excessive sweating, loss of muscle coordination, blurred vision, numbness or tingling, convulsions, and fainting. Fig. 9.3 shows some of the important organs affected after sting bite.

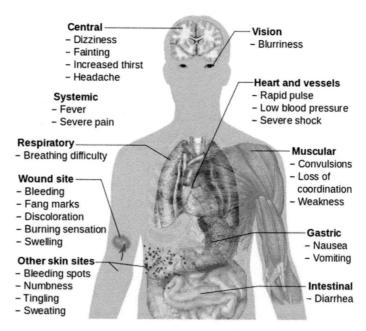

FIGURE 9.3

General symptoms observed after bite of a venomous snake.

Available at Wikimedia Commons. https://upload.wikimedia.org/wikipedia/commons/a/a4/Snake_bite_symptoms.svg.

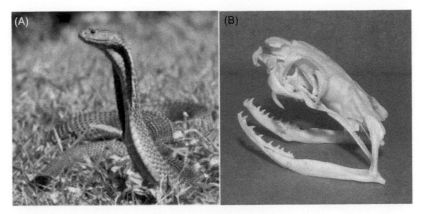

FIGURE 9.4

Naja philippinensis in defensive posture (A) and skull (B).

(A) Available at Wikimedia Commons. https://en.wikipedia.org/wiki/Philippine_cobra. (B) Available at Wikimedia commons. https://upload.wikimedia.org/wikipedia/commons/8/87/Ophiophagus_hannah_skull.jpg.

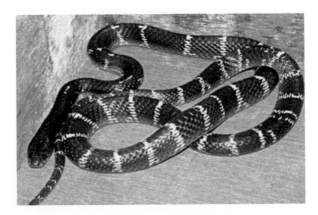

FIGURE 9.5

Venomous snake: Krait.

Available at Wikimedia Commons. https://en.wikipedia.org/wiki/Common_krait.

Q. Describe the order in which muscles are affected after the bite of neurotoxic venomous snake.

The neurotoxic symptoms are common in Elapidae snakes, e.g., krait and cobra (Figs. 9.4 and 9.5).

The toxins act like curare affecting mainly the motor nerve cells and results in muscular paralysis. The muscles are affected in the following order:

First—muscles of mouth

Second—muscles of the throat

Finally—muscles of respiration

Q. What are the local actions of neurotoxic snakebite?

Local manifestations of neurotoxic venoms are severe burning at bite site, rapid edema, and inflammatory changes followed by oozing of serum may be observed.

Q. What are the systemic actions of neurotoxic snakebite?

Systemic action: Within 15—30 minutes to 2 hours of biting, convulsions may be seen with cobra venom, whereas krait venom produces only paralysis. Recovery is complete from paralysis, if patient survives. The flowchart presents the neurotoxic effects of venom produced by neurotoxic venomous snakes (Fig. 9.6). The patient shows giddiness, weakness, lethargy, muscle weakness followed by paralysis and death:

Q. What are the local actions of hemotoxic venomous snakes?

Hemotoxic symptoms are common in Viperidae snakes (Fig. 9.7), e.g., pit viper (Crotalidae); pit-less viper (Russell's viper, saw-scaled viper/phoorsa/*Echis/Echis carinatus*), and bamboo snake (common green pit viper). Local actions are severe pain at bite site, followed by swelling, ecchymosis, cellulitis, and severe hemorrhage.

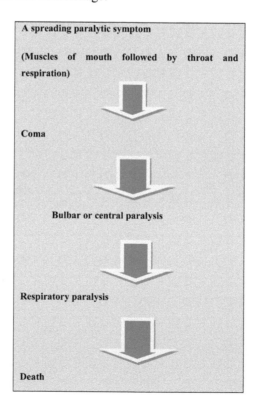

FIGURE 9.6

Schematic representation of symptoms produced by neurotoxic venom.

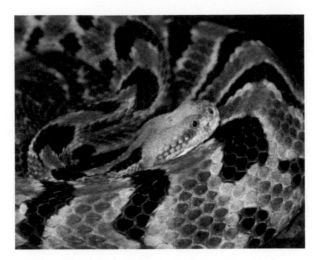

FIGURE 9.7

Hemotoxic venomous snake *Crotalus horridus.*

Wikimedia Commons. https://commons.wikimedia.org/wiki/File:Crotalus_horridus_(1).jpg.

Q. What are the local actions of hemotoxic venomous snakes?

Systemic actions are due to hemolytic effect on heart and blood vessels resulting in cardiovascular collapse and death. If the patient survives suppuration, sloughing with infection at the site of bite, hemorrhage from the mucosa of rectum, other natural orifice, etc., and gangrene of the parts involved can occur. The venom acts by cytolysis of endothelium of blood vessels, lysis of red cells, and other tissue cells and coagulation disorders. This can lead to severe swelling with oozing of blood and spreading cellulitis at bite site. Blood from such patients fails to clot even on adding thrombin, because of very low level of fibrin. This is followed by necrosis of renal tubules and functional disturbances like convulsions, due to intracerebral hemorrhage.

9.3 VENOMOUS ARTHROPODS

Q. Classify arthropods.

There are more than a million species of arthropods, generally divided into 25 orders, of which at least 12 are of importance to humans from an economic standpoint. However, medically, the following orders of venomous or poisonous animals are of importance. These include:

1. Arachnids (scorpions, spiders, whip scorpions, solpugids, mites, and ticks)
2. Myriapods (centipedes and millipedes)

3. Insects—Heteroptera (true bugs), Hymenoptera (ants, bees, wasps, and hornets), Formicidae (ants), Apidae (bees), Vespidae (wasps), Lepidoptera (caterpillars, moths, and butterflies) (water bugs, assassin bugs, and wheel bugs)

4. Beetles (blister beetles).

Q. Define nature of toxins produced by scorpions.

Many scorpions' (Fig. 9.8) venoms contain low-molecular-weight proteins, peptides, amino acids, nucleotides, and salts, among other components. Venom (toxalbumin) having two components, a hemolytic and a neurotoxic fraction.

Q. What are the signs and symptoms of scorpion?

Victim presents with nausea, vomiting, restlessness, fever followed by convulsions, paralysis, coma, and death (due to respiratory paralysis). Neurotoxic factor can mimic strychnine poisoning. Hemolytic factors can mimic viperine snakebite (Fig. 9.8).

Q. Why the stinger is lost due to stinging and results in death of honeybee?

The stinger in honeybees is barbed which gets struck in the victim's skin along with venom sac (Fig. 9.9). Hence, stinger apparatus is lost and results in death of the insect. Wasps can withdraw the stinger as it is not barbed and can sting multiple times (Fig. 9.10).

Q. What is tick paralysis?

Tick paralysis is the only tick-borne disease that is not caused by an infectious organism. The illness is caused by a neurotoxin produced in the tick's salivary gland. For example, ticks such as *Dermacenter* sp. and *Riphicephalus* sp. (Fig. 9.11), after prolonged attachment, the engorged tick transmits the toxin to its host.

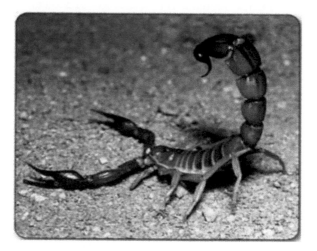

FIGURE 9.8

Poisonous insect: Scorpion.

Available at Robert Frost Middle School. https://room42.wikispaces.com/Desert1Animals.

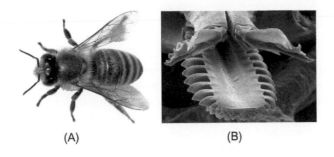

(A)　　　　　　　　　(B)

FIGURE 9.9

Honeybee (A) and stinger of honeybee (barbed) (B).

(A) Reproduced from Shutterstock (https://thumb1.shutterstock.com/display_pic_with_logo/278821/524883124/
stock-photo-detail-of-bee-or-honeybee-in-latin-apis-mellifera-european-or-western-honey-bee-isolated-on-the-
524883124.jpg. (B) Reproduced from American Association for the Advancement of Science. (http://www.
sciencemag.org/sites/default/files/styles/article_main_large/public/images/sn-ticks.jpg?itok=sqYE42-k).

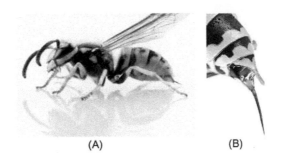

(A)　　　　　　　　　(B)

FIGURE 9.10

Insect wasp (A) and stinger of wasp (unbarbed) (B).

(A) Reproduced from Irabia Plagas (https://encrypted-tbn0.gstatic.com/images?q=tbn:
ANd9GcSACSKPU7ZWc-jd6HvZFmqnyJ6kIUt4TcibUvtaafoV3OqOViTe). (B) Reproduced from Shutterstock
(https://www.shutterstock.com/image-photo/thorn-flesh-81929605?src=AZ3pYVsWXI7S6HsaPOyisA-1-13).

(A)　　　　　　　　　(B)

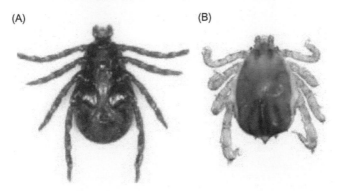

FIGURE 9.11

Important ticks causing tick paralysis. *Dermacenter* sp. (A) and *Riphicephalus* sp. (B).

(A) http://www.vetbook.org/wiki/dog/index.php?title = Dermacentor_spp. (B) https://encrypted-tbn0.gstatic.
com/images?q = tbn:ANd9GcRjSaaOxZsy34Ifw2K8Gjtnm2E_Qj26sSHghORonEZa2eCEgcM4.

Q. Define in brief the nature of toxins of ants.

Fire ant (Fig. 9.12) is the common name for several species of ants in the genus *Solenopsis*. Ant venom is any of, or a mixture of, irritants and toxins inflicted by *ants*. Most *ants* spray or inject a venom, the main constituent of which is formic acid only in the case of subfamily Formicinae. The ants get a grip and then sting (from the abdomen) and inject a *toxic* alkaloid venom called solenopsin, a compound from the class of piperidines.

Q. What are the signs and symptoms of toxicity by fire ants?

In human being signs of toxicity include sterile pustules on the body (Fig. 9.13).

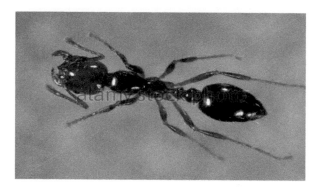

FIGURE 9.12

Fire ant (*Solenopsis*).

http://l7.alamy.com/zooms/0ee1cd49640d458088d931783f8add2d/fire-ants-solenopsis-invicta-adult-close-up-sting-and-bite-causing-d1kpfj.jpg.

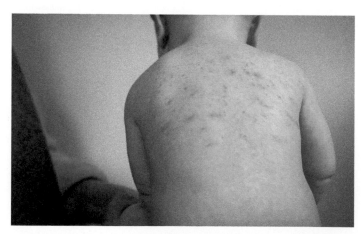

FIGURE 9.13

Sterile pustule—fire ant bite.

Reproduced from Shutterstock (https://thumb1.shutterstock.com/display_pic_with_logo/1334698/682741516/stock-photo-allergies-pimples-on-the-baby-s-skin-food-allergy-skin-diseases-symptoms-682741516.jpg).

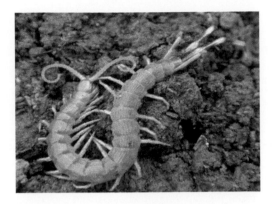

FIGURE 9.14

Poisonous insect: centipede in peat marshland.

Available at Wikimedia Commons. https://en.wikipedia.org/wiki/Centipede.

Q. What are myriapods (Centipedes, chilopoda)?

Myriapods are found worldwide; these elongated, many-segmented (Fig. 9.14), brownish yellow arthropods have a pair of walking legs on most segments. They are fast-moving, secretive, and nocturnal. They feed on other arthropods and even small vertebrates and birds. Centipede venoms contain high-molecular-weight proteins, proteinases, esterases, 5-hydroxytryptamine, histamine, lipids, and polysaccharides. Such venom contains a heat-labile cardiotoxic protein of 60 kDa that produces, in humans, changes associated with acetylcholine release.

Centipedes belong to the class Arthropods and are organic animal irritants. They have a long, segmented, dark to brownish black body with a pair of legs in each segment.

9.4 FISH POISONING

Q. Define fish poisoning.

Fish poisoning is an acute illness resulting from the consumption of fish:
1. Illness due to eating fish that normally contain neurotoxins in their flesh
2. Illness due to eating stale fish either due to histamine or bacterial food poisoning
3. Erysipeloid (dermatitis of the hands due to bacterial infection, occurring mainly among handlers of meat and fish products).

Q. How do we get fish poisoning?

Eating of contaminated fish and seafoods is responsible for fish poisoning. The most common of these are ciguatera poisoning (*Gambierdiscus toxicus*, barracuda fish, Fig. 9.15), scombroid poisoning (mackerel and tuna fish, Fig. 9.16), tetrodotoxins (puffer fish, Fig. 9.17), and various shellfish poisonings (mussels, clams, oysters, and scallops, Fig. 9.18). For example, ciguatera is a

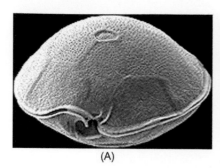
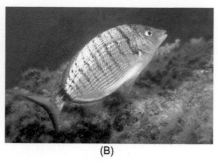

FIGURE 9.15

Source of ciguatoxin toxin: *Gambierdiscus toxicus* (A) and Diplodus puntazzo (B).

(A) Reproduced from National Museum of Natural History Smithsonian Institution under Fair Use (https:// encrypted-tbn0.gstatic.com/images?q=tbn:ANd9GcTCcpRATzugo3Hnl85FVepxm9Stj- zuBNPpSpUYzbdr_xuGi47V), (B) Reproduced from https://commons.wikimedia.org/wiki/File: Diplodus_puntazzo_Guido_Picchetti.jpg.

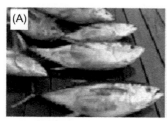
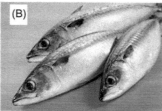

FIGURE 9.16

Source of scombroid poisoning: tuna fish (A) and mackerel fish (B).

(A) https://encrypted-tbn3.gstatic.com/images?q = tbn: ANd9GcQAdx3p2SSNrn4em3rRDmPDkekH1ZELb73kOf3ENOQ3t6Rgg37U. (B) https://encrypted-tbn3. gstatic.com/images?q = tbn:ANd9GcT58jbYvCirjl3ExQbHoyr1UwVZRO_-Rq33QBJirqP9luYfV5CJ1Q.

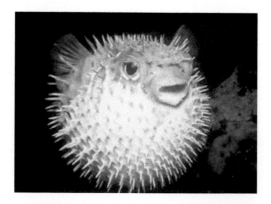

FIGURE 9.17

Puffer fish—source of tetrodotoxin.

https://encrypted-tbn3.gstatic.com/images?q = tbn: ANd9GcToUYbnlfA6iO3v_miJm7puHj3v3xqv70YVYS5G4ASQML8WYfDjQA.

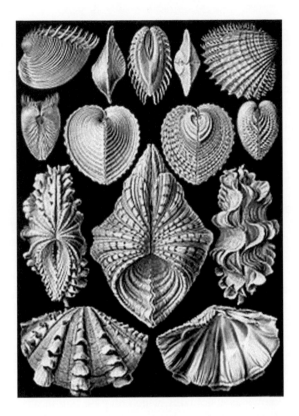

FIGURE 9.18

Paralytic poisoning by shellfishes, the most commonly known to cause poisoning are bivalve shellfishes like mussels, oysters, scallops, cockles, and penshell.

Reproduced from Wikipedia (https://upload.wikimedia.org/wikipedia/commons/thumb/3/31/ Haeckel_Acephala.jpg/220px-Haeckel_Acephala.jpg).

food-borne illness (food poisoning) caused by eating fish that is contaminated by ciguatera toxin. Ciguatera toxin is a heat-stable lipid-soluble compound, produced by dinoflagellates and concentrated in fish organs, that can cause nausea, pain, cardiac, and neurological symptoms in humans when ingested.

Q. What is diarrheic shellfish poisoning (DSP)?

DSP is caused by chemicals of the okadaic acid family (okadaic acid + four related compounds) produced by several species of *Dinophysis dinoflagellates*.

Q. What is ciguatera fish poisoning (CFP)?

CFP is caused by the ciguatoxin family (ciguatoxin + three or more related compounds) and produced by several species of dinoflagellates including *Gambierdiscus*, *Prorocentrum*, and *Ostreopsis*.

9.5 MARINE BITES AND STINGS

Q. What are marine bites and stings?

Some marine bites and stings are toxic, all create wounds at risk for infection with marine organisms, most probable are *Vibrio* and *Mycobacterium* spp. Shark bites result in jagged lacerations with near-total or total amputations, e.g., cnidaria, stingrays, mollusks, and sea urchins.

9.6 MOLLUSKS

Q. What are mollusks?

Mollusks of human interest are known due to their beautiful patterns on their shells. Cone snails were known to Roman scholars and natural history collectors, because the shells were often made into jewelry. The genus *Conus* is a group of approximately 500 species of carnivorous predators found in marine habitats that use venom as a weapon for prey capture. Cone snails (Fig. 9.19) may be divided into three groups depending on preferred prey. The largest group contains worm-hunting species that feed on polychaetes (segmented marine worms in the phylum Annelida).

The second group is molluscivorous and hunts other gastropods. The final group is piscivorous and has venoms that rapidly immobilize fish. There are probably more than 100 different venom components per species. Components have become known as conotoxins, which may be rich in disulfide bonds and conopeptides. Some components have enzymatic activity. Conopeptides also target ligand-gated ion channels that mediate fast synaptic transmission, resulting in poisoning.

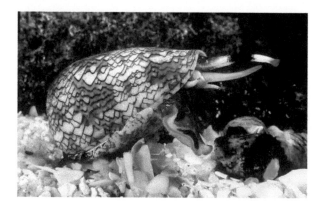

FIGURE 9.19

Australian cone snail.

Available at David Paul, Melbourne University, AAP Image. http://www.australiangeographic.com.au/news/2014/03/cone-snail-pain-drug-is-non-addictive.

9.7 QUESTION AND ANSWER EXERCISES

9.7.1 SHORT QUESTIONS AND ANSWERS

Exercise 1

Q.1 What does the word "predator" mean?

An animal that eats other animals.

Q.2 What does the word "prey" mean?

An animal that is eaten by other animals.

Q.3 Who is usually poisonous, the predator or the prey?

The prey.

Q.4 How is a poisonous animal different from a venomous animal?

Poisonous animal is different from a venomous animal because venomous animals inject their poison into their victim. A predator comes in contact with the poison of a poisonous animal if it touches or eats the animal.

Q.5 Why alcohol is contraindicated in cleaning the area of snakebite?

Alcohol causes vasodilation promoting the spread of the venom in the body.

Q.6 What are the local actions of myotoxic venomous snakes?

Myotoxic venomous snakes produce minimal swelling and pain.

Q.7 What are the systemic actions of myotoxic venomous snakes?

Myotoxic symptoms are common with hydrophidae or sea snakes. The venom produces generalized muscular pain, myalgia, muscular stiffness, myoglobinuria, renal tubular necrosis, and death usually occurs due to respiratory failure.

Q.8 Why snakebite in human beings and dogs is fatal compared to large animals?

Human beings and dogs are relatively smaller in size compared to other large animals like horses and cattle. Hence, the bite is fatal in smaller subjects than the larger ones.

Q.9 Why avoiding reef fish consumption is the only way to avoid ciguatera?

The detection of ciguatoxin is difficult as it does not produce any change in organoleptic properties of fish. Further, ciguatoxin is not destroyed by temperature or gastric acid. Hence, avoiding eating of reef fish is the only way to prevent ciguatera.

Q.10 Why puffer fish are resistant to tetrodotoxin?

Puffer fish have sodium channels with altered structure due to mutation, which are resistant to tetrodotoxin action.

Exercise 2

Q.1 Define toxin.

Toxin (biological definition)—A toxin is a poisonous substance produced within living cells or organisms. Toxins can be small molecules, peptides, or proteins that are capable of causing immune reaction.

Q.2 Define poison.

They are substances that cause disturbances to organisms, usually by chemical reaction or other activity on the molecular scale, when a sufficient quantity is absorbed by an organism.

Q.3 Define venom.

Venoms are toxins that are injected by a bite or sting, this is exclusive to animals.

Q.4 What is cytotoxin?

A *cytotoxin* is any substance that has a toxic effect on cells. Some common examples of cytotoxins include chemical agents and certain snake venoms. Cytotoxins typically attack only a specific type of cell or organ, rather than an entire body.

Q.5 What is cardiotoxins?

Cardiotoxins are components that are specifically toxic to the heart. They bind to particular sites on the surface of muscle cells and cause depolarization, the toxin prevents muscle contraction. These toxins may cause the heart to beat irregularly or stop beating, causing death. Snake example: mambas and some cobra species.

Q.6 What is hemotoxins?

Hemotoxins cause hemolysis, the destruction of red blood cells (erythrocytes), or induce blood coagulation (clotting). Snake example: most vipers and many cobra species. The tropical rattlesnake *Crotalus durissus* produces convulxin, a coagulant.

Q.7 How millipedes do protect themselves?

Millipedes protect themselves by oozing sticky droplets when attacked. These droplets are poisonous.

Q.8 What is amnesic shellfish poisoning (ASP)?

ASP is caused by domoic acid produced by several species of *Pseudonitzschia* diatoms.

Q.9 What is paralytic shellfish poisoning (PSP)?

PSP is caused by the saxitoxin family (saxitoxin + 18 related compounds) produced by several species of *Alexandrium dinoflagellates*.

Q.10 What is neurotoxic shellfish poisoning (NSP)?

NSP is caused by the brevetoxin family including dinoflagellate, *Karenia brevis*, and *Gymnodinium breve*.

9.7.2 FILL IN THE BLANKS

Exercise 3

Q.1 The order under the class Insecta, which includes greatest number of poisonous insect species, is _____.

Q.2 The antigenic component of honeybee venom, which can cause allergies or anaphylactic shock is _____.

Q.3 The drug of choice for treatment of systemic reactions produced by stinging from bees or wasps is _____.

Q.4 The potent cytotoxin present in ant venom is _____.

Q.5 The piperidine alkaloid component of fire ant venom is _____.

Q.6 Focal necrotic ulcers of cornea and conjunctiva in calves are caused by the bite of _____ insect.

Q.7 The most potent neurotoxin present in the venom of black widow spider (*Latrodectus mactans*) is _____.

Q.8 The most dangerous species of scorpion is _____.

Q.9 The most common tick species which are responsible for the development of tick paralysis are _____.

Q.10 Tick paralysis is caused by the injection of _____ which is neurotoxic.

Answers

1. HYMENOPTERA (the important families are Apidae [honeybees]; Vespidae [wasps], and Formicidae [ants]. Stinging from wasps is more common as they dwell in human and animal settlements); 2. MELLITIN; 3. EPINEPHRINE (ADRENALINE); 4. FORMIC ACID; 5. SOLENOPSIN (piperidine alkaloids are also known as hemolytic factors and induce histamine release); 6. FIRE ANTS (*Solenopsis invicta*); 7. α-LACROTOXIN; 8. *LEIURUS QUINQUESTRIATUS* (the venom contains potent neurotoxins); 9. *RIPHICEPHALUS* and *DERMACENTOR* (other species of ticks which can cause tick paralysis include *Ixodes*, *Amblyomma*, and *Ornithodorus*); 10. SALIVA.

Exercise 4

Q.1 The most susceptible species for tick paralysis is _____.

Q.2 The type of paralysis seen in tick paralysis is of _____ type.

Q.3 *Dermacentor* species toxin acts by blocking _____ channels, whereas Ixodidae ticks block the release of _____ in motor nerves.

Q.4 Diagnosis of tick poisoning is made by the detection of _____ sex ticks on the animal body along with the symptoms of paralysis.

Q.5 The venom in toads is produced by _____ glands.

Q.6 The most toxic among the toads is _____.

Q.7 The principal component of toad venom is _____.

Q.8 The animal species which is more prone for toad poisoning is

_____.

Q.9 Treatment of toad poisoning involves the use of _____ drug to control cardiac arrhythmia and fibrillation.

Q.10 Snakebite is commonly observed in _____ and species of animals.

Answers

1. DOG; 2. ASCENDING; 3. SODIUM, ACETYLCHOLINE; 4. FEMALE; 5. PAROTOID; 6. BUFO MARINUS; 7. BUFODIENOLIDES (cardiac glycosides). (the symptoms involve cardiac arrhythmia, ventricular fibrillation, and heart failure); 8. DOG; 9. PROPRANOLOL; 10. DOGS, HORSES.

Exercise 5

Q.1 The type of toxins present in the venom of Elapidae snakes (cobra, krait, mamba, coral snakes) are _____.

Q.2 The type of toxins present in the venom of Viperidae snakes (viper, rattle snake, adder) are _____.

Q.3 α-Bungarotoxin is the neurotoxin present in the venom of _____ snakes.

Q.4 In snakes, the venom glands are homologues to _____ glands in other animals.

Q.5 The symptoms in elapine snakebite are predominantly _____.

Q.6 Diagnosis of snakebite is possible by observing _____ marks on the body of the animal.

Q.7 The main treatment for snakebite is _____.

Q.8 The only poisonous lizard known to cause poisoning in animals and humans is _____.

Q.9 The inclusion of _____ component in feeds can expose animals to fish poisons.

Q.10 The most potent among all marine toxins is _____.

Answers

1. NEUROTOXINS; 2. HAEMOTOXINS; 3. KRAIT; 4. PAROTID; 5. NEUROLOGICAL; 6. FANG; 7. MONOVALENT/POLYVALENT ANTIVENIN (if snake is identified, monovalent antivenin is sufficient otherwise polyvalent antivenin is necessary. Further, during treatment with antivenin, the development of allergic reactions should be controlled using epinephrine); 8. HELODERMA SUSPECTUM (*Gila monster*); 9. FISH MEAL; 10. TETRODOTOXIN (TTX) (TTX is 10 times more toxic than snake venom; 100 times more toxic than black widow spider; 10,000 times more toxic than cyanide).

Exercise 6

Q.1 The eating of _____ fish is commonly associated with tetrodotoxin poisoning.

Q.2 The organs in which tetrodotoxin (TTX) primarily accumulates in puffer fish are _____ and _____.

Q.3 Tetrodotoxin is produced by the bacteria _____, which live symbiotically with puffer fish.

Q.4 Tetrodotoxin acts as a potent neurotoxin through blocking of _____ channel in central and peripheral nervous system.

Q.5 Ciguatera is a fish-borne poisoning resulting from the consumption of _____ fish.

Q.6 The toxin responsible for ciguatera poisoning is _____.

Q.7 Ciguatoxin is produced by the dinoflagellate _____ present in reef fish.

Q.8 Consumption of tuna and mackerel fish is associated with _____ poisoning.

Q.9 Scombroid poisoning is caused by _____ which is produced from histidine by bacterial action.

Q.10 Local toxic effects are more prominent after snakebite of _____.

Answers

1. TETRAODON (puffer)/FUGU; 2. LIVER and OVARY; 3. PSEUDOALTEROMONAS TETRADONIS; 4. SODIUM; 5. REEF FISH (such as barracuda and eel); 6. CIGUATOXIN (CTX); 7. *GAMBIERDISCUS TOXICUS* (similar to TTX, reef fish do not produce CTX, they only possess the toxin); 8. SCOMBROID; 9. HISTAMINE (other compounds such as putrescine and cadaverine are also involved in triggering histamine toxicity); 10. RATTLE SNAKE (the venom in Viperidae (vipers, rattle snake, etc.) snakes is hemotoxic and contains enzymes such as hyaluronidase. Hence, local reactions predominate).

9.7.3 MATCH THE STATEMENTS

Exercise 7

Q. Match the statements in Column A and B

Column A	Column B
1. *Escherichia coli*	a. Mahi mahi
2. Ciguatera poisoning	b. GRAS substance
3. Endotoxin	c. Gram-negative bacteria toxin
4. Emetic toxin	d. Enzyme
5. Fluoride	e. Apple products
6. Scombroid poisoning	f. Beets
7. Iron oxide	g. *Bacillus cereus*
8. Rennet	h. Dinoflagellates
9. Patulin	i. Contaminant in hamburger, meat, raw vegetables
10. High nitrates	j. Osteosclerosis

Answers

Column A	Column B
1. *Escherichia coli*	i. Contaminant in hamburger, meat, raw vegetables
2. Ciguatera poisoning	h. Dinoflagellates
3. Endotoxin	c. Gram-negative bacteria toxin
4. Emetic toxin	g. *Bacillus cereus*
5. Fluoride	j. Osteosclerosis
6. Scombroid poisoning	a. Mahi mahi
7. Iron oxide	b. GRAS substance
8. Rennet	d. Enzyme
9. Patulin	e. Apple products
10. High nitrates	f. Beets

FURTHER READING

Gupta, P.K., 1988. Veterinary Toxicology. Cosmo Publications, New Delhi, India, Chapter 5.

Gupta, P.K., 2014. Essential Concepts in Toxicology. BSP Pvt Ltd, Hyderabad, India, Chapter 28.

Gupta, P.K., 2016. Fundamental in Toxicology: Essential Concepts and Applications in Toxicology. Elsevier/BSP, USA, Chapter 28.

Gwaltney-Brant, S.M., Dunayer, E., Youssef, H., 2012. Terrestrial zootoxins. In: Gupta, R.C. (Ed.), Veterinary Toxicology: Basic and Clinical Principles, second ed. Academic Press/Elsevier, Amsterdam, pp. 969—992.

Merck Veterinary Manual, 2016. Poisonous and Venomous Animals. Merck Research Laboratories, Merck & Co. Inc, Kenilworth, NJ, pp. 3157—3165.

Pillay, V.V., 2008. Comprehensive Medical Toxicology., second ed. Paras Medical Publisher, Hyderabad, India, Chapter 20.

Rao, G.N., 2010. Textbook of Forensic Medicine & Toxicology. Jaypee Brothres Medical Publishers, New Delhi, India, Chapter 33.

Sharma, R.P., Salunkhe, D.K., 2010. Animal and plant toxins. In: second reprint Gupta, P.K. (Ed.), Modern Toxicology: The Adverse Effects of Xenobiotics, vol. 2. PharmaMed Press, Hyderabad, India, pp. 252—316.

Watkins III, J.B., 2013. Properties and toxicities of animal venoms. In: Klaassen, C.D. (Ed.), Casarett and Doull's Toxicology: The Basic Science of Poisons, eighth ed. McGraw-Hill, New York, NY, pp. 1083—1102.

Poisonous foods and food poisonings

10.1 DEFINITIONS

Q. What is food poisoning?

Food poisoning is a vague term. It includes illnesses resulting from ingestion of all foods containing nonbacterial or bacterial products. The nonbacterial products include poisons delivered from plants and animals, and certain naturally occurring toxins. Foods containing such products are, by convention, known as poisonous foods.

Q. Define microbial toxins.

Microbial toxins are toxins produced by microorganisms, including bacteria and fungi. Microbial toxins promote infection and disease by directly damaging host tissues and by disabling the immune system. Some bacterial toxins, such as botulinum neurotoxins, are the most potent natural toxins known.

Q. Define biotoxins.

Biotoxins are the substances which are both toxic and have a biological origin. They come in many forms and can be produced by nearly every type of living organism: there are mycotoxins (made by fungi), zootoxins (made by animals), and phytotoxins (made by plants).

Q. What do you mean by poisonous plant toxins?

The large array of toxic chemicals produced by plants, usually referred to as secondary plant compounds, are often have chemicals that are used as defense

Illustrated Toxicology. DOI: http://dx.doi.org/10.1016/B978-0-12-813213-5.00010-9

mechanisms against herbivorous animals, particularly insects and mammals. For example, a bitter alkaloid poison resembling strychnine and extracted from nuxvomica; hemlock, a poisonous drug derived from a Eurasian plant of the genus *Conium*; mycotoxin, a toxin produced by a fungus.

10.2 MICROBIAL TOXINS

Q. Name at least four toxins and bacteria involved.

Name of Toxin	Bacteria Involved
Botulinum toxin	*Clostridium botulinum*
Tetanus toxin	*Clostridium tetani*
Diphtheria toxin (Dtx)	*Corynebacterium diphtheria*
Exotoxin A	*Pseudomonas aeruginosa*

Q. Define bacterial toxins.

Bacteria generate toxins which can be classified as either exotoxins or endotoxins.

1. Exotoxins are generated and actively secreted.

2. Endotoxins remain part of the bacteria. Usually, an endotoxin is part of the bacterial outer membrane, and it is not released until the bacterium is killed by the immune system. The body's response to an endotoxin can involve severe inflammation. In general, the inflammation process is usually considered beneficial to the infected host, but if the reaction is severe enough, it can lead to sepsis.

Q. What is toxinosis?

Toxinosis is a pathogenesis caused by the bacterial toxin alone, not necessarily involving bacterial infection (e.g., when the bacteria have died, but have already produced toxin, which are ingested). It can be caused by *Staphylococcus aureus* toxins.

Q. What are the three important types of food poisonings?

Microbial food poisoning is of three types:

1. Infectious type

2. Toxic type

3. Botulism

Q. What is infectious type of food poisoning?

In infectious type, the food poisoning results from ingestion of viable microorganisms that multiply in gastrointestinal (GI) tract producing a true infection, e.g., *Salmonella* and *Shigella* group of organisms.

Q. What is toxic type of food poisoning?

In toxic type, the food poisoning results from poisonous substances produced by multiplying organisms that have gained access to the prepared food, e.g., enterotoxin produced by the *Staphylococcus*.

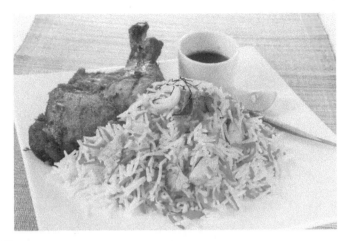

FIGURE 10.1

Food exposed outside may get contaminated and lead to food poisoning.

Reproduced from Shutterstock https://thumb9.shutterstock.com/display_pic_with_logo/4474768/
537424228/stock-photo-a-nicely-served-hyderabadi-chicken-biryani-with-hint-of-lemon-and-chutney-
garnished-with-roasted-537424228.jpg.

Q. What is botulism type of food poisoning?

In botulism type, the food poisoning results from the ingestion of preformed botulinum toxin in the preserved food. The toxin is produced by *C. botulinum.*

Q. What is ptomaine poisoning?

Ptomaine poisoning due to advanced decomposition of food is not common. Ptomaine is proteolytic degradation products formed in decomposing carcasses. Sometimes food exposed outside may get contaminated and lead to food poisoning (Fig. 10.1). There are several main bacteria indicated in ptomaine poisoning, when the term is used interchangeably with food poisoning.

Q. Give three examples of bacteria and germs responsible for food poisoning.

Bacteria and germs responsible for food poisoning are *Escherichia coli, Salmonella* (Fig. 10.2), and listeria. *E. coli* is probably the most dangerous bacterium, usually caused by eating improperly cooked ground beef. Even a little bit of pink in a hamburger can mean possible exposure to *E. coli.*

Q. What are the symptoms of *E. coli* poisoning?

E. coli tends to cause watery diarrhea with no fever. In about 5% of cases, significant kidney failure can develop. The risk is higher in children under age 5 years. When this kidney failure develops, it can cause death. Those who recover may require kidney transplantation or regular dialysis while waiting for a transplant. This very serious complication, though rare, is reason enough to use caution when cooking, preparing, or serving ground beef.

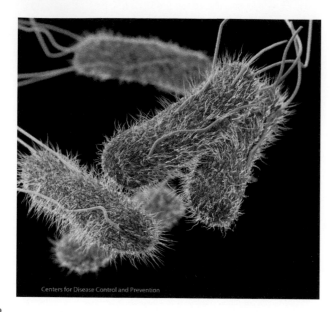

Centers for Disease Control and Prevention

FIGURE 10.2

Salmonella organisms responsible for food poisoning.

Reproduced from Center for Disease Control and Prevention (https://www.cdc.gov/media/subtopic/library/DiseaseAgents/img18.jpg).

Q. Describe the common signs and symptoms of food poisoning.

There is a great variation in the susceptibility of individuals to *Salmonella* food poisoning. Hence, while some participants may remain free from symptoms, others may be severely affected. It is usually self-diagnosable. Food poisoning symptoms may include cramping, nausea, vomiting, or diarrhea. Three characteristics that help to differentiate this poisoning with *staphylococcal* enterotoxin are muscular weakness, fever, and very foul-smelling persistent diarrhea. Severe poisoning may show convulsions, muscle paralysis, and death (Fig. 10.3).

10.3 MYCOTOXINS

The toxicity of mycotoxins is also covered in Chapter 15, Veterinary Toxicology.

Q. What are common mycotoxins that cause poisoning?

They include:

1. The ergot alkaloids produced by *Claviceps* sp.
2. Aflatoxins and related compounds produced by *Aspergillus* sp.
3. The tricothecenes produced by several genera of fungi imperfecti, primarily *Fusarium* sp.

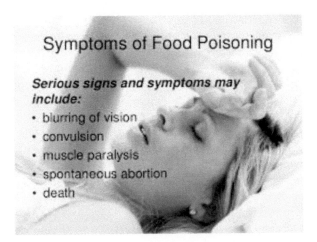

FIGURE 10.3

Symptoms of food poisoning.

https://encrypted-tbn0.gstatic.com/images?q = tbn:ANd9GcRLMa4L9ey91wMInzkqhXmSBsq-Cy9OBGDhwSGdpkIbp1uTdPkvSg

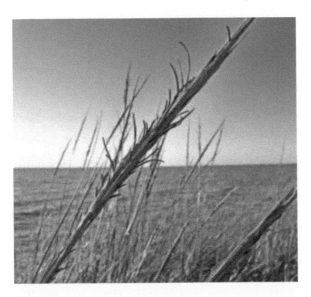

FIGURE 10.4

Fungus *C. purpurea* on rye.

https://media4.picsearch.com/is?I8VTp7WpHIz326esVHyJorSwavwiJWIqIZ0Uj-JnoA4&height=281.

Q. Describe the common name and properties of ergot.

The common name of ergot is mother of rye. Ergot is an alkaloid. It is the sclerotium (mycelium) of a fungus *Claviceps purpurea*, which grows on many cereals like rye, barley, wheat, and oat. Fungus gradually replaces the whole grain to a dark purple mass, which on drying yields ergot (Fig. 10.4).

Q. What are the toxic principles of ergot?

    The active toxic principles are ergotamine, ergotoxin, and ergometrine. They are known to contract arterioles which can lead to gangrene of the part supplied.

Q. What are the acute toxicity signs and symptoms of ergot?

    Acute poisoning is very rare. Some of the common symptoms include irritation of throat, dryness, severe thirst, nausea and vomiting, diarrhea, pain in abdomen, tingling in hands and feet, cramps in muscles (all due to contraction of smooth muscles), dizziness, and feeling of coldness. Sometimes symptoms of hypoglycemia, anuria, abortion, and hemorrhages in a pregnant woman may be seen. Death is usually slow.

Q. What are the chronic toxicity signs and symptoms of ergot?

    Chronic poisoning is called ergotism and is quite common.

    It occurs in two forms:

1. Convulsive form: *Shows* painful toxic contraction of voluntary muscles followed by drowsiness, headache, giddiness, madness, etc. Victim may complain of feeling of itching/numbness and ant crawling sensation under the skin.

2. Gangrenous form: Begins as pustules and swelling of limbs and feet, followed by intense hot feeling, severe pain, numbness, etc. followed by gangrenous changes (resemble Raynaud's disease). Recovery is possible, if ergot is withheld.

    The ergot alkaloids are known to affect the nervous system and cause vasoconstriction. The ergot alkaloids are derivatives of ergotine, the most active being, more specifically, amides of lysergic acid.

Q. How are tricothecenes produced?

    Tricothecenes are produced particularly by members of the genera *Fusarium* and *Tricoderma*.

Q. What do you know about *Penicillium* fungi?

    Penicillium fungi are often blue. They are responsible for food spoilage and are commonly known as molds. They are excellent at growing in low humidity environments, while allows for them to remain alive in food storage. Many of these species produce toxins that may cause food poisoning. However, *Penicillium* fungi also are of some benefit to humans (besides production of the antibiotic). They are used in the production of certain cheeses, including Roquefort, Brie, Camembert, and Stilton. *Penicillium* spores were among the most prevalent spores in indoor air. The indoor spore levels were higher even than outdoor levels (Figs. 10.5 and 10.6).

Q. How are rubratoxins produced?

    Rubratoxins are produced by *Penicillium rubrum*.

Q. Describe in brief three main *Aspergillus* sp. that are potentially toxic.

    Mycotoxins are fungal secondary metabolites that are potentially harmful to animals or humans. The word "aflatoxin" came from "*Aspergillus flavus*

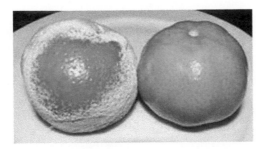

FIGURE 10.5

Some *Penicillium* mold on mandarin oranges.

*https://upload.wikimedia.org/wikipedia/commons/thumb/d/d4/Penicilliummandarijntjes.jpg/440px-
Penicilliummandarijntjes.jpg.*

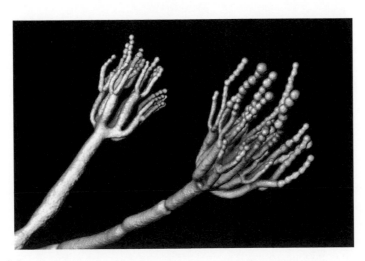

FIGURE 10.6

View of *Penicillium* fungi.

*Reproduced from Shutterstock https://image.shutterstock.com/z/stock-photo-fungi-penicillium-which-cause-
food-spoilage-and-are-used-for-production-of-the-first-antibiotic-727124323.jpg.*

toxin." Three predominant species responsible for aflatoxin poisoning are (Figs. 10.7–10.9):

1. *Aspergillus flavus*
2. *Aspergillus parasiticus*
3. *Aspergillus fumigatus*

Q. What are aflatoxins?

Aflatoxins are the products of species of the genus *Aspergillus*; common fungi found as a contaminant of grain, maize, peanuts, and so on.

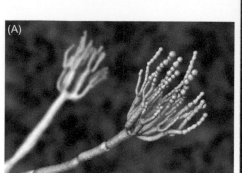
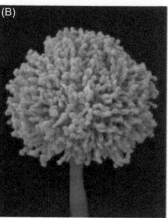

FIGURE 10.7

Aspergillus parasiticus (A) and *Aspergillus flavus* (B).

(A) Reproduced from Shutterstock (https://www.shutterstock.com/th/image-illustration/fungi-penicillium-which-cause-food-spoilage-728468668)

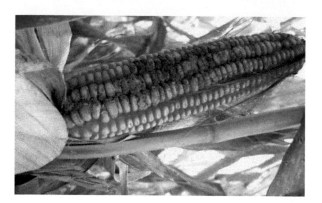

FIGURE 10.8

Aspergillus flavus on maize—source of aflatoxins.

Reproduced from United States Department of Agriculture.

Q. What are the main toxic potentials of aflatoxins?

Aflatoxins are extremely potent liver toxins and carcinogens, and are considered the most hazardous of all the mycotoxins. The compounds are resistant to destruction by heat, and ingestion can be dangerous since the toxins can build up if ingested regularly.

Q. What are four major aflatoxins and metabolic derivatives?

There are four major aflatoxins:

Aflatoxin B1, B2, G1, and G2.

Additionally, there are two metabolic derivatives:

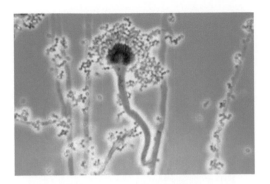

FIGURE 10.9

A. fumigatus.

http://upload.wikimedia.org/wikipedia/commons/4/4f/Aspergillus.jpg.

Aflatoxin M1 (derivative of B1)
Aflatoxin M2 (derivative of B2)

Q. Name the hormone that is inhibited by zearalenone, which is involved in ovarian follicle maturation.

Follicle-stimulating hormone (FSH). Due to this the characteristic symptom of follicular atresia is observed in ovaries.

10.4 MUSHROOM TOXICITY

Q. What do you mean by mushroom toxicity?

Mushrooms are fungi with umbrella-shaped tops and stems, e.g., *Stropharia semiglobata*, *Hypholoma fasciculare*, and *Lactarius vellereus* are among the poisonous varieties of mushrooms. The toxic mushroom *Amanita muscaria*, commonly known as "fly agaric," is shown in Fig. 10.10.

Mostly "poisonous" mushrooms effect GI tract but usually does not cause any long-term damage. However, there are a number of recognized mushroom toxins with specific, and sometimes deadly, effects.

Q. Describe in brief mushroom poisoning symptoms.

The symptoms usually appear within 20 minutes to 4 hours of ingesting the mushrooms, and include nausea, vomiting, cramps, and diarrhea, which normally pass after the irritant had been expelled. Some mushrooms contain Psilocybin which may cause hallucinations, tachycardia, and hypertension. Some mushrooms cause muscarinic symptoms such as miosis, diarrhea, and bradycardia. Members of *Amanita* genera cause hypoglycemia, hepatic and renal failures. Severe cases may require hospitalization.

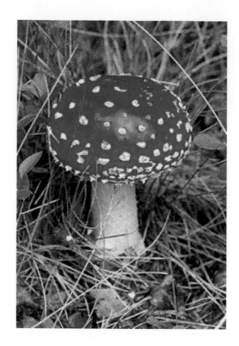

FIGURE 10.10

The toxic mushroom *A. muscaria*, commonly known as "fly agaric."

https://upload.wikimedia.org/wikipedia/commons/thumb/c/c2/Amanita_muscaria_%28fly_agaric%29.JPG/
330px-Amanita_muscaria_%28fly_agaric%29.JPG.

10.5 ALGAL INTOXICATION

Q. Define algal toxins.

Algal toxins are broadly defined to represent the chemicals derived from many species of *cyanobacteria* (blue-green bacteria), *dinoflagellates*, and *diatoms*. The toxins produced by these freshwater and marine organisms often accumulate in fish and shellfish inhabiting the surrounding waters, causing both human and animal poisonings, as well as overt fish kills (Fig. 10.11). Unlike many of the microbial toxins, algal toxins are generally heat stable and, therefore, not altered by cooking methods, which increases the likelihood of human exposures and toxicity.

Q. What are cyanobacterial (blue-green bacteria) toxins?

Cyanobacterial (blue-green bacteria) toxins are produced (biotoxins and cytotoxins) by several species of cyanobacteria.

Q. What are Ambush predator toxins?

Ambush predator (*Pfiesteria piscicida* and toxic *Pfiesteria* complex) toxins are produced by several dinoflagellate species.

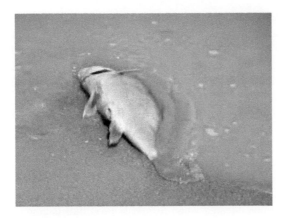

FIGURE 10.11

A dead fish surrounded by algae.

http://www.regions.noaa.gov/great-lakes/wp-content/uploads/2015/07/dead-fish-algal-bloom-1024x774.jpg.

Q. Define harmful algal bloom (HAB).

Harmful algal blooms or HABs are algal blooms composed of phytoplankton known to naturally produce biotoxins; they can occur when certain types of microscopic algae grow quickly in water, forming visible patches that may harm the health of the environment, plants, or animals.

Q. Describe the mode of action of tetrodotoxin.

Tetrodotoxin causes paralysis by affecting the sodium ion transport in both the central and peripheral nervous systems. A low dose of tetrodotoxin produces tingling sensations and numbness around the mouth, fingers, and toes. Higher doses produce nausea, vomiting, respiratory failure, difficulty walking, extensive paralysis, and death.

Q. List four methods by which chemicals enter our food and give an example of each.

   1. *Packaging materials*: Substances such as plasticizers, stabilizers, and inks can enter our food through migration from the packaging, e.g., antimony from chipped enamel container, cadmium from trays and containers, and lead from the solder of metal containers and cans.

   2. *Agricultural application of pesticides and fertilizers*: Organochlorides, such as dichlorodiphenyltrichloroethane (DDT), which is used to control insects and fungi.

   3. *Food additives for preservation and coloring*: Monosodium glutamate (MSG) to enhance flavor in Chinese food, nitrates which give meat their taste and color, and colorings, i.e., Red Dye No. 2 which may be a carcinogen.

   4. *Industrial processes*: Mercury as a by-product of many processes is an acute toxin which causes neurological complications and birth defects, and polychlorinated biphenyls, PCBs.

Q. The rise of many new and old food-borne pathogens coincides with changes in diet and food processing. Describe at least four of these changes.

1. Processing of milk has caused a decrease in certain competitive bacteria, thereby increasing the chances of survival for *Salmonella* and *Campylobacter*.

2. Water polluted with raw sewage and manure, carrying harmful microbes, comes in contact with food.

3. Abuse of antibiotics has allowed some bacteria to acquire antibiotic resistance.

4. Increase in demand for packaged food supports anaerobic pathogens such as *Clostirida*.

5. Ready-to-eat foods that only require minimal heating increases the survivability of bacteria by not destroying the pathogen.

Q. Describe the life cycle of the pork tapeworm, *Taenia solium*.

A pig becomes infested when it ingests food that is contaminated with human fecal matter that contains tapeworm eggs. The larvae excyst in the intestine and migrate through the bloodstream where they encyst in the muscles. Here they develop into cysterici which contain a scolex, or inverted head of the worm. Humans then ingest undercooked pork and the larvae excyst in the intestine where the scolex attaches to the intestine wall. Here it grows and produces a chain of proglottids. Each mature proglottid produces eggs, which are carried in human fecal matter. If a person ingests the eggs from an infected person, the eggs can then enter the bloodstream and migrate throughout the body to the brain, eyes, and muscles of the human.

Q. List at least five factors commonly found to be the cause of food-borne illness, which are largely preventable.

1. Improperly refrigerated food

2. Improperly heated or cooked food

3. Food handlers with poor hygiene

4. Lapse of time (more than a day) between preparing and serving food

5. Improper storage of foods at temperatures ideal for bacteria growth. Introducing raw (or contaminated) materials into a food that will not undergo further cooking.

1. Failing to properly heat previously cooked foods to temperatures that will kill bacteria.

2. Cross-contamination of foods with raw foods, contaminated utensils, or mishandling of foods.

10.6 QUESTION AND ANSWER EXERCISES

10.6.1 SHORT QUESTIONS AND ANSWERS

Exercise 1

Q.1 How does food poisoning spread?

- The food can be contaminated during growth, production, processing, shipping, and preparation; this preparation can include slaughtering of the animal, cutting into small parts which can become contaminated by the feces of the animal.

- There could also be "cross-contamination," a situation in which the platform used for cutting poultry for example is used for cutting vegetables and fruits without thorough cleansing first.
- Food can be contaminated by flies, by infected food handlers, or by food handlers whose hands became contaminated by touching items previously handled by infected persons and forgetting to wash their hands thoroughly with soap and water.

Q.2 What is "cross-contamination"?

The process by which bacteria or other microorganisms are unintentionally transferred from one substance or object to another, with harmful effect is known as cross-contamination. Cross-contamination between raw and cooked food is the cause of most infections.

Q.3 When do you suspect you may have food poisoning?

One can suspect food poisoning if:

1. one develops vomiting and/or diarrhea with severe abdominal pains a few hours after eating at a gathering foods such as vegetable salads, fairly cooked meat/poultry, or canned food;
2. if the stooling and/or vomiting are severe.

Q.4 What can put you at risk of food poisoning?

The following can put you at risk:

1. Age (more severe and commoner in old age and childhood)
2. Pregnancy
3. Chronic diseases with reduced immunity.

Q.5 How can you prevent food poisoning?

You can prevent food poisoning by:

1. Being careful about what you eat at parties, avoid salads
2. Preparing your food hygienically
3. Cooking your meat/poultry thoroughly and eat your food while hot
4. Always washing your hands with soap and water before preparing food
5. Covering your food if not ready to eat
6. Reading carefully the label on canned food
7. Cleaning your work top after dealing with animal products (meat, poultry) before preparing vegetables and fruits
8. Always boiling your milk before consumption.

Q.6 Only a large amount of harmful bacteria can cause food poisoning. Write whether statement is right or wrong, give explanation.

Wrong. Some food poisonings can be caused by very tiny amounts of bacteria in the food.

Q.7 Is it possible to get food poisoning from ice cubes?

Yes. Deep freezing or freezing does not even nearly kill all harmful microbes in food or water even though some microbes may die. If there are harmful microbes in an ice machine or in water being used in ice cubes, they may also appear in the ice cubes and possibly cause food poisoning.

Q.8 Does temperature affect the reproduction of microbes?

Temperature is one of the factors affecting the reproduction of microbes. The reproduction of microbes becomes more effective when the temperature is favorable for them.

Q.9 What is the source of tetrodotoxin?

Tetrodotoxin is a naturally occurring toxin that has been responsible for human intoxications and fatalities. Its usual route of toxicity is via the ingestion of contaminated puffer *fish* which are a culinary delicacy, especially in Japan.

Q.10 What do you mean by chemical poisoning?

Chemical food poisoning is caused by eating plant or animals that contain a naturally occurring toxin containing chemicals such as acetylcholine, alkaloids, serotonin, histamines, sulfur, lipids, phenols, and glycosides. Chemical food poisoning often involves mushrooms, poisonous plants, or marine animals.

Q.11 List the SEVEN key principles of HACCP (hazard critical control point).

1. Assessing hazards
2. Identifying critical control points (CCPs)
3. Setting up procedures and standards for CCPs
4. Monitoring CCPs
5. Taking corrective actions
6. Setting up record-keeping system
7. Verifying that system works.

10.6.2 MULTIPLE CHOICE QUESTIONS (CHOOSE THE BEST STATEMENT, IT CAN BE ONE, TWO OR ALL OR NONE)

Exercise 2

Q.1 Which of the following is NOT true regarding *Amanita phalloides* mushrooms?

a. Toxic components are phalloidin and amatoxins.
b. Produces liver and GI toxicity.
c. Cardiovascular toxicity is responsible for mortality.
d. Common name is "death cap."
e. No specific antidotal treatment of poisoning is available.

Q.2 The following feed stuff supports growth of aflatoxins:

a. Groundnut cake
b. Soybean cake
c. Cotton seed meal
d. All

Q.3 Aflatoxin has the following character(s):

a. Carcinogenic
b. Mutagenic

c. Teratogenic

d. Immunosuppressive

Q.4 Which of the following forms of aflatoxicosis is most common?

   a. Per acute

   b. Acute

   c. Subacute

   d. Chronic

Q.5 Rubratoxins are destroyed at the following temperature:

   a. Freezing

   b. Room temperature

   c. 50–60°C

   d. 85–100°C

Q.6 The site of action of ochratoxins in the nephron is

   a. proximal convoluted tubule

   b. loop of Henle

   c. distal convoluted tubule

   d. collecting duct

Q.7 Which of the following serotype(s) of botulinum is/are most commonly implicated in animals and poultry?

   a. A-type

   b. B-type

   c. C-type

   d. D-type

Q.8 Which of the following toxicities are infectious?

   a. Botulism

   b. Tetanus

Q.9 The type of skeletal muscle contractions seen in tetanus are

   a. Clonic

   b. Tonic

   c. Both

   d. Twitching

Q.10 What is the correct temperature that frozen food should be kept at?

   a. 0°C

   b. 15°C or lower

   c. 18°C or lower

   d. 20°C or lower

Answers

1. c; 2. d; 3. d (hence aflatoxins are considered more dangerous than other myco-toxins); 4. d. (chronic form occurs due to continuous intake of low level of afla-toxins); 5. d (85–100°C for 2 hours can destroy rubratoxins); 6. a (proximal convoluted tubule. Inhibits anion transport and damages renal brush border); 7. c and d (type C and D botulinum toxins are mostly implicated in animals and birds); 8. b (tetanus can spread from one animal to another, whereas botulism is a

food-borne toxicity); 9. b (tonic muscle contraction without twitching seen in tetanus is called tetany); 10. c.

Exercise 3

Q.1 In the case history of the young woman who was finally diagnosed with parasitic diseases, what was the screening test used to finally discover her illness?
  a. Pap smear
  b. Cardiography
  c. Rectal smear
  d. X-ray

Q.2 A major mode of transmission of food-borne illnesses is
  a. via mosquito transmission
  b. via fecal−oral route
  c. via person to person contact
  d. via hypodermic syringes

Q.3 Which of the following is/are economic consequence(s) of food-borne illness?
  a. Medical costs
  b. Investigative costs
  c. Loss of wages
  d. Litigation costs
  e. All of the above

Q.4 Of those listed below, which is not a food-borne pathogen?
  a. Lectins
  b. Nematodes
  c. Bacteria
  d. Protozoans

Q.5 Which of the following chemicals in food can cause significant neurological complications (may choose more than one)?
  a. Mercury
  b. Lead
  c. Cadmium
  d. Antimony

Q.6 GRAS substances are those substances added to food that are
  a. generally responsible for acute sickness
  b. government reported assumed safe
  c. general response acidosis sickness
  d. generally recognized as safe

Q.7 All of the following are gram-negative bacteria except
  a. *Staphylococcus aureus*
  b. *Escherichia coli*
  c. *Salmonella typhimurium*
  d. *Vibrio cholerae*

Q.8 Acidic conditions will leach all but which of the following from packaging material?
   a. Lead
   b. Cadmium
   c. Antimony
   d. Mercury

Q.9 *T. solium* (pork tapeworm) has more serious consequences than *Taenia saginata* (beef tapeworm) because
   a. it has a hooked rostellum that attaches it to the intestine wall
   b. it can migrate to the brain, eyes, and muscles
   c. it can be ingested from the waste of another human
   d. all of the above

Q.10 Of those listed below, which is not a protozoan?
   a. *Cryptosporidium*
   b. *Entamoeba histolytica*
   c. *Penicillium* spp.
   d. *Giardia lamblia*

Answers

1. c; 2. b; 3. e; 4. a; 5. a and b; 6. d; 7. a; 8. d; 9. d; 10. c.

Exercise 4

Q.1 *Hepatitis A* can be transferred via
   a. the fecal oral route
   b. shellfish from polluted water
   c. intravenous drug users
   d. food handling by infected workers
   e. all of the above

Q.2 Heterocyclic amines and acrylamide are food contaminants which
   a. are produced by microorganisms
   b. are produced by the process of cooking
   c. are considered as GRAS
   d. are residues from animal feeds

Q.3 The concepts of "de minimis" as applied to food safety means
   a. find the smallest harmful dose
   b. only food colors 1/100 of the no-observed adverse-effect level (NOAEL) can be used
   c. pesticide residues can be present at the acceptable daily intake (ADI)
   d. the risk is so small it is of no concern

Q.4 The primary reason for adding nitrates and nitrites to food is to
   a. prevent the growth of *C. botulinum*
   b. give the meat a characteristic flavor
   c. turn the meat a brown-red color
   d. sweeten the food product

Q.5 Where should raw meat be stored in a refrigerator?
  a. At the top
  b. In the middle
  c. At the bottom, below all other food

Q.6 What is the ideal temperature for pathogens to flourish?
  a. 10°C
  b. 37°C
  c. 55°C
  d. 90°C

Q.7 Which of the following is true about bacteria?
  a. Bacteria multiplies and grows faster in warm environments.
  b. Bacteria needs air to survive.
  c. Every type of bacteria can give people food poisoning.
  d. By freezing food you can kill bacteria.

Q.8 How can you tell if food has enough bacteria to cause food poisoning?
  a. It will smell.
  b. You cannot, it will appear normal.
  c. It will have a different color.
  d. It will taste different.

Q.9 Which of the following do bacteria need to assist it to grow and multiply?
  a. Water
  b. Food
  c. Warm temperatures
  d. All of the above

Answers

1. e; 2. b; 3. d; 4. a; 5. c (it should be covered to stop juices dripping from it onto other food stuff); 6. b; 7. a; 8. b (contaminated food CANNOT be identified by smell, taste, or looks, unless it is under a microscope); 9. d.

10.6.3 FILL IN THE BLANKS

Exercise 5

Q.1 The secondary metabolites of fungus which cause deleterious effects to animal and human life is called as _____.

Q.2 Molds generally grow in stored fed stuffs containing a moisture content more than _____.

Q.3 Mycotoxins are classified based on _____ affected.

Q.4 Turkey X disease is caused by mycotoxins _____.

Q.5 Aflatoxins are produced by _____ and _____.

Q.6 The most potent among the aflatoxins is _____.

Q.7 Aflatoxins are heat resistant but are unstable in _____.

Q.8 Aflatoxin producing molds grow in stored feed stuffs which contain moisture content more than ------------------------.

Q.9 The domestic species of animal which is highly susceptible for aflatoxicosis are ------------- and ------------------.

Q.10 The metabolite of aflatoxins that is excreted in milk and urine is --------------------.

Answers

1. MYCOTOXINS; 2. 15% (the other factors being a relative humidity of >85% and optimum temperature of 25–30°C, i.e., without refrigeration); 3. ORGAN SYSTEM (hepatotoxic—aflatoxins, rubra toxins; nephrotoxic—ochratoxin, citrinin; estrogenic—zearalenone (F-2); cytotoxic—trichothecenes (T-2); neurotoxic—tremorgens); 4. AFLATOXIN; 5. *ASPERGILLUS FLAVUS, A. PARASITICUS*; 6. AFB1 (the other being AFB2, AFG1, and AFG2. The letters B (blue) and G (green) represent the type of light under which the respective toxin exhibits the fluorescence); 7. UV LIGHT; 8. 15%; 9. DOG and DUCKLINGS; 10. AFM1.

Exercise 6

Q.1 The aflatoxins content in cattle feeds should not exceed _____.

Q.2 The carcinogenic metabolite formed in the body from aflatoxins is _____.

Q.3 Aflatoxins causes defective protein synthesis by binding with _____ residue of DNA causing mispairing of nucleotides.

Q.4 Aflatoxin epoxide causes carcinogenic and mutagenic effect by causing _____ of the strands of DNA. (alkylation forms cross-bridges between DNA strands).

Q.5 Hemorrhage in aflatoxicosis is due to the decrease in _____ and _____.

Q.6 The type of carcinoma caused by aflatoxins is _____.

Q.7 Aflatoxins can be detected by _____ method.

Q.8 Hemorrhagic syndrome in poultry is caused by _____ mycotoxins.

Q.9 Rubratoxins are produced by _____ and _____.

Q.10 The most toxic metabolite of rubratoxins is _____.

Answers

1. 20 ppb; 2. AFLATOXIN 8, 9-EPOXIDE (aflatoxins need biological activation to produce their toxic effects, i.e., lethal synthesis); 3. N-7 GUANINE; 4. ALKYLATION; 5. PROTHROMBIN and VITAMIN K; 6. HEPATOCELLULAR CARCINOMA; 7. THIN LAYER CHROMATOGRAPHY; 8. RUBRATOXINS; 9. *PENICILLIUM RUBRUM* and *PENICILLIUM PURPUROGENUM*; 10. RUBRATOXIN B (rubratoxin B is hepatotoxic, mutagenic, and teratogenic).

Exercise 7

Q.1 Ruminant's facial eczema is caused by _____ mycotoxicosis.

Q.2 The most potent nephrotoxic mycotoxins which cause mold nephrosis or mycotoxic nephropathy are _____.

Q.3 Ochratoxins are produced by _____ and _____.

Q.4 The most toxic among the ochratoxins is _____.

Q.5 The most susceptible species for ochratoxicosis are _____ and _____.

Q.6 The level of ochratoxin in feed should not exceed _____.

Q.7 An example for estrogenic mycotoxin which can cause reproductive disorders is _____.

Q.8 Zearalenone (F-2) toxins are produced by _____ mold.

Q.9 The most susceptible species for zearalenone toxicosis is _____.

Q.10 Vulvovaginitis of hyperestrogenic syndrome in pigs is caused due to _____ mycotoxin.

Answers

1. SPORIDESMIN; 2. OCHRATOXINS; 3. *ASPERGILLUS OCHRACEUS* and *PENICILLIUM VIRIDICATUM*; 4. OCHRATOXIN A; 5. BIRDS and PIG; 6. 10 ppb; 7. ZEARALENONE (F-2); 8. *FUSARIUM ROSEUM*; 9. PIG; 10. ZEARALENONE.

Exercise 8

Q.1 The maximum permitted level of zearalenone in feed is _____.

Q.2 The histological picture of uterus and vaginal in zearalenone toxicosis is _____.

Q.3 Alimentary toxic aleukia (ATA) in human being is caused by _____ mycotoxins.

Q.4 The mycotoxins that were used as biological warfare agents are _____.

Q.5 The species of animal which is more susceptible to trichothecenes is _____.

Q.6 An example for neurotoxic mycotoxin is _____.

Q.7 The most potent among the tremorgens is _____.

Q.8 The most susceptible species for tremorgen mycotoxins are _____ and _____

Q.9 Staggers syndrome in cattle is produced by _____ mycotoxins.

Q.10 Ergotoxins are produced by the mold _____.

Answers

1. 10 ppb; 2. METAPLASIA; 3. TRICHOTHECENES (trichothecenes commonly includes T-2 toxin, DON, and DAS. DON—deoxy-nevalenol (vomition) and DAS—diacetoxy-scirpenol); 4. TRICHOTHECENES (alleged "yellow rain" attacks of Vietnam on local tribes, which were supported by United States);

5. CAT; 6. TREMORGENS (the name "tremorgens" indicates muscle tremors produced by the toxins due to CNS effects); 7. PENITREM A; 8. CATTLE and DOG;9. TREMORGEN; 10. *CLAVICEPS PURPUREA* (important ergot alkaloids are ergotamine and ergometrine).

Exercise 9

Q.1 Feeding of _____ grass most commonly causes ergotism in cattle.

Q.2 Ergot alkaloids are partial agonist for _____ receptors.

Q.3 The ergot alkaloid which has oxytocic effect on uterus is _____ or _____.

Q.4 Acute egotism is manifested as NERVOUS form while chronic ergotism is manifested as _____ form.

Q.5 The type of ergotism commonly found in cattle is _____ form.

Q.6 In buffaloes, fusarium mycotoxins produce symptoms resembling chronic ergot poisoning known as _____.

Q.7 Botulin exotoxins are produced by _____ microorganism.

Q.8 Botulism is most common in _____ species.

Q.9 The food-borne toxicity caused due to preformed toxins is _____.

Q.10 Limber neck in birds due to paralysis of neck muscles is caused by _____ toxins.

Answers

1. RYE (*C. purpurea* grows mainly on rye grass. The fungi forms a dense sclerotia around the seeds); 2. ALPHA (hence, vasoconstriction is seen in ergotism leading to gangrene in extremities); 3. ERGOMETRINE or ERGONOVINE; 4. GANGRENOUS; 5. GANGRENOUS ERGOTISM; 6. DEGNALA DISEASE (in 2012, an epidemic of degnala disease was reported in southeast Asia due to feeding of rice straw contaminated with fusarium species); 7. *CLOSTRIDIUM BOTULINUM*; 8. CHICKEN; 9. BOTULISM (anaerobic environment favors the production of botulinum toxin. Hence, tinned foods are more likely to contain botulinum toxins); 50. BOTULINUM.

Exercise 10

Q.1 The practice of using chicken manure as cattle feed or fertilizer can cause _____ toxicosis.

Q.2 Botulinum acts as a neurotoxin by inhibiting the release of _____ neurotransmitter.

Q.3 The specific treatment for botulism is _____.

Q.4 Tetanus toxin (also called tetanospasmin) is produced by _____.

Q.5 The most susceptible species of animal for tetanus is _____.

Q.6 "Saw horse" or "Wooden horse" condition in horses is caused by _____.

Q.7 Spinal stimulation in botulism is caused mainly due to inhibition of
_____ neurotransmitter.

Q.8 The specific treatment for tetanus is administration of _____.

Answers

1. BOTULINUM; 2. ACETYLCHOLINE (due to inhibition of ACh release, flaccid paralysis is seen); 3. POLYVALENT BOTULINUM ANTITOXIN; 4. *CLOSTRIDIUM TETANI*; 5. HORSE; 6. TETANUS (due to spasms and stiffness in neck, back, and leg muscles, the animal assumes wooden horse appearance. Prolapse of third eyelid is also observed); 7. GLYCINE; 8. TETANUS ANTITOXIN.

10.6.4 TRUE OR FALSE STATEMENTS (WRITE T FOR TRUE AND F FOR FALSE STATEMENT)

Exercise 11

Q.1 Radiation can be introduced into the food chain naturally from cosmic rays entering the atmosphere.
Q.2 Nitrates and nitrites prevent the growth of *Salmonella*.
Q.3 Lectins and saponins are two plant sources of food poisoning.
Q.4 *E. coli* stains gram-negative because it has 90% peptidoglycan in its cell wall.
Q.5 *S. aureus* is difficult to destroy because it is heat stable.
Q.6 HACCP is used to assess hazards by following the flow of foods.
Q.7 Virtually any food can serve as a vehicle for bacterial infection if handled carelessly by food workers.
Q.8 The vaccine that can be used for immunization against tetanus is *C. purpurea*.
Q.9 Spinal stimulation in botulism is caused mainly due to inhibition of glycine neurotransmitter.
Q.10 Botulin exotoxins are produced by *C. purpurea* microorganism.

Answers

1. T; 2. F; 3. T; 4. F; 5. T; 6. T; 7. T; 8. F; 9. T; 10. F.

FURTHER READING

Kotsonis, F.N., Burdock, G.A., 2013. Food toxicology. In: Klaassen, C.D. (Ed.), Casarett and Doull's Toxicology: The Basic Science of Poisons, eighth ed. McGraw-Hill, New York, NY, pp. 1305–1356.
Gupta, P.K., 2014. Essential Concepts in Toxicology. BSP Pvt Ltd, Hyderabad, India (Chapter 27).

Gupta, P.K., 2016. Fundamental in Toxicology: Essential Concepts and Applications in Toxicology. Elsevier/BSP, USA (Chapter 27).

Gupta, P.K., Singh, Y.P., 2010. Mycotoxins. In: second reprint Gupta, P.K. (Ed.), Modern Toxicology: The Adverse Effects of Xenobiotics, vol. 2. PharmaMed Press, Hyderabad, India, pp. 317–341.

Nageshkumar, R.G., 2010. Textbook of Forensic Medicine & Toxicology. Jaypee Brothers Medical Publishers, New Delhi, India (Chapter 39).

Pillay, V.V., 2008. Comprehensive Medical Toxicology, second ed. Paras Medical Publisher, Hyderabad, India.

Püssa, T., 2013. Principles of Food Toxicology, second ed. CRC Press, p. 414.

Thompson, L.J., 2012. Enterotoxins. In: Gupta, R.C. (Ed.), Veterinary Toxicology: Basic and Clinical Principles, second ed. Academic Press/Elsevier, Amsterdam, pp. 950–952.

Poisonous plants

CHAPTER OUTLINE

11.1 POISONOUS PLANTS

Poisonous/toxic plants have also been discussed in Chapter 15, Veterinary Toxicology.

Q. Define poisonous plants.

A poisonous plant is defined as a plant that when touched or ingested in sufficient quantity can be harmful or fatal to an organism or any plant capable evoking a toxic and/or fatal reaction.

Q. List some common poisonous plants.

Abrus precatorius, azalea, castor bean, chinaberry, European bittersweet, wild or black cherry, oleander, berries of holly and mistletoe, dieffenbachia,

Illustrated Toxicology. DOI: http://dx.doi.org/10.1016/B978-0-12-813213-5.00011-0

horse chestnuts, poison hemlock, laurel, death cup, black nightshade or deadly nightshade, rhododendron, belladonna, foxglove, rhubarb leaves, poison oak, and so on.

11.2 *ABRUS PRECATORIUS*

Q. Describe in brief some properties of *A. precatorius* plant.

Abrus precatorius is grown in many parts of the world. It is commonly known as jequirity bean, rosary pea, Buddhist rosary bead, rosary bead, Indian bead, Indian liquorice, Seminole bead, prayer head, crab's eye, weather plant, lucky bean, gulagunchi, rati, etc. It belongs to the family Leguminosae. It is a slender vine and climber, with compound leaves having 10−15 pairs of narrow leaves, small pinkish flowers with seedpods which split open when ripe exposing four to six seeds within. These seeds are bright red in color with black spot in one pole and weigh about 105 mg (Fig. 11.1).

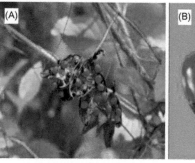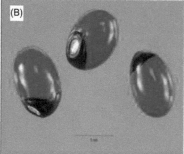

FIGURE 11.1

Abrus precatorius plant leaves with seeds (A) and seeds (B).

Available at Wikimedia Commons. https://en.wikipedia.org/wiki/Abrus_precatorius.

Q. Name the active toxic principle(s) of *A. precatorius*.

Active principles are *N*-methyltryptophan, Glycyrrhizin (lipolytic enzyme—the active principle of liquorice), abrin (toxalbumin also known as phytotoxin), abrine (amino acid), abralin (glucoside), and abric acid.

Q. What are the local toxic effects of *A. precatorius*?

The plant can lead to dermatitis, conjunctivitis, rhinitis, asthma, etc. Oral ingestion can produce severe gastroenteritis, hemorrhagic gastritis with severe pain, copious vomiting, and diarrhea that may become bloody, severe thirst, and circulatory collapse. Death is reported to be due to persistent gastroenteritis.

Q. What are the systemic toxic effects of *A. precatorius*?

Whole plant is poisonous; however, seeds are more often used. Toxicity occurs only when the seed is masticated and swallowed. When implanted as "suis" or the seed extract is injected parenterally, the person can develop cardiac manifestations like a viperine snakebite, with the site of injection turning edematous and hemorrhagic. Victim (animal/human) then turns drowsy, unable to move, goes into coma, followed by convulsions and death. Abrin can lead to the development of cardiac arrhythmias, convulsions, and cerebral edema.

11.3 CASTOR (*RICINUS COMMUNIS*, CASTOR OIL PLANT)

Q. Describe in brief some properties of castor plant.

The common names are castor, arandi, and moleean. It belongs to the family Euphorbiaceae. The plant is a large shrub with greenish-red leaves. Fruits are in clusters and are soft-spined greenish/brownish capsules with seeds. Seeds are oval/round in shape and are of two types: larger in size, red in color with brown blotches (yields 40% oil) and second variety small in size, gray in color with glossy bright, polished, brown mottling (yields 37% oil) (Fig. 11.2).

Q. Describe in brief some toxic principles of castor plant.

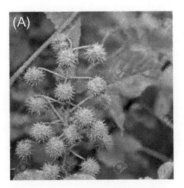 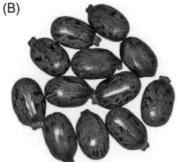

FIGURE 11.2

Castor plant leaves and pods (A) and seeds (B).

(A) Available at Horseback Riding worldwide. http://www.horsebackridingworldwide.com/the-castor-oilplant-ricinus/. (B) Available at Indo Exports. http://indoexports.tradeget.com/F38632/castor_bean_seeds.html.

Toxic part is the seeds, especially the seed oil (castor oil) extract which is pale yellow in color with faint odor. Leftover cake after the extraction of oil is also highly toxic. The oil extract of the seeds has an acid called ricinoleic acid and the leftover cake has the toxalbumin called ricin. Ricin is one of the most toxic parenteral substances in the plant kingdom. It contains two polypeptide chains held together by a single disulfide bond. Both these chains can bind with cell surface facilitating toxin entry into the cell and then disrupt the protein synthesis. Since the cell binding and protein disruption needs some time, its toxic effects are usually delayed but are widespread. Ricin is more poisonous than cobra venom and is classified as super-toxic poison.

Q. What are the local toxic effects of castor plant?

Local effects include dermatitis, conjunctivitis, rhinitis, and asthma. Castor bean dust is highly allergenic and may cause anaphylaxis.

Q. What are the systemic toxic effects of castor plant?

Orally, seeds if masticated and swallowed produce burning pain in the throat, followed by nausea, vomiting, colicky pain in the abdomen, and bloody purging. Ultimately it lead to dehydration and muscular cramps.

11.4 CROTON

Q. Describe in brief some properties of croton plant.

Croton plant grows all over, especially in wastelands. Grown in many varieties for their brightly colored foliage. The common names are croton, jamalgota, naepala. It belongs to the family Euphorbiaceae. Plant is an evergreen tree with smooth ash-colored bark. The leaves of the tree are ovate-lanceolate. Flowers are small and oblong. Fruits are three lobed containing oval, dark brown seeds, with brownish black color and longitudinal striations. Seeds though resemble castor seeds, the longitudinal striations mark the difference from castor seeds, which has mottling (Fig. 11.3).

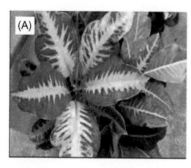 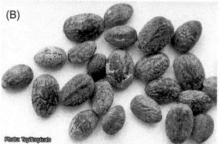

FIGURE 11.3

Croton plant leaves (A) and seeds (B).

(A) Indian Nursery. http://indiannursery.in/indoor-plants/Codiaeum.html. (B) Available at Prota 11(1): Medicinal plants/Plantes médicinales1. http://database.prota.org/PROTAhtml/Croton%20sylvaticus_En.htm.

Q. Name the active toxic principle(s) of croton plant.

Seed oil extracted from the seeds is extremely toxic. Seed oil is known to have tumor-promoting diesters. Active principles are crotin (toxalbumin) and crotonoside (glycoside).

Q. What are the local toxic effects of croton plant?

Local effects include dermatitis, conjunctivitis, rhinitis, and asthma. Castor bean dust is highly allergenic and may cause anaphylaxis.

Q. What are the systemic toxic effects of croton plant?

Orally, seeds if masticated and swallowed produce burning pain in the throat, followed by nausea, vomiting, colicky pain in the abdomen, and bloody purging. Both can ultimately lead to dehydration, muscular cramps, etc. After parenteral, it can produce same manifestation as after oral ingestion, but symptoms are more rapidly than the oral route.

11.5 *CALOTROPIS*

Q. Describe the common properties of *Calotropis* plant.

Calotropis grows all over, especially in wasteland and deserts. The common name is Madar. It has two species and belongs to the family Asclepiadaceae:

1. *Calotropis gigantea*, which is a purple flowered plant
2. *Calotropis procera*, which is a white flowered plant.

It is a tall shrub with yellowish-white bark, and oblong thick leaves and purplish or white flowers (Fig. 11.4). When stem, branches, and leaves are cut, crushed, or incised, they yield milky white latex, which is an acrid juice called madar juice.

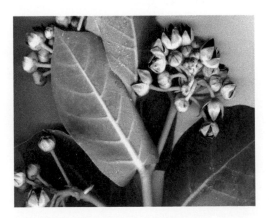

FIGURE 11.4

Calotropis leaves and flowers.

Available at Wikimedia Commons. https://commons.wikimedia.org/wiki/Calotropis_procera.

Q. What are the toxic principles of *Calotropis* plant?

Toxic parts include stem, branches, leaves, and the milky white latex (madar juice). Important toxic principles are uscharin, calotoxin, calotropin, and gigantin.

Q. What are the local toxic signs and symptoms of *Calotropis*?

It can give rise to lesions resembling bruises on skin (called fabricated injuries), which at times can lead to the formation of pustules and vesicles. Juice when instilled into the eyes or come in contact with eyes can result in severe conjunctivitis.

Q. What are the systemic toxic signs and symptoms of *Calotropis* plant?

The plant is bitter in taste. It produces burning pain in the throat, salivation, nausea, vomiting, etc. followed by diarrhea, pain abdomen, mydriasis, tetanic convulsions, delirium, collapse, and death.

11.6 *SEMECARPUS ANACARDIUM*

Q. Describe in brief some common properties of *S. anacardium*.

Semecarpus grows all over, especially in wasteland and deserts. The common names are marking nut, bhilawan, bibva, bhela, and oriental cashew. It belongs to the family Anacardiaceae.

It is a small tree having flowers which are dull/greenish yellow in color. Fruit is black, heart-shaped with hard ring within which is a thick fleshy pericarp (Fig. 11.5) which yields brown oily resinous fluid. This turns black on exposure to air. This fluid is often used as "marking ink," on linen and cotton clothes by the washermen (dhobis).

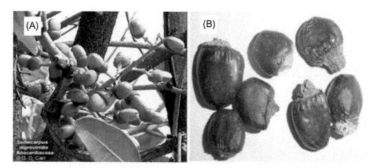

FIGURE 11.5

Semecarpus plant (A) and seeds (B).

(A) Available at Dr. Gerlad Carr, University of Hawaii. http://www.botany.hawaii.edu/faculty/carr/images/ sem_nig_2319.jpg. (B) Available at Wikimedia Commons. https://commons.wikimedia.org/wiki/.

Q. What are the important toxic principles of *S. anacardium*?

Semicarpol (monohydroxy phenol compound) and bhilawanol (alkaloid).

Q. What are the local toxic symptoms of *S. anacardium*?

On skin it produces bruise-like lesions which are actually raised blackish blisters or vesicular eczematous eruptions, which are itchy and scratching of which can cause similar lesions on the tip of fingers, on the nail beds, below the nail tips. These can lead to pain, fever, and stranguria with excretion of brownish urine.

Q. What are the systemic symptoms of toxicity of *S. anacardium*?

Orally, large dose can produce blisters in mouth and throat, with gastroenteritis. It can also produce dyspnea, cyanosis, tachycardia, coma, and death.

11.7 *CAPCICUM ANNUM*

Q. Describe in brief some characteristics of *C. annum*.

The plant belongs to the genus *Capcicum* and family Solanaceae. The common names are chillies, lal mirchi, red pepper, and cayenne pepper. The fruit (chilly) contains a number of small, flat, yellowish seeds, which bear a superficial resemblance to datura seeds (Fig. 11.6).

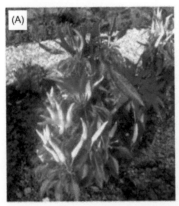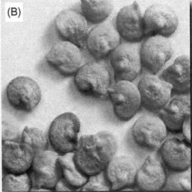

FIGURE 11.6

Capsicum annuum plant (A) and seeds (B).

(A) https://en.wikipedia.org/wiki/Capsicum_annuum#/media/File:Piment_fort.jpg. (B) Available at Indoor Gardening Club. http://indoorgardeningclub.com/product/giant-marconi-hybrid-sweet-pepper-seeds-capsicumannuum-0-2-grams-approx-30-gardening-seeds-vegetable-garden-seed/.

Q. What are the important principles of *C. annum*?

Capsaicin (8-methyl-*N*-vanillyl-6-nonenamide) is an active component of chili peppers. It is an irritant for mammals, including humans, and produces a sensation of burning in any tissue with which it comes into contact.

Q. Describe the local toxic signs of *C. annum*.

Locally it can produce irritation resulting in burning and redness of skin; and burning, redness, and lacrimation of eyes.

Q. Describe systemic signs and symptoms of toxicity of *C. annum*.

Large quantity can produce burning and fiery hot sensation in the mouth, salivation, excessive perspiration, abdominal pain, vomiting, and diarrhea. Urine may also turn dark.

11.8 *EUCALYPTUS GLOBUS*

Q. Describe some properties of *E. globus* plant.

The plant is commonly known as eucalyptus, blue gum, etc. It is a tall tree with smooth bark, long curved leaves, and large flowers. Eucalyptus oil is obtained by steam distillation of the extract derived from the leaves.

Q. What is the toxic principle of *E. globus* plant?

Eucalyptol (cineole).

Q. Describe the signs and symptoms of toxicity of *E. globus* plant.

Common symptoms include burning pain in the mouth, nausea, vomiting, diarrhea, abdominal pain, bronchospasm, tachypnea, chemical pneumonitis, respiratory depression, headache, vertigo, drowsiness, slurred speech, ataxia, convulsions, and coma. Breath and urine may smell of eucalyptus oil.

11.9 COLCHICUM (*COLCHICUM AUTUMNALE*)

Q. Describe some properties of *Colchicum* plant.

The plant is common in Eurasia and Africa. The common names are autumn crocus, meadow saffron, and naked ladies. It belongs to the family Liciacea; height 15–30 cm, with basal, slender leaves; and long, tubular, flowers are pink, violet/lavender, or white in color (Fig. 11.7). All parts of plant are highly poisonous and may be fatal if eaten.

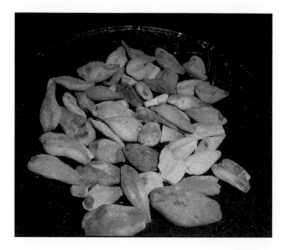

FIGURE 11.7

Colchicum plant seeds.

Imran Usman Enterprises. http://iue.weebly.com/colchicum-bitter.html.

Q. What are the important toxic principles of *Colchicum* plant?

Alkaloid colchicines and demecolcin.

Q. What are the signs and symptoms of toxicity of *Colchicum* plant?

The prominent symptoms are:

- Gastrointestinal (GI) system: Vomiting, diarrhea, abdominal pain, cramping, and hepatic dysfunction.
- Cardiovascular system: increased blood pressure. Rarely, it can produce disseminated intravascular coagulation and bone marrow failure.
- Respiratory system: Rarely it can produce respiratory failure.
- Urinary system: It may also cause signs and symptoms of renal dysfunction.
- Hairs: It can produce alopecia.

11.10 OLEANDERS

Q. Describe in brief oleander plants.

Oleanders are widely cultivated in various parts of world for their ornamental flowers. A general view of the plant is shown in Fig. 11.8.

Q. What are the important oleander plants?

1. *Nerium odorum*: Common names are white/pink oleander, kaner.

2. *Cerbera thevetia*: Common names are yellow oleanders, peela kaner, exile, bastard oleander.

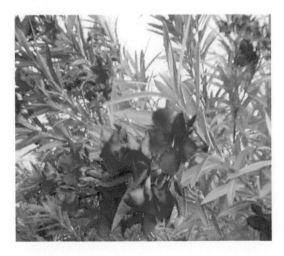

FIGURE 11.8

Oleander plant.

3. *Cerbera odollam*: Common names are Dabur, Dhakur, Pilikibir. All parts of the plant are poisonous, especially fruit with kernels or seeds and the nectar from the flowers, which yields poisonous honey.

Q. What are the toxic principles of *Nerium odorum*?

Nerium odorum has nerin, containing cardiac glycosides: (1) neriodorin, (2) neriodorein, (3) karabin, (4) oleandrin, (5) folinerin, and (6) rosagerin.

Q. What are the toxic principles of *C. thevetia*?

Cerbera thevetia has glycosides: (1) thevetin (one-eighth as potent as ouabain which is similar in action to digitalis, (2) thevitoxin is less toxic than thevetin, and (3) nerifolin, which is more potent than thevetin, (4) peruvoside, (5) ruvoside, and (6) cerberin.

Q. What are the toxic principles of *C. odollam*?

Cerbera odollam contains glycoside, cerberin.

Q. Describe in brief the mode of action of oleander plants.

Oleanders act like digitalis, toxic doses can produce malignant dysrhythmias and cardiac failure, cardiac arrest, and convulsions. Oleanders are absorbed easily via skin and GI route.

Q. Describe the signs and symptoms of toxicity of oleander plants.

In general, oleander poisoning closely resembles digitoxin poisoning with predominantly GI and cardiac symptoms. Severe toxic effects result from cardiotoxicity and specifically from ventricular ectopy and cardiovascular collapse. Digitalis toxicity is characterized by increased ectopy and conduction delay which may persist for 3–6 days (e.g., supraventricular tachycardia with atrioventricular block).

11.11 ACONITE

Q. Describe in brief the properties of aconite plant.

The plant (Fig. 11.9) is grown in the garden and the common names are monkshood, blue rocket, wolf's bane, mithazaha/mitha vish (meaning "sweet poison" in Hindi), etc. The whole plant is poisonous; however, roots are highly toxic.

Q. What are the toxic principles of aconite plant?

The toxic principles are diterpene alkaloids known as:

1. Aconitine

2. Misaconitine

3. Hypaconitine.

These alkaloids are sparingly soluble in water and considered as most virulent poison with sweetish taste. Other alkaloids present in small quantities in the plant are picraconitine, pseudoaconitine, and aconine.

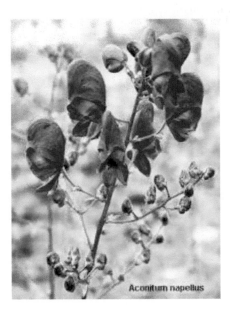

Aconitum napellus

FIGURE 11.9

Aconite plant with leaves and flowers.

Available at Antosh, G., 2012. Aconite Plant: How to Grow Monkshood Plants. Plant-Care.com.
http://www.plant-care.com/aconite-plant.html.

Q. What is the mode of action of aconite toxins?

Diterpene alkaloids are known as cardiac and neurotoxins that can cause conduction block and paralysis through their action on voltage-sensitive sodium channels in the axons. This can result in initial neurological stimulation, followed by depression of myocardium, smooth and skeletal muscles, central nervous system (CNS), and peripheral nervous system. Aconite is absorbed via skin and oral route. Symptoms generally appear within 30–90 minutes after ingestion of the poison and last up to approximately 30 hours.

Q. Describe in brief the signs and symptoms aconite toxicity.

Some of the typical features of poisoning are:

Cardiovascular: palpitation, hypertension, ventricular ectopics/arrhythmias.

GI tract (GIT): nausea, salivation, pain in stomach, vomiting, and diarrhea.

Neurological: Paraesthesia, tingling, and numbness in the lips, mouth, tongue, and pharynx. It may extend to all parts of the body, followed by profuse sweating, weakness impending paralysis of the extremities and/ seizers. Typical symptoms in the forehead include band-like sudden violent bursting (Fig. 11.10). Deep tendon reflexes may be absent.

Eye: There may be difficulty in vision due to hippus, which means initially there is alternate dilatation and constriction of pupils, followed by complete dilatation.

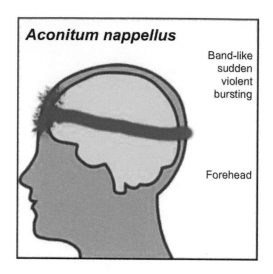

FIGURE 11.10

Effects of *Aconitum napellus* on forehead.

Available at Bisciotti, K., 2014. 9 Homeopathic Remedies for 9 Common Headaches. Musings of a Modern Hippie. http://musingsofamodernhippie.com/2014/02/homeopathyforheadaches.html.

11.12 NICOTINE (TOBACCO)

Q. Describe in brief the properties of nicotine (tobacco) plant.

Nicotine grows in all tropical regions of the world. The common name is tobacco plant, botanical name is *Nicotiana tobacum* (Fig. 11.11). Dried leaves

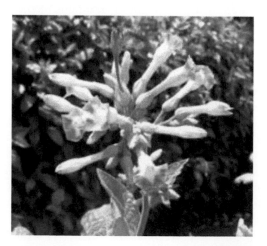

FIGURE 11.11

Nicotine plant with flowers.

Available at GeoChemBio.com. http://www.geochembio.com/biology/organisms/tobacco/#top.

and stems of *Nicotiana* sp. include *N. tobacum* (cultivated tobacco), *N. attenuate* (wild tobacco,), *N. glauca* (tree tobacco), and *N. trigonophylla* (dessert tobacco).

Q. What are the toxic principles of nicotine plant?

Lobeline is the chief constituent of nicotine plant (Indian tobacco), obtained from the leaves and tops of *Lobelia inflata*, an alkaloid similar to nicotine, but less potent than nicotine, and is used in antismoking tablets and lozenge.

Q. What are the signs and symptoms of toxicity of nicotine?

In general nicotine affects a wide range of systems such as CNS, heart, lungs, GIT, muscles, joints, and endocrine system. Side effects induced by smoking are shown in Fig. 11.12.

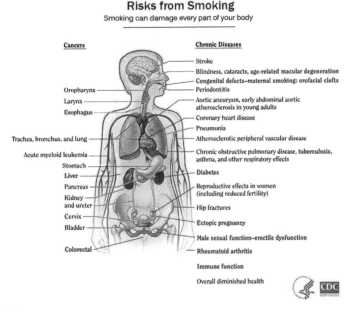

FIGURE 11.12

Side effects of smoking on various systems of the body.

https://www.cdc.gov/tobacco/infographics/health-effects/images/he-infographic1.jpg?s_cid=bb-osh-effects-image-005.

Brain symptoms include stimulation and depression followed by paralysis of cells of peripheral autonomic ganglia, midbrain, spinal cord, muscles, etc. Mild poisoning frequently occurs by chewing the dried leaves producing dizziness, nausea, vomiting, headache, perspiration, weakness, cardiac irregularities, etc. and victim usually turns to normal in a few hours. The available evidence indicates that nicotine is a highly addictive substance.

11.13 STRYCHNINE

Q. What is the source of strychnine?

Strychnine is a spinal poison caused by *Strychnos nux-vomica*, kuchila plant (Fig. 11.13). It contains alkaloids such as *strychnine*, *brucine*.

Q. What is the mode of action of strychnine?

For the toxic potential of strychnine, the seeds (bitter in taste) must be *masticated* and swallowed, and the site of action is anterior horn cells of spinal cord. It acts by competitive antagonism of inhibitory neurotransmitter glycine at the postsynaptic motor neurons of the spinal cord.

Q. What are the signs and symptoms of strychnine toxicity?

After ingestion of seeds, within 15 minutes to 1 hour it produces epigastric pain followed by stiffness in the muscles and typical type of strychnine convulsions which are initially clonic (intermittent), followed by tonic type (sustained), affecting both the flexor and extensor muscles of the body simultaneously. The clinical picture after strychnine poisoning is shown in Fig. 11.14.

- Facial muscles get fixed in a "grin" clinically called *Risus sardonicus* and prolonged spasm of the jaw muscles producing "lockjaw" called *trismus*.
- Other muscles of the body may contract and get fixed in one of the following postures.
    1. *Opisthotonus*, i.e., the body is bent backward (hyperextension of spine) making it rest on the occiput and heels like a bow.
    2. *Emprosthotonus*, i.e., the body is bent forward.
    3. *Pleurothotonos*, i.e., the body is bent laterally (to left/right).

Q. Other symptoms are cyanosis, dilated pupils, frothy salivation, respiratory distress, and failure, leading to death. Consciousness is retained, resulting in an agonizing death.

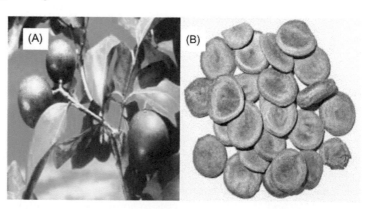

FIGURE 11.13

Strychnine plant along with fruits (A) and seeds (B).

(A) Available at The Poison Diaries. http://thepoisondiaries.tumblr.com/post/36597628648/strychnosnux-vomica. (B) Available at Wikimedia Commons. https://en.wikipedia.org/wiki/Strychnos_nux-vomica.

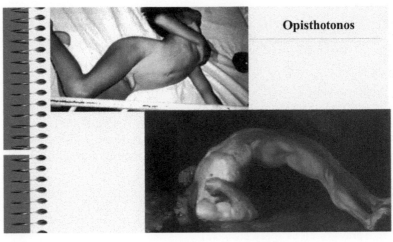

FIGURE 11.14

Uncontrolled muscle contractions and seizures are symptoms of strychnine poisoning.

Available at Adnan, A., 2015. Treating strychnine poisoning, Part 1. In: Prodding Physiology.
http://www.proddingphysiology.com/?p5182.

11.14 OTHER PLANTS

Q. What are invasive plants?

Invasive plants are plant species that can be harmful when introduced to new environments. These plants can reproduce quickly and thrive in different habitats. Invasive plants can grow in natural areas (forests, grasslands, and wetlands), managed areas (cultivated fields, gardens, lawns, and pastures), and areas where the soil and vegetation have been disturbed (ditches, rights of way, and roadsides).

Q. Why are invasive plants a problem?

A plant that looks harmless can invade agricultural and natural areas, causing serious damage to economy and environment. These plants can negatively affect the ecosystems. They create an imbalance in nature by competing for the same resources that native species need to survive. Human health can also be affected as some invasive plants are toxic, or cause skin reactions or allergies. In some cases, animal health may also be affected.

Q. Why phenothiazine tranquilizers are contraindicated in datura intoxication?

In datura intoxication, anticholinergic symptoms are seen. As phenothiazines also possess anticholinergic activity, they are contraindicated for controlling CNS excitation in datura intoxication.

11.15 QUESTION AND ANSWER EXERCISES
11.15.1 SHORT QUESTIONS AND ANSWERS

Exercise 1

Q.1 What is a poison?

A poison is anything that can harm someone if it is (1) used in the wrong way, (2) used by the wrong person, or (3) used in the wrong amount. Poisons may harm you when they get in your eyes or on your skin. Other poisons may harm you if you breathe them in or swallow them.

Q.2 What are the different forms of poison?

Poison comes in four forms:

1. Solids (such as medicine pills or tablets)

2. Liquids (such as household cleaners including bleach)

3. Sprays (such as spray cleaners)

4. Gases (such as carbon monoxide).

Q.3 Name a few lilies that can cause kidney failure in felines.

The following lilies have been shown to cause kidney failure in cats:
Common name (scientific name)
Easter lily (*Lilium longiflorum*)
Tiger lily (*Lilium tigrinum*)
Rubrum lily (*Lilium speciosum*)
Japanese show lily (*Lilium lancifolium*)
Day lily (*Hemerocallis* sp.)

Q.4 Why would a cat ever eat a lily?

Cats are naturally curious and often chew on plants. All parts of the lily are considered toxic to cats, and consuming even small amounts can be deadly.

Q.5 What are the common signs and symptoms of lily poisoning?

Within a few hours of ingestion, the cat may vomit, become lethargic, or develop a lack of appetite. These signs are initially vague, but continue and worsen as kidney damage progresses. The cat may develop kidney failure. The actual cause of kidney failure is still unknown.

Q.6 What is photodynamic substance?

A substance which absorbs UV light and emits energy while coming to ground state is called *photodynamic substance*.

Q.7 What is secondary/hepatogenous photosensitization?

The type of photosensitivity which is produced due to hepatic damage consequent to ingestion of hepatotoxic substances is called secondary/hepatogenous photosensitization.

Q.8 Name at least three plants that can cause secondary/hepatogenous photosensitization.
1. Pyrrolizidine alkaloid containing plants—*Senecio* sp.
2. *Heliotropium* sp.; *Lantana camara*
3. Mycotoxins—sporodesmins; blue-green algae—*Microcystis* sp.

Q.9 Why lesions in photosensitization are seen only in few areas of the body?
Melanin pigment protects skin from UV light. Hence, in light pigmented areas or in areas devoid of fur/wool, more UV light is absorbed leading to sunburn lesions. Light pigmented areas and areas devoid of hair/wool-like face, eyelids, muzzle, coronary band, udder, etc. are more prone to photosensitization.

Q.10 Why swallowing of seeds of abrus and castors is not "toxic" to animals?
Abrus and castor seeds have tough outercoating which resists digestion and hence are passed through GIT without causing any toxicity. However, crushing or chewing prior to swallowing will produce toxicity.

Q.11 Why strychnine is least toxic to chicken and pigeons?
In chickens and pigeon, strychnine is absorbed very slowly. Hence, strychnine is least toxic to chicken and pigeons. However, other avian species are easily affected.

11.15.2 MULTIPLE CHOICE QUESTIONS (CHOOSE THE BEST STATEMENT, IT CAN BE ONE, TWO OR ALL OR NONE)

Exercise 2

Q.1 Consumption of milk from goats which have grazed on lupine plants containing the alkaloid, anagyrine, may cause
a. birth defects when ingested by women during early pregnancy
b. severe liver damage characterized by centrilobular necrosis
c. dizziness, nausea, headaches, and hallucinations
d. numbness of the extremities
e. aphrodisia and a general increase in sexual awareness

Q.2 During expression of oil from castor seeds, the toxic principle of ricin is only present in
a. oil
b. seed cake
c. both
d. none

Q.3 Intoxication from consumption of wild cherry or apricot pits would best be treated by
a. hyperbaric oxygen
b. artificial respiration
c. inhalation of amyl nitrite
d. intravenous sodium nitrite and sodium thiosulfate
e. oral sodium nitrate

Q.4 The imbalance of the following electrolyte is observed in oleander poisoning:
  a. Sodium
  b. Potassium
  c. Magnesium
  d. Calcium

Q.5 The contraindications in strychnine poisoning are
  a. ketamine
  b. morphine
  c. emesis
  d. all

Q.6 Toxic part of castor seed is
  a. seeds
  b. oil
  c. stem
  d. leaves

Q.7 The active toxic principle of croton plant is
  a. calotoxin
  b. calotropin
  c. crotin (toxalbumin)
  d. none of the above

Q.8 Which one is toxic part of *Calotropis* plant?
  a. Stem
  b. Branches
  c. Milky white latex
  d. All of the above

Q.9 The toxic principle of *Nerium odorum* is
  a. nerin
  b. capsaicin
  c. calotoxin
  d. gigantin

Q.10 Which one is/are toxic principle(s) of aconite plant?
  a. Aconitine
  b. Misaconitine
  c. Hypaconitine
  d. All of the above.

Answers

1. a; 2. b (ricin is not extracted in oil but is retained in seed cake); 3. d; 4. b (hyperkalemia produced in cardiac glycoside toxicity is fatal); 5. d (ketamine causes motor stimulation; morphine—respiratory depression, and emesis leads to seizure development); 6. a; 7. c; 8. d; 9. a; 10. d.

11.15.3 FILL IN THE BLANKS

Exercise 3

Q.1 *Abrus precatorius* is commonly known as _____ or _____.

Q.2 The toxicity due to seeds of *A. precatorius* is commonly referred to as _____ poisoning.

Q.3 The toxic principle present in the seeds of *A. precatorius* is _____.

Q.4 *Ricinus communis* is commonly referred to as _____.

Q.5 The toxic principle present in the seeds of *R. communis* is _____.

Q.6 The toxic principles of abrin and ricin belong to the class of glycoproteins known as _____.

Q.7 The toxic principle present in castor bean which causes hemagglutination and hemolysis is _____.

Q.8 The species of animal that is more susceptible to abrin and ricin poisoning is _____.

Q.9 At the cellular level, lectins (abrin and ricin) acts by inhibiting _____ preventing protein synthesis.

Q.10 The toxic plant whose flowers are known as "angel's trumpets" or "moonflowers" is _____.

Answers

1. ROSARY PEA or RATHI; 2. SUI/NEEDLE (needles made from abrus seeds are inserted under the skin of the animal, causing poisoning, hence sui/needle poisoning); 3. ABRIN; 4. CASTOR BEAN; 5. RICIN; 6. LECTINS; 7. RCA (*R. communis* agglutinin) (however, RCA is not absorbed through GIT; it needs parenteral administration); 8. HORSE; 9. RIBOSOMES (one molecule of abrin inhibits up to 1500 ribosomes per second); 10. DATURA STRAMONIUM (thorn apple).

Exercise 4

Q.1 The major tropane alkaloids present in *Datura stramonium* are _____ and _____.

Q.2 The toxic principles in datura are present in _____ and _____.

Q.3 The plant that is known as "deadly nightshade" is _____.

Q.4 The species of animal which is resistant to *Atropa belladonna* is _____.

Q.5 Tropane alkaloids (atropine) acts by inhibiting _____ receptors in the body.

Q.6 The symptoms of datura toxicity are termed as _____.

Q.7 Urine from datura intoxicated animals produces _____ in cat, which is used for diagnosis.

Q.8 The competitive inhibitor of acetyl choline esterase, which is used for treating datura (atropine) intoxication is _____.

Q.9 The active toxic principles of *A. precatorius* is _____.

Q.10 The leftover cake after the extraction of oil is also _____.

Answers

1. HYOSCINE (scopolamine), ATROPINE (DL-hyoscyamine); 2. SEEDS, FLOWERS; 3. *ATROPA BELLADONNA* (Italian: Bella, beautiful; Donna, lady; atropine causes dilatation of pupil (mydriasis) when instilled into eyes. In ancient, women used to beautify their eyes through atropine-induced mydriasis. Hence the name bella-donna. The same reason is behind "candlelight dinners" of modern times, where dull light induces mydriasis, beautifying one's appearance); 4. RABBIT (rabbits contain atropinase enzyme, which destroys atropine); 5. MUSCARINIC; 6. ANTICHOLINERGIC DELIRIUM; 7. MYDRIASIS; 8. PHYSOSTIGMINE; 9. ABRIN; 10. HIGHLY TOXIC.

Exercise 5

Q.1 *Ipomoea turpethum* (Indian jalapa or morning glory) contains the toxic principle of _____.

Q.2 The toxic principle present in *Ipomoea orizabensis* is _____.

Q.3 The main symptom in ipomoea plant poisoning is _____.

Q.4 The toxic principles present in *Nerium oleander* (white oleander) is _____.

Q.5 The toxic principle present in *N. odorum* is _____.

Q.6 *Cerbera thevetia* contains the toxic glycosides _____ and _____.

Q.7 The steroidal glycoside present in *Nerium indicum* is _____.

Q.8 The most toxic part of *Nerium* sp. of plants is _____.

Q.9 The species of animal most susceptible to oleander glycoside poisoning is _____.

Q.10 Oleander glycosides act by inhibiting _____ enzyme in cardiac cells.

Answers

1. TURPETHIN; 2. CAMMONIN (jalapin); 3. DIARRHEA (the toxic resins present in ipomoea species produce drastic purgation); 4. OLEANDRIN; 5. NERIN; 6. THEVETIN, CEREBRIN; 7. ODOROSIDE; 8. LEAF (a leaf can kill a human and two to three leaves can kill a sheep. Leaf is effective even when dry); 9. HORSE; 10. Na^+-K^+ ATPase.

Exercise 6

Q.1 The toxic principle present in *S. nux-vomica* is _____.

Q.2 The toxic principle of strychnine is present in _____ part of *S. nux-vomica*.

Q.3 Strychnine produces spinal stimulation through inhibition of _____ neurotransmitter.

Q.4 The major site for action of strychnine in spinal cord is _____ cells.

Q.5 In strychnine toxicity, the characteristic symptom is of _____ appearance.

Q.6 The preferred sedative for strychnine poisoning is _____.

Q.7 The toxic principle present in cotton seeds is _____.

Q.8 Gossypol produces anemia by inhibiting heme synthesis by binding with _____.

Q.9 Inhibition of the testicular enzyme _____ is responsible for the development of reproductive toxicity in males.

Q.10 Intake of high amounts of _____ is protective in gossypol toxicity.

Answers

1. STRYCHNINE; 2. SEEDS; 3. GLYCINE; 4. RENSHAW (recurrent inhibitory interneuron cells of reflex arc of spinal cord); 5. SAW HORSE (saw horse appearance is due to continuous tetanic seizures which lead to rigidity giving saw horse appearance. Tetanus also produces similar saw horse appearance); 6. PENTOBARBITONE (barbiturate); 7. GOSSYPOL; 8 IRON; 9. LACTATE DEHYDROGENASE (LDH); 10. PROTEIN.

FURTHER READING

Gopalakrishnakone, P., Carlini, C.R., Ligabue-Braun, R. (Eds.), 2017. Plant Toxins. Springer, USA.

Gupta, P.K., 1988. Veterinary Toxicology. Cosmo Publications, New Delhi, India (Chapter 5).

Gupta, P.K., 2014. Essential Concepts in Toxicology. BSP Pvt Ltd, Hyderabad, India (Chapter 26).

Gupta, P.K., 2016. Fundamental in Toxicology: Essential Concepts and Applications in Toxicology. Elsevier/BSP, San Diego, USA (Chapter 26).

Norton, S., 2013. Toxic effects of plants. In: Klaassen, C.D. (Ed.), Casarett and Doull's Toxicology: The Basic Science of Poisons, eighth ed. McGraw-Hill, New York, NY, pp. 1103–1116.

Nelson, L.S., Shih, R.D., Balick, M.J., 2007. Handbook of Poisonous and Injurious Plants, second ed. Springer, New York, NY, p. 339.

Pillay, V.V., 2008. Comprehensive Medical Toxicology, second ed. Paras Medical Publisher, Hyderabad, India (Chapter 18).

Rao, G.N., 2010. Textbook of Forensic Medicine & Toxicology. Jaypee Brothes Medical Publishers, New Delhi, India (Chapter 33).

Sharma, R.P., Salunkhe, D.K., 2010. Animal and plant toxins. In: second reprint Gupta, P.K. (Ed.), Modern Toxicology: The Adverse Effects of Xenobiotics, vol. 2. PharmaMed Press, Hyderabad, India, pp. 252–316.

Drugs of use, dependence, and abuse

12

CHAPTER OUTLINE

12.1 DEPENDENCE, ABUSE, AND HABITUATION

Q. Define drug dependence.

Drug dependence is defined as a psychic and physical state of the person characterized by behavioral and other responses resulting in compulsions to take a drug, on a continuous or periodic basis in order to experience its psychic effect and at times to avoid the discomfort of its absence.

Q. Define drug abuse.

Compulsive, excessive, and self-damaging use of habit-forming drugs or substances, leading to addiction or dependence, serious physiological injury (such as damage to kidneys, liver, heart), and/or psychological harm (such as dysfunctional behavior patterns, hallucinations, memory loss), or death. Also called substance abuse

Illustrated Toxicology. DOI: http://dx.doi.org/10.1016/B978-0-12-813213-5.00012-2

Q. List the drugs that are commonly abused.

Hashish, marijuana, barbiturates, benzodiazepines (BDZ), flunitrazepam (Rohypnol), γ-hydroxybutyrate, methaqualone (Quaaludes), phencyclidine, lysergic acid diethylamide (LSD), codeine, heroin, morphine, opium, amphetamine, cocaine, ecstasy (MDMA), methamphetamine, methylphenidate (Ritalin), nicotine, anabolic steroids, inhalants, prescription medications.

Q. Define withdrawal symptoms (abstinence syndrome).

The withdrawal symptoms are self-explanatory. They develop in 6–48 hours of withdrawal of drugs to which an individual has become an addict and are characterized by the presence of restlessness, a feeling of anxiety, vague pain in abdomen and limbs, diarrhea and increased libido, etc. These symptoms last for variable periods, depending on the drug used, dose consumed, and duration of the drug.

Q. Define drug habituation.

Drug habituation is defined as a condition resulting from repeated consumption of a drug, which produces a psychological or emotional dependency on the drug such as caffeine and nicotine.

Q. What is the mode of drug habituation?

Like drug addiction, the measures of drug habituation are obscure. However, the following facts are true:

It is common in people with an imitative curiosity.

Communicable from one person to other.

Q. What are the signs and symptoms of drug habituation?

Person habituated to drug is called a drug habituate, and presents with the following:

1. A desire, but not irresistible to continue to take the drugs

2. Little or no tolerance

3. Hence, little or no tendency to increase the dose

4. Some degree of psychic, but no physical dependence

5. A detrimental effect only on the person if any, but not on society

6. Absence of withdrawal symptoms.

Q. Define drug addiction.

Drug addiction is defined as a state of periodic or chronic intoxication harmful to the individual and to society resulting from repeated consumption of a drug such as opium and its derivatives, pethidine, cannabis, heroine, alcohol, barbiturates, cocaine, LSD, amphetamine, and chloral hydrates.

Q. Describe the mode of drug addiction.

The mode of drug addiction is obscure. The diagrammatic representation of drug addiction is presented in Fig. 12.1.

Q. Describe in brief the signs and symptoms of drug addiction.

Signs and symptoms of drug addiction include the following:

• Irresistible desire to continue to take the drug

• Development of tolerance

• Thus a tendency to increase the dose

• Physical dependence on drug

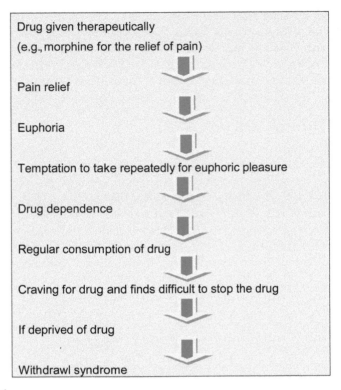

Drug given therapeutically

(e.g., morphine for the relief of pain)

Pain relief

Euphoria

Temptation to take repeatedly for euphoric pleasure

Drug dependence

Regular consumption of drug

Craving for drug and finds difficult to stop the drug

If deprived of drug

Withdrawl syndrome

FIGURE 12.1

Diagrammatic representation of steps that leads to drug addiction.

- Desire to obtain drug by any means (even using criminal ways)
- Withdrawal symptoms when the drug is stopped.

Q. What is the difference between a habit and a dependence?

Addiction is a state of dependence, physical and/or psychological, produced by the habitual taking of drugs. Withdrawal symptoms occur if the drug is stopped. These can be very severe and in the worst scenario can result in death.

Habit is the condition of being psychologically dependent on a drug (or an activity such as gambling) following repeated intake. The drug induces reliance upon it not unlike that of an addiction. However, in this case withdrawal produces no physical withdrawal symptoms although psychological symptoms can be very severe producing an almost overwhelming desire to continue taking the drug.

Q. What is meant by the term avoidance therapy?

Avoidance therapy is a form of behavioral control in which adverse conditions are produced if a drug is taken. This type of therapy may be by administering electric shocks to an individual who takes a drug or could be specific as in the use of disulfiram in alcohol addiction. The aim is to produce an unpleasant stimulus related to taking an addicting or habit-producing drug.

Q. Would one consider nicotine chewing gum as an alternative to smoking for clients with severe cardiovascular disease? Give reasons for your answer.

Nicotine stimulates the release of catecholamines from the adrenal medulla, which in turn have an inotropic and chronotropic effect on the heart. This would not be considered desirable in one with cardiovascular disease.

12.2 PSYCHOACTIVE DRUGS

Q. What are the toxic effects of psychoactive drugs?

Most psychoactive drugs (especially those used on the club scene) are toxic to the liver, kidneys, and central nervous system (CNS). While infrequent use of these drugs may pose little threat to the healthy person, repeated exposure over a period of time can have long-term consequences. Unfortunately, the toxic effects of such drugs may not be apparent for months or years after the damage is done. As an example, effects of alcohol drinking are shown in Fig. 12.2 (toxic effects of alcohol are also discussed in

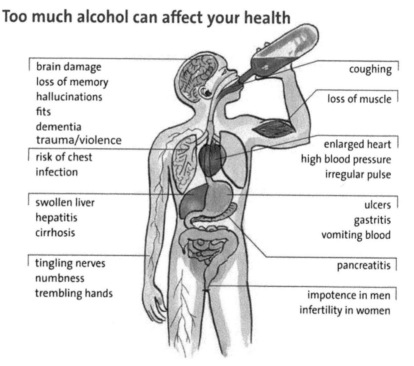

FIGURE 12.2

Effects of alcohol drinking in human beings.

Reproduced from Abuse-Drug.com https://abuse-drug.com/wp-content/uploads/2016/02/Effects-Of-Alcohol-
Long-Term-Effects.jpg.

Chapter 8: Solvents, Vapors, and Gases, dealing with solvents, vapors, and gases).

Some drugs of abuse may affect only higher nervous functions (change mood, reaction time, and coordination); many produce physical dependence and have serious physical effects, with fatal overdoses being a frequent occurrence.

12.3 COCA ALKALOIDS/COCAINE/COKE/CRACK

Q. What is cocaine?

Cocaine is a *deliriant cerebral neurotoxic*.

Q. What are the slang names of cocaine?

The slang names for cocaine are *snuff*, *rock*, *crack*, *coke*, *snow*, *cadillac*, *white lady*, etc. Cocaine hydrochloride is a white, colorless, crystalline substance, which has a bitter numbing taste.

Q. What is the source of coca alkaloids/cocaine/coke/crack?

Coca alkaloids/cocaine/coke/crack are obtained from the dried leaves of *coca plant* (*Erythroxylum coca*). *Coca plant* (Fig. 12.3), however, may not be confused for *cocoa plant* which contains *caffeine* rather than cocaine.

Q. Describe the characteristics of cocaine.

It is slightly soluble in water, but freely soluble in alcohol, chloroform, and glycerin. After oral consumption it gives feeling of numbness to tongue

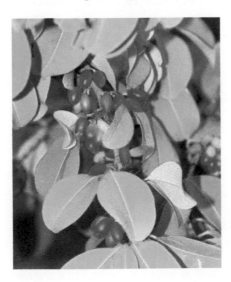

FIGURE 12.3

Coca leaves and flowers (*E. coca*).

Available at enthroloy.com. http://entheology.com/plants/erthroxylum-coca-coca-bush/.

and mucosa of the mouth. It has synthetic substitutes, namely novocaine and nupercaine, which are used frequently as local anesthetics. It cannot be used as such for smoking as it gets decomposed in heating. Crack cocaine is a cocaine preparation which has been separated from its hydrochloride base (free base) by adding baking soda and water, followed by heating and then drying, which can be mixed with tobacco and smoked. The name "*crack*" arises from the noise made when it is being prepared, as well as due to the *fissured* appearance of heated cocaine. Chronic consumption can develop addiction to cocaine.

Q. What is the mechanism of action of coca alkaloids?

It is usually snorted. It has a potent stimulating action on CNS. It interferes with the transport of the neurotransmitter dopamine.

Q. What are the signs and symptoms of cocaine?

The adverse effects of cocaine depend upon the chronic use of cocaine. It effects on CNS, lungs, heart, and other organs. Coca alkaloids produce a sense of euphoria, excitement, and increase in energy. Excessive dosage of cocaine can cause hallucinations.

Q. What are the side effects of cocaine?

There are many slangs used for these drugs in different places and different countries. The cocaine is available in different forms (powder, liquid, ash, crystalline, etc.). With small doses, peak "high" effect appears and weans off after some interval. However, in fatal cases, onset and progression of symptoms is accelerated and death may occur in minutes. It has a stage of initial stimulation of CNS followed by depression characterized by loss of reflexes, muscle paralysis, pulmonary edema, feeble respiration, circulatory and respiratory failure followed by death. The side effects of cocaine are shown in Fig. 12.4.

Q. What are the complications of acute cocaine poisoning?

Complications include:

- Stroke, including subarachnoid and intracerebral hemorrhage and cerebral infarcts
- Cardiovascular complications such as myo cardial infarction, ventricular arrhythmias, and cardiac arrest
- Intestinal ischemia.

Q. What is cocainism?

It is also known as chronic cocaine poisoning (cocainophagia, cocainomania, cocaine addiction, cocainism). For the euphoric effects of cocaine, addicts usually take cocaine by subcutaneous injection or eat in *paan* or inhale it as snuff. A comparison of illicit drug abuse of different drugs is presented in Fig. 12.5.

Q. What is Magnan's symptom (cocaine bugs)?

Magnan's symptom is a type of tactile hallucination that makes the addict feel as if insects (bugs) are crawling under the skin of the part of their body. One may even complain of presence of sand grain under the skin. In chronic consumers, the teeth and tongue are black.

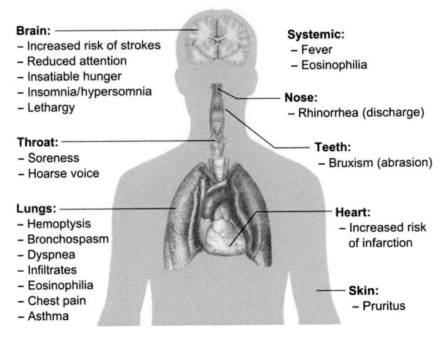

Brain:
- Increased risk of strokes
- Reduced attention
- Insatiable hunger
- Insomnia/hypersomnia
- Lethargy

Systemic:
- Fever
- Eosinophilia

Nose:
- Rhinorrhea (discharge)

Throat:
- Soreness
- Hoarse voice

Teeth:
- Bruxism (abrasion)

Lungs:
- Hemoptysis
- Bronchospasm
- Dyspnea
- Infiltrates
- Eosinophilia
- Chest pain
- Asthma

Heart:
- Increased risk
  of infarction

Skin:
- Pruritus

FIGURE 12.4

Side effects of chronic use of cocaine.

Available at Häggström, M., 2014. Medical gallery of Mikael Häggström. Wikiversity J. Med. 1 (2). https://commons.wikimedia.org/wiki/File:Side_effects_of_chronic_use_of_Cocaine.png.

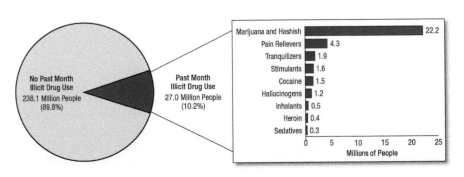

FIGURE 12.5

Comparison of different illicit drugs of abuse.

Reproduced from Substance Abuse and Mental Health Services. (https://www.samhsa.gov/data/sites/default/files/NSDUH-FRR1-2014/images/NSDUH-FFR1-fig1.png).

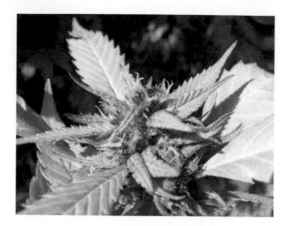

FIGURE 12.6

Cannabis plant with flowers.

Available at Grow Weed Easy. http://www.growweedeasy.com/advanced-breeding-techniques.

12.4 MARIJUANA, HASHISH/HASH, CHARAS, AND GANJA

Q. What are the sources of marijuana, hashish/hash, charas, and ganja?

Marijuana, hashish/hash, charas, and ganja are cannabinoids obtained from inflorescences of the plant *Cannabis sativa* (hemp). Cannabis is classified under delirium cerebral neurotic plant poison. It has a mild hallucinogen or sedative or a narcotic effect. In fact the drug is believed to produce all these effects in various individuals in a different way. It is the *most abused drug* all over the world. The slang terms for cannabis include *hash*, *grass*, *pot*, *ganja*, *spliff*, and *refer*.

The flower tops, leaves, and the resin of cannabis plant are used in various combinations to produce marijuana, hashish/hash, charas, and ganja (Fig. 12.6).

Q. Which is a recreational drug?

Hashish, or hash, is a cannabis-family recreational drug that is consumed by oral ingestion or smoking; typically in a pipe, vaporizer or joints, where it is normally mixed with cannabis or tobacco, as pure hashish will not burn if rolled alone.

Q. What is the active ingredient of *hashish*?

Hash is an extracted cannabis product composed of compressed or purified preparations of stalked resin glands, called trichomes, from the plant. It contains the same active ingredients as marijuana—such as tetrahydrocannabinol (THC) and other cannabinoids—but often in higher concentrations than the unsifted buds or leaves from which the marijuana is made.

Hashish may be solid or resinous depending on the preparation; pressed hashish is usually solid, whereas water-purified hashish—often called "bubble melt hash"—is often a paste-like substance with varying hardness and pliability; its color, most commonly light to dark brown, can vary from transparent to yellow, tan, black, or red. This all depends on the process and amount of solvent left over.

Q. What is the source of *ganja?*

Ganja is obtained from the top leaves and unfertilized flower of young female plant. These are generally taken by inhalation or orally.

Q. Describe in brief the signs and symptoms of cannabis poisoning.

In acute poisoning, the clinical features vary with dose consumed. With low dose, there is an initial euphoria associated with overtalkativeness, perceptual alterations followed by relaxation, drowsiness, hypertension, tachycardia, slurred speech, ataxia, excessive appetite and eating food with great relish, etc.

At higher dose, there is *conjunctival congestion and miosis, acute paranoid psychosis, anxiety, depersonalization, confusion, hallucinations (especially of sexual character, hence cannabis is considered as an aphrodisiac), and disorientation to time and space may be observed. This may be followed by* giddiness, confusion, drowsiness, dilated pupils, tingling, and numbness in the extremities, generalized anesthesia (may be seen in severe cases). The victim will then go into deep sleep and can be woken up soon without depression, nausea, or any hangover effects. Rarely the victim may lead to paralysis of muscles, loss of reflexes, coma, and death. However, a few individuals may turn violent and go into state called "run amock."

12.5 LYSERGIC ACID DIETHYLAMIDE

Q. What are the synonyms of LSD?

LSD is lysergic acid diethylamide. It is the most potent and widely abused hallucinogen. Some of the common popular street names for LSD are *acid, blotter acid, blue caps, blue dots, brown caps, crackers, deeda, green caps, orange wedges, Paisley caps, pink dots, pink chief, the ghost, the Hawk, white lighting, window panes, yellow caps, yellow dots, 25,* etc.

Q. What is the source of LSD?

It is synthesized from rye ergot. Ergot is a biological product of fungus *Claviceps purpurea*, a parasite of cereal grain (especially rye type). LSD is tasteless, odorless, and most potent hallucinogen in minute doses. These can be supplied illicitly on sugar cubes, though it is available in the form of pills of varying colors, sizes, and shapes, and also in ampoules.

Q. What are the acute signs and symptoms of LSD poisoning?

The signs of acute LSD poisoning include mydriasis, hippus, large pupils, nystagmus may occur, vertigo, vomiting, diarrhea, sweating, piloerection, tachypnea and bronchiolar smooth muscle constriction (at high doses), muscle weakness, cerebral artery spasm followed by coma.

Psychologically there may be euphoria, anxiety and behavioral changes, tremors and incoordination. There may be bizarre perpetual changes.

Q. What are the chronic signs and symptoms of LSD poisoning?

Prolonged psychotic reactions which are mainly schizophrenic in nature, severe depression, flashback phenomenon, a perceptual disorder (such as seeing images on floor or walls, floating faces hovering in space), aeropsia (visualization of vibrating pinpoint-sized dots), etc. are the common features observed in chronic intoxication. The patient may enter the stage of bad trips.

Q. What are bad trips?

It is defined as the adverse effects experienced by a person after consuming LSD. LSD mainly acts by interfering with filtering mechanism of the mind. The victim's sense of perception alters uniquely resulting into effect such as:

- Patient will hear noises with total disturbance of sense of time, space, and distance, and will get into a dream-like state with loss of awareness of body boundaries.
- He or she will be experiencing fantasies and hallucinations of varied nature and might present with a flight of ambivalent emotions such as depression and elation, happiness and sadness, etc. simultaneously.

Q. What are the complications of bad trips?

Bad trips might give a "flashback" of all the events of dreamy state for several months even up to 2 years or so requiring a long-term therapy for total cure. There will be hangover or aftereffects.

Though aftereffects with any hallucinogen are rare, however, there may be insomnia, headache, vertigo, and psychotic reactions.

Prolonged consumption of hallucinogens may lead to permanent damage of brain cells, and chromosomal damage in the peripheral blood smears (especially with LSD).

12.6 PEYOTE

Q. What is the source of peyote?

It is obtained from a variety of cactus plants (peyote), *Lophophora williamsii* or *peyote* (/pə'jouti/) which is a small, spineless cactus (Fig. 12.7). Peyote contains psychoactive alkaloids, particularly mescaline. Synthetic mescaline is also available.

Q. What is the active principle of peyote?

The toxic principle is in its button-shaped growth of the plant. Peyote (Fig. 12.7) contains 1%−6% mescaline. Each button contains about 45 mg of mescaline. They are just rolled into balls and kept in capsules. It is not as potent as LSD.

Q. What are the signs and symptoms of peyote poisoning?

The common symptoms of peyote poisoning are unusual bizarre behavior, hilarity, emotional swings, and suspiciousness. The patient may complain of nausea and vomiting. There may be dilated pupils and tremors.

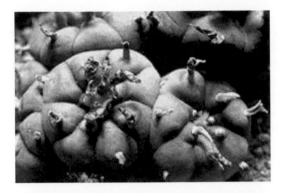

FIGURE 12.7

Cactus plant (peyote): *L. williamsii.*

https://upload.wikimedia.org/wikipedia/commons/thumb/6/6d/Peyote_Cactus.jpg/330px-Peyote_Cactus.jpg.

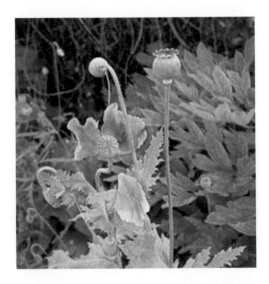

FIGURE 12.8

Leaves and seeds of opium plant.

Available at Wikimedia Commons. https://en.wikipedia.org/wiki/Papaver_somniferum.

12.7 OPIUM (AFIM)

Q. What is the source of opium (afim) and its derivatives?

The common name is white poppy plant, opium (afim) plant. Opium is a gray mass with bitter taste, obtained on drying the milky latex of unripe seed capsule of poppy plant, *Papaver somniferum* (Fig. 12.8).

Q. What are the uses of opium?

Opium is used extensively as a sedative and painkiller. The various derivatives are also habit-forming narcotics. Seeds inside are nonpoisonous and called khaskhas which constitute a condiment in Indian cooking.

Q. Describe in brief the opium alkaloids and its derivatives.

The milky latex juice of poppy plant has opium alkaloids. An alkaloid is a complex substance with nitrogenous base and behaves like an alkali and unites with acid-forming salts. The crude opium has about 25 alkaloids, which belongs to two groups, namely phenanthrene derivatives and benzyl isoquinoline derivatives. Phenanthrene derivatives generally have the alkaloids with sedative and analgesic properties, while the benzyl isoquinoline derivatives have the alkaloids with antitussive and smooth muscle relaxant effects.

Q. What is the difference between pethidine (meperidine) and opium?

Pethidine is an opioid, narcotic analgesic drug, which is a synthetic derivative of opium.

Pethidine addiction is quite severe, difficult to treat, and has a high mortality rate than opium.

Q. What is the difference between opium and heroin?

Opium comes straight out of the *P. somniferum* as a liquid latex. You do not have to do anything to it—just slit the green part under the flower and collect the opium. Heroin is processed from opium into a semisynthetic. Opium comes as a reddish blob. Heroin is usually a brown, white, or yellow powder (there is also "black tar" predominantly in some areas). Opium is more culturally acceptable in most parts of the world—an almost sophisticated ritual. Heroin is stigmatized as having thieves and lowlifes as its main consumer.

12.8 HEROIN

Q. What is the source of heroin?

Heroin commonly called smack is a white, odorless, bitter crystalline compound obtained by acetylation of morphine.

Q. What are the slangs used for heroin?

There are many slangs used for every different form (powder, liquid, ash, crystalline, etc.) at every particular place. Since heroin is mixed with other drugs too, it also has slang names like dope, H, big H, white, white lady, china white, Mexican mud, horse, scag, black tar, brown crystal, brown sugar, nod, chiba, chiva, tar, snowball, junk, black pearl. It is taken by snorting and injection.

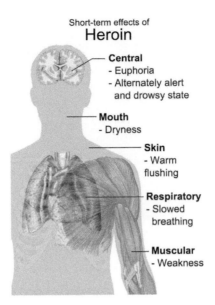

Short-term effects of
Heroin

Central
- Euphoria
- Alternately alert
  and drowsy state

Mouth
- Dryness

Skin
- Warm
  flushing

Respiratory
- Slowed
  breathing

Muscular
- Weakness

FIGURE 12.9

Heroin addict.

Reproduced from Wikipedia https://upload.wikimedia.org/wikipedia/commons/8/87/Short-term_effects_of_heroin.png.

Q. What are the symptoms of heroin poisoning?

People use heroin to get "high." But if they overdose on it, they get extremely sleepy or may become unconsciousness and stop breathing (Fig. 12.9).

Symptoms of a heroin overdose in different parts of the body are given as follows:

- *Airways and lungs*: no breathing, shallow breathing, slow and difficult breathing
- *Eyes, ears, nose, and throat*: dry mouth, extremely small pupils, sometimes as small as the head of a pin (pinpoint pupils), discolored tongue
- Heart and blood: low blood pressure, weak pulse
- Skin: bluish-colored nails and lips
- Stomach and intestines: constipation, spasms of the stomach and intestines
- Nervous system: coma, delirium, disorientation, drowsiness, uncontrolled muscle movements.

12.9 DATURA

Q. Describe in brief datura.

The common name of datura is thorn apple, stinkweed, angel's trumpet, and Jamestown weed. It is a vegetable deliriant type of cerebral poison. The botanical

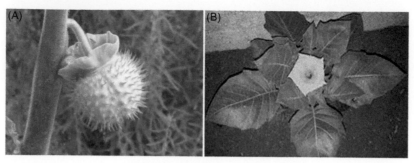

FIGURE 12.10

Datura plant with fruit (A) and plant flower (B).

Available at Wikipedia Commons. https://en.wikimedia.org /wiki/Datura.

name is *Datura stramonium.* Commonly there are two varieties of plants: *Datura alba* (with white flower) and *Datura nigra* (with blackish or purple flowers). A view of the plant along with fruits, seeds, and flower is shown in Fig. 12.10.

Q. What are the active principles of datura plant?

The active principles are alkaloids such as hyoscine (scopolamine), hyoscyamine, and atropine.

Q. What is the mode of action of datura?

Poisoning occurs only if seeds are masticated and swallowed. It is bitter in taste and can initially lead to stimulation of higher centers of brain. Later the vital centers are depressed followed by death due to respiratory paralysis.

Q. Describe in brief the signs and symptoms of datura.

It produces characteristic manifestations of anticholinergic poisoning (remember as six Ds):

* Dryness of mouth, nausea, vomiting
* Dysphagia
* Dysarthria (all the three, a—c, are due to inhibition of salivation)
* Diplopia (due to dilated pupil)
* Dry, hot (due to inhibition of sweat secretion), and red (due to the dilation of cutaneous blood vessels), skin, especially in the face/chest
* Drowsiness leading to coma.

Other symptoms are: The patient is in a confused state, i.e., deliriant (muttering delirium) and hallucinating, exhibiting typical pill rolling movements, or with movements like pulling imaginary threads from fingertips. There may be urinary retention or dysuria. Death is usually due to respiratory failure or cardiac arrhythmias.

In short, the clinical features of datura poisoning are described in its classic phrase as blind as bat, hot as hare, dry as bone, red as beet, and mad as hen.

12.10 AMPHETAMINES

Q. Define toxic symptoms of amphetamines (CNS stimulant, hallucinogen).

Intoxication with amphetamines leads to flushed face, sweating, excitement, restlessness, insomnia, tremors, ventricular tachycardia, hypertension, delirium, hallucinations, convulsions, and deep unconsciousness. Toxic psychosis is seen in chronic poisoning.

12.11 CARBON TETRACHLORIDE

Toxicity of carbon tetrachloride is also discussed in Chapter 8, Solvents, Vapors, and Gases, dealing with solvents, vapors, and gases.

Q. Describe in brief toxicity of carbon tetrachloride.

Carbon tetrachloride is both hepatotoxic and nephrotoxic. Inhalation of carbon tetrachloride leads to irritation of eyes and throat, headache, nausea, vomiting, mental confusion, loss of consciousness, arrhythmia, slow respirations, convulsions, etc. When ingested can cause dizziness, headache, nausea, vomiting, colic, tremors, convulsions, coma. The chemical is hepatotoxic as well as nephrotoxic.

12.12 ASPIRIN AND PARACETAMOL

Q. What are the toxic effects of aspirin?

The most common symptoms of aspirin poisoning include vomiting, flushed face, edema of face, skin rash, tinnitus, deafness, hyperpnea, nausea, hematemesis, hypoprothrombinemia, acute renal failure, pulmonary edema, and respiratory arrest.

Q. What are the toxic effects of paracetamol?

Paracetamol (acetaminophen) is a nonnarcotic analgesic and antipyretic. It acts by the inhibition of prostaglandin synthesis. It can produce severe liver damage due to the accumulation of a highly toxic intermediate metabolite: N-acetyl-p-benzoquinoneimine (NAPQ). Initially within the first 24 hours the drug can produce anorexia, nausea, vomiting, and epigastric pain. This is followed by disappearance of all discomforts giving a false sense of relief followed by progressive hepatic encephalopathy as is evidenced by vomiting, jaundice, hepatic pain, confusion, coma, and coarse flapping tremors of hands (asterixis), gastrointestinal (GI) hemorrhage, cerebral edema, renal tubular necrosis, etc. There may be cardiac arrhythmias, hemorrhagic pancreatitis, disseminated, intravascular coagulation, etc.; death often taken place in this stage.

Table 12.1 Classification of Barbiturates

Ultrashort acting (duration of action <15−20 minutes)	Thiopentone sodium, methohexitone, pentothal sodium, hexobarbital sodium, kemithal sodium, thiamylal sodium, etc.
Short acting (duration of action <3 hours)	Cyclobarbitone, pentobarbitone, amobarbitone, aprobarbitone, butobarbitone, hexabarbitone, etc.
Intermediate acting (duration of action 3−6 hours)	Amylobarbitone, butobarbitone, probarbitone sodium, amobarbitone, aprobarbital, vinbarbital, allobarbitone, etc.
Long acting (duration of action 6−12 hours)	Barbitone, phenobarbital, mephobarbitone, methyl phenobarbital, diallylbarbituric acid, etc.

12.13 BARBITURATES

Q. Describe in brief abuse of barbiturates.

Barbiturates belong to a class of sedative−hypnotic drugs with abuse potential and a recognized withdrawal syndrome. Toxic manifestations of barbiturates vary with the amount of ingestion, type of drug, and time elapsed since ingestion. The lower doses of short-acting barbiturates (e.g., pentobarbital) than the long-acting barbiturates (e.g., phenobarbital) generally cause toxicity, but fatalities are more common with the latter (Table 12.1). Mild intoxication resembles that of alcohol intoxication. Moderate intoxication is characterized by greater depression of mental status and severe intoxication causes coma.

12.14 QUESTION AND ANSWER EXERCISES

12.14.1 SHORT QUESTIONS AND ANSWERS

Exercise 1

Q.1 What is the difference between heroin, cocaine, and ganja?

Heroin is an opiate, i.e., a derivation from the opium plant. Heroin is an intravenous drug and instils a feeling of euphoria upon use.

Cocaine is a stimulant, i.e., it excites the activity of neurons in the brain. It is generally snorted at use. Crack is a form of cocaine that can be smoked. Cocaine is extracted from the coca plant. Ganja is the leaves and buds of the plant marijuana. Marijuana prominently consists of THC, which is a mild psychedelic. It can be smoked or consumed orally after extracting the THC in oil or fat.

Q.2 What is drug addiction?

Drug addiction is the point at which the user has developed a psychological or physiological dependence on a substance and can no longer make the choice whether or not to use.

Q.3 What is drug abuse?

Drug abuse is using any drug for something other than its intended purpose, or using it improperly. This can include using too much prescription medication, or using it too often, other than the prescribed way as directed by the doctor. It is using alcohol to the point where you get intoxicated. Drug abuse is a conscious choice.

Q.4 Do *all* people who use drugs for recreation become addicts?

No. There are many factors that go into addiction, such as genetics, personality, and of course the substance itself. Not everybody who drinks is an alcoholic and not everybody who uses heroin for recreation will become an addict. It is an individual occurrence. People are born with the inclination to abuse and become addicted, but it is not until the substance is introduced to the brain that the cycle begins.

Q.5 Is drug addiction a disease?

Yes. Drug addiction and alcoholism are diseases of the brain. It also causes moral changes and affects a person's whole being.

Q.6 Is drug addiction a choice?

No. Nobody sets out in life to become an addict. But there is an ongoing debate about this and there are strong arguments on both sides of the issue. The insanity of drug addiction and alcoholism is in the self-destructive nature of the disease, as people will use regardless of the consequences. They will ignore reason, medical fact, and all forms of warning. Bottom line, people do have to make free will decisions to act in their own best interest.

Q.7 Is there a cure for drug addiction?

No. Drug addiction and alcoholism are chronic diseases for which there is no cure. However, the disease can be managed and people can live healthy, productive lives with treatment and support.

Q.8 Does drug addiction damage the brain?

It can. Prolonged use of drugs and alcohol can cause permanent brain damage. In some cases treatment and recovery can lead to the reversal of negative effects. These are controversial drug addiction questions and answers but this represents the opinion of this website.

Q.9 Is the brain damage induced due to drug addiction a permanent one?

Prolonged use of drugs can cause irreversible damage to the brain, including but not limited to the ability to reason, memory, physical coordination, and a host of physiological maladies.

Q.10 How drug addiction happens?

Drug addiction is the end result of a sequence of events. Imagine a cycle of events. When people have a pleasurable experience with a drug, they want to repeat that experience. Over time they build a tolerance to the drug. Over time they can develop a psychological and physiological dependence.

Exercise 2

Q.1 What drugs are abused the most?

In the United States, by far the most abused drug is alcohol, followed closely by nicotine (cigarettes, chewing tobacco, etc.). The most widely abused illegal drug is marijuana.

Q.2 What are the long-term effects of alcohol on the body?

Alcohol is extremely toxic. In long term it will cause liver, kidney, and heart disease, hypertension, respiratory distress, and contribute significantly to the deterioration of the alcoholic's overall state of health and well-beings.

Q.3 What causes an overdose?

As people continue to use a drug they will build up a tolerance to it. For example, regardless of the substance, cocaine, alcohol, whatever may be, it will take more of that substance to achieve the desired effects. They will use more. In some point, the brain can only take so much, or there is alcohol poisoning, or other side effects come into play such as heart attack, stroke, or respiratory failure.

If a person has built up a tolerance and they quit for a period of time, the body will lose the tolerance. If they go back to using at the same level, that might cause overdose. Everybody is different. Some people will overdose on a seemingly small amount of the drug the first time they take it.

Q.4 What is the best way to pass a drug screening test?

Do not use the drug.

Q.5 Is marijuana addictive?

According to the National Institute on Drug Abuse, yes it is.

Q.6 Can you overdose on marijuana?

No. There is no proof that it is possible.

Q.7 Who is most likely to use illegal drugs?

Teenagers from suburban, middle-class families. Young middle-class adults are also high on the list.

Q.8 What is the botanical name of datura?

The botanical name of datura is *D. stramonium*.

Q.9 What are the uses of opium?

Opium is used extensively as a sedative and painkiller.

Q.10 What is the source of heroin?

Heroin is an opiate and is obtained from the opium plant.

Exercise 3

Q.1 How does alcohol adversely affect the pregnant women?

Alcohol can permeate the placenta and enter fetal circulatory system, thereby causing developmental abnormalities. Ethanol impairs placental blood flow to the fetus by constricting blood vessels: inducing hypoxia and fetal malnutrition.

Q.2 During which period alcohol has its greatest effect in pregnant women?

In the first 4 weeks of pregnancy.

Q.3 What is the consequences of continued or excessive exposure to alcohol in pregnant women?

Fetal alcohol effect, progressing to fetal alcohol syndrome (FAS). FAS does seem to be dose-dependent in that greater amounts of alcohol consumed increase the chances of having an FAS child.

Q.4 What kind of syndrome is caused by ethanol in pregnant women?

FAS. FAS is seen in approximately 3 in 1000 live births, depending upon culture and socioeconomic status.

Q.5 What are the symptoms of FAS?

FAS include a range of facial deformities (small head, small eye openings, thin upper lip) and severe growth, developmental and intellectual retardation.

Q.6 What is the estimate of the number of children affected by thalidomide?

5000 to greater than 10,000.

Q.7 What is the source of datura?

Datura stramonium.

Q.8 What are the effects of morphine?

Morphine is a very effective sedative and painkiller and is very useful in patients who have undergone surgery but is harmful if used as an opioid. It is a depressant, slows down the body functions, and affects the CNS and GI tract.

Q.9 How opium is collected from the plant?

The opium is usually collected after all the flower petals have fallen off from the capsule, by making slits along its circumference, allowing the milky latex to ooze out and harden. After the plastic gummy opium is removed, it can be refined into heroin, morphine, and codeine.

Q.10 Is there a difference between opium and opiates?

Opium is the "raw material" that you get from the opium poppy (*P. somniferum*). Opiates are group of drugs you can create from opium, such as morphine or codeine.

12.14.2 MULTIPLE CHOICE QUESTIONS (CHOOSE THE BEST STATEMENT, IT CAN BE ONE, TWO OR ALL OR NONE)

Exercise 4

Q.1 Toxicity associated with any chemical substance is referred to as

a. poisoning

b. intoxication

    c. overdose

    d. toxicology

Q.2 Clinical toxicity which is secondary to accidental exposure is

    a. toxicology

    b. intoxication

    c. poisoning

    d. overdose

Q.3 Chest pain is related to

    a. neurological examination

    b. cardiopulmonary examination

    c. GI examination

    d. both cardiopulmonary examination and GI examination

Q.4 Technique in which anticoagulated blood is passed through a column containing activated charcoal or resin particles is referred to as

    a. whole bowel irrigation

    b. forced dieresis

    c. hemodialysis

    d. hemoperfusion

Q.5 Which of the following substances is not easily adsorbed by activated charcoal?

    a. Iron

    b. Ethanol

    c. Methanol

    d. All of the above

Q.6 The effect of syrup ipecac starts within 30 minutes of administration and lasts for approximately

    a. 30 minutes

    b. 1 hour

    c. 1 hour and 30 minutes

    d. 2 hours

Q.7 Which of the following procedure(s) is/are contraindicated for patients who have ingested strong acids?

    a. Emesis

    b. Gastric lavage

    c. Whole bowel irrigation

    d. Both emesis and gastric lavage

Q.8 Which of the following technique is helpful in removing ethanol from the body?

    a. Dialysis

    b. Activated charcoal

    c. Diuresis

    d. Hemoperfusion

Q.9 Q.9. The most effective treatment in GI decontamination with acetaminophen is
    a. emesis
    b. gastric lavage
    c. activated charcoal
    d. dialysis

Q.10 Drug X is available as a 2.5% solution for intravenous administration. The desired dosage of this drug is 5 mg/kg. What volume of drug should be injected if the patient weighs 50 kg?
    a. 0.2 mL
    b. 1.0 mL
    c. 2.0 mL
    d. 10 mL
    e. 20 mL

Answers

1. b; 2. c; 3. b; 4. d; 5. d; 6. d; 7. a and b; 8. a; 9. c; 10. d.

Exercise 5

Q.1 Thalidomide was accidentally discovered as
    a. cardiotoxic agent
    b. liver tonic
    c. a sedative/tranquilizer
    d. cough mixture

Q.2 With barbiturate and BDZ abuse and dependency, sedative intoxication generally associated with
    a. slurred speech
    b. uncoordinated motor movements
    c. impairment attention
    d. all of the above

Q.3 A target organ of toxicity is
    a. lung
    b. heart
    c. reproductive system
    d. kidney
    e. liver

Q.4 A single large dose of *N*-nitrosodimethylamine fails to induce cancer in rats, but repeated dosing induces cancer because
    a. the single large dose is lethal, while the threshold for cancer induction can be exceeded by repeated smaller doses
    b. the main DNA lesion from a single large dose can be repaired readily by methyltransferase, while repeated smaller doses can deplete the available repair enzyme, induce mutations in DNA, and effectively induce cancer
    c. the enzyme system involved in detoxification of *N*-nitrosodimethylamine is depleted after repeated doses, allowing

       N-nitrosodimethylamine to build up and exceed the threshold for cancer induction

  d. the enzyme system involved in the conversion of *N*-nitrosodimethylamine to the active carcinogen is induced and on subsequent repeated doses more active carcinogen is produced

  e. the initial dose of *N*-nitrosodimethylamine causes cell damage and, thus, high mitotic rates; subsequent small doses induce mutations in DNA and effectively induce cancer

Q.5 Allergic contact dermatitis is

  a. a nonimmune response caused by a direct action of an agent on the skin

  b. an immediate type I hypersensitivity reaction

  c. a delayed type IV hypersensitivity reaction

  d. characterized by the intensity of reaction being proportional to the elicitation dose

  e. not involved in photoallergic reactions

Q.6 Duration of ultrashort-acting barbiturate is

  a. 6 hours

  b. 3 hours

  c. 15−20 minutes

  d. 0 minutes

Q.7 For each of the following substances, indicate which of the substances would result in increased androgen production in a male athlete?

  a. Cortisol

  b. Dehydroepiandrosterone

  c. Growth hormone

  d. Luteinizing hormone

  e. Salbutamol

Q.8 For each of the following drug or drug groups, which has been established for wrestling, boxing, or horse riding use?

  a. Diuretics

  b. β-Blockers

  c. AASs (androgenic−anabolic steroids)

  d. Streptomycin

Q.9 For each of the following drug or drug groups, which has been established for precision sports, yatching, soccer, and modern pentathalon use?

  a. Diuretics

  b. β-Blockers

  c. AASs

  d. Streptomycin

Q.10 For each of the following drug or drug groups, which has been established for weightlifting, track and field, bodybuilders, footballers use?
  a. Diuretics
  b. β-Blockers
  c. AASs
  d. Streptomycin

Answers

1. c; 2. d; 3. d; 4. b; 5. c; 6. c; 7. b and d; 8. a; 9. b; 10. c.

Exercise 6

Q.1 Which of the following drugs does NOT cause a prolonged QRS?
  a. Thioridazine
  b. Propranolol
  c. Quinine
  d. Metoprolol

Q.2 Which of the following antidotes is NOT used in cyanide poisoning?
  a. Dicobalt EDTA
  b. Hydroxocobalamin
  c. Sodium nitrite
  d. Dimercaprol

Q.3 Regarding "Tests for Drugs" in Toxicology, which statement is FALSE?
  a. Bedside electrocardiogram (ECG) and serum-paracetamol are regarded as routine toxicology screening tests.
  b. Fluorescence polarization immunoassay on urine or blood samples is used for "drug screening."
  c. Gas chromatography/mass spectrometry is performed as "confirmatory test" on blood or urine samples.
  d. Thin layer/paper chromatography used on urine and blood samples assists in "drug screening."

Q.4 Extracorporeal elimination of drugs may be of use in all of the following EXCEPT:
  a. ethylene glycol
  b. salicylates
  c. atenolol
  d. organophosphates

Q.5 The following statements about Digibind are true EXCEPT:
  a. indicated when there is a history of ingestion of greater than 10 mg
  b. 40 mg binds approximately 0.6 mg digoxin
  c. serum digoxin levels increase following its administration
  d. indicated for use if serum digoxin level is greater than 10 nmol/L in acute overdose

Q.6 The following is contraindicated to treat theophylline seizures:
   a. diazepam
   b. phenobarbitone
   c. chloral hydrate
   d. phenytoin

Q.7 Following aspirin overdose the initial acid–base derangement is usually
   a. respiratory acidosis
   b. metabolic acidosis
   c. respiratory alkalosis
   d. metabolic alkalosis

Q.8 Which of the following pairs is FALSE regarding drugs and their appropriate antidotes?
   a. β-Blockers–glucagon
   b. Chloroquine–diazepam
   c. Isoniazid–pralidoxime
   d. Methanol–ethanol

Q.9 With regard to sympathomimetic toxicity, which of the following is TRUE?
   a. Coingestion of cocaine and alcohol results in greater neurological toxicity than cocaine alone.
   b. There is no difference between intravenous or oral amphetamine use and the incidence of rhabdomyolysis.
   c. Patients with psychomotor acceleration and psychosis should initially be reviewed by the psychiatric team.
   d. Auditory hallucinations are uncommon.

Q.10 The maximum safe dose for paracetamol every 24 hours is
   a. 90 mg/kg in children
   b. 150 mg/kg in children
   c. 200 mg/kg in children
   d. in an adult up to 5 g

Answers

1. d; 2. d; 3. d; 4. d; 5. d; 6. d; 7. c; 8. c; 9. d; 10. a.

Exercise 7

Q.1 Theophylline toxicity
   a. often presents with abdominal pain, hematemesis, and drowsiness
   b. causes its effects by blockade of voltage-sensitive calcium channels in cardiac muscle and CNS
   c. is rarely fatal with good supportive care
   d. may cause refractory seizures

Q.2 Which statement is FALSE regarding antihistamine toxicity?
   a. Doxylamine overdose may result in nontraumatic rhabdomyolysis.
   b. The first-generation antihistamine is a common cause for patients presenting with anticholinergic toxicity in ED.

    c. Phenytoin is indicated for managing seizures.

    d. Diphenhydramine and dimenhydrinate may cause cardiac conduction delays similar to tricyclic antidepressant (TCA) overdose.

Q.3 Which statement is FALSE regarding colchicine poisoning?

    a. Colchicine is rapidly absorbed following oral administration.

    b. The multiorgan failure phase typically occurs 24 hours after ingestion.

    c. A rebound leukocytosis occurs 3 weeks after poisoning in survivors, signaling recovery of bone marrow function.

    d. Charcoal is indicated for gut decontamination.

Q.4 Which statement is TRUE regarding anticonvulsant drug poisoning?

    a. Chronic toxicity with therapeutic dosing is uncommon with phenytoin.

    b. A poisoning with sodium valproate at 100 mg/kg is likely to result in coma.

    c. Cardiac monitoring is not required where phenytoin is the only agent ingested.

    d. Carbamazepine levels are not useful in the management of carbamazepine poisoning.

Q.5 Regarding antimicrobial toxicity, the following are often fatal EXCEPT

    a. isoniazid

    b. neomycin

    c. chloroquine

    d. quinine

Q.6 Regarding isoniazid toxicity, all of the following are true EXCEPT

    a. metabolic acidosis are common

    b. treatment of seizures is best treated with high-dose BDZ

    c. acidosis is thought to be secondary to seizures

    d. toxicity is seen early post ingestion (within 1−2 hours)

Q.7 Which is FALSE regarding quinine poisoning?

    a. Deliberate overdose is often fatal.

    b. Significant overdose may result in cardiovascular collapse.

    c. Deliberate overdose may result in permanent blindness.

    d. PR interval prolongation is a major ECG change seen.

Q.8 In overdose the following are true EXCEPT

    a. penicillins and cephalosporins are associated with seizures

    b. seizures in isoniazid toxicity are due to pyridoxine disruption

    c. a farmer presenting with hallucinations, dementia, and exquisitely painful legs may well have ergot poisoning

    d. a patient presenting after ingestion of colchicine presenting with minimal symptoms can be safely discharged after a short period of observation

Q.9 In a patient with a history of unknown psychiatric medication, which of the following is TRUE?

    a. Hyperreflexia, rigidity, and hyperthermia would likely represent a dose-related effect of olanzapine.

    b. Extrapyramidal effects make it more likely to be a typical than atypical antipsychotic.

    c. Positive ECG changes in TCA toxicity are highly predictive of likely arrhythmias.

    d. If you suspect serotonin syndrome in an intubated patient, then midazolam and fentanyl sedation would be a good choice due to its short duration of action.

Q.10 Which of the following is LEAST likely to be helpful in a calcium channel?

    a. Blocker overdose

    b. Atropine

    c. Intra-aortic balloon counterpulsation

    d. Insulin

    e. Resonium

Answers

1. d; 2. c; 3. c; 4. c; 5. b; 6. b; 7. d;8. d; 9. b; 10. d.

FURTHER READING

Bischoff, K., 2018. Toxicity of drugs of abuse. In: Gupta, R.C. (Ed.), Veterinary Toxicology: Basic and Clinical Principles, third ed. Academic Press/Elsevier, San Diego, pp 385–410.

Bischoff, K., 2018. Toxicity of over-the-counter drugs. In: Gupta, R.C. (Ed.), Veterinary Toxicology: Basic and Clinical Principles, third ed. Academic Press/Elsevier, San Diego, pp 357-384.

Gregory, C.W., Leidy, R.B., Hodgson, E., 2004. Classes of toxicants: use classes. A Textbook of Modern Toxicology. John Wiley & Sons, Hoboken, NJ, pp. 49–73.

Gupta, P.K., 2014. Essential Concepts in Toxicology. BSP Pvt Ltd, Hyderabad, India (Chapter 24).

Gupta, P.K., 2016. Fundamental in Toxicology: Essential Concepts and Applications in Toxicology. Elsevier/BSP, USA (Chapter 24).

Papich, M.G., 1990. Toxicosis from over-the-counter human drugs. Vet. Clin. North Am. Small Anim. Pract. 20, 431–451.

Pillay, V.V., 2008. Comprehensive Medical Toxicology, second ed. Paras Medical Publisher, Hyderabad, India (Chapter 21).

Rao, G.N., 2010. Textbook of Forensic Medicine & Toxicology. Jaypee Brothers Medical Publishers, New Delhi, India (Chapter 40).

Radioactive materials

13

CHAPTER OUTLINE

13.1 DEFINITIONS

Q. Define ionization.

Ionization is the process by which an atom or a molecule acquires a negative or positive charge by gaining or losing electrons to form ions, often in conjunction with other chemical changes. Ionization can result from the loss of an electron after collisions with subatomic particles, collisions with other atoms, molecules and ions, or through the interaction with light.

Q. Define radiation.

Radiation is the emission and propagation of energy through space or tissue in the form of waves.

Q. Define alpha particle.

Alpha particle is an electrically charged (+) particle emitted from the nucleus of some radioactive chemicals, cf. plutonium. It contains two protons and two neutrons, and is the largest of the atomic particles emitted by radioactive chemicals. It can cause ionization.

Illustrated Toxicology. DOI: http://dx.doi.org/10.1016/B978-0-12-813213-5.00013-4

Q. Define beta particle.

Beta particle is an electrically charged (−) particle emitted from some radioactive chemicals. It has the mass of an electron. Krypton 85, emitted from nuclear power plants, is a strong beta emitter. Beta particles can cause ionization.

Q. Define curie.

The curie is a unit of ionizing radiation (radioactivity), symbolized as Ci and is equal to 37 billion (3.7×10^{10}) disintegrations or nuclear transformations per second. This is approximately the amount of radioactivity emitted by 1 g of radium-226. The unit is named after Pierre Curie, a French physicist. Ci is the symbol used.

Q. What is microcurie?

Microcurie is one-millionth of a curie (3.7×10^{4} disintegrations per second). Symbol: μCi, mCi, μc.

Q. What is picocurie?

Picocurie is one-trillionth of a curie. Thus, a picocurie (abbreviated as pCi) represents 2.2 disintegrations per minute. One can also say it is one-millionth of a microcurie (3.7×10^{2} disintegrations per second). Symbol: pCi.

For those interested in the numbers, a picocurie is 0.000,000,000,001 (one-trillionth) of a curie, an international measurement unit of radioactivity. One pCi/L means that in 1 L of air, there will be 2.2 radioactive disintegrations each minute.

Q. Define dose energy.

Dose energy imparted to matter by nuclear transformations (radioactivity). Rad = 100 ergs per gram; 1 gray = 100 rad = 10,000 ergs per gram.

Rem = rads $\times$ Q, where Q is a quality factor that attempts to convert rads from different types of radioactivity into a common scale of biological damage (100 rad = 1 Sv).

Q. Compare older units of measure with standard international unit system of radiation energy.

The units, which are used to describe the exposure and dose of ionizing radiation, have changed to an international system (SI), which stands for Systeme Internationale. Table 13.1 compares the previous unit, the older system, and the SI system. Recommended limits on radiation exposure are expressed in sievert.

Q. Define gamma ray.

Gamma ray is a short wavelength electromagnetic radiation released by some nuclear transformations. It is similar to X-ray and will penetrate through the human body. Iodine 131 emits gamma rays. Both gamma and x-rays cause ionization.

Q. Define half-life (biological).

Half-life is biological time required for the body to eliminate one-half of an administered quantity of a radioactive chemical.

Table 13.1 Comparison of Older Units of Measures With Standard International Unit System of Radiation Energy

Item	Previous Unit	SI Unit	Ratios
Activity (i.e., quantity rays or particles)	Curie (Ci)	Becquerel (Bq)	(Ci) 1 Ci = 3.7 × 10^{10} Bq 1 mCi = 37 MBq 1 µCi = 37 KBq U78
Exposure Absorbed dose	Roentgen (R) Rad	X (Coul/kg) Gray (Gy) Gy = 1 J/kg	1 R = 2.58 × 10^{-4} Coul/kg 1 Gy = 100 rad 1 rad = 10 mGy
Gray (Gy)	Gray (Gy) Rem Sievert (Sv)	1 Sv = 100 Rem	1 rem = 10 mSv

m = milli = 1/1000; SI = International System of Units (Systeme Internationale).

Q. Define half-life (physical).

Half-life is physical time required for half of a quantity of radioactive material to undergo a nuclear transformation. The chemical resulting from the transformation may be either radioactive or nonradioactive.

13.2 CLASSIFICATION OF RADIATION BY ITS FREQUENCY

It usually refers to electromagnetic radiation, classified by its frequency:
1. radio
2. infrared
3. visible
4. ultraviolet
5. x-ray
6. gamma ray
7. cosmic rays

Q. What is natural background radiation?

Natural background radiations are emissions from radioactive chemicals, which are not man-made. These chemicals include uranium, radon, potassium, and other trace elements. They are made more hazardous through human activities such as mining and milling because this makes them more available for uptake in food, air, and water.

Q. What is background radiation?

Background radiation includes emissions from radioactive chemicals, which occur naturally, and those that result from the nuclear fission process.

Q. Define Atomic Bomb Casualty Commission (ABCC).

ABCC is now called Radiation Effects Research Foundation (RERF).

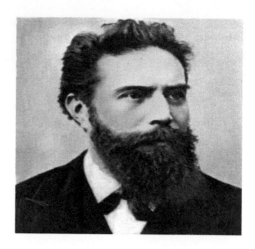

FIGURE 13.1

Wilhem Conrad Roentgen (1845–1923).

http://nautilus.fis.uc.pt/wwwfi/figuras/fisicos/img/roentgen.jpg.

Q. Who discovered X-ray?

In 1895, Wilhem Conrad Roentgen discovered x-rays, and in 1901 he was awarded the first Nobel Prize for physics (Fig. 13.1). These discoveries led to significant advances in medicine.

Q. Who is Marie Curie and what are her contributions?

Marie Skłodowska Curie (7 November 1867 – 4 July 1934) was a Polish and naturalized-French physicist and chemist who conducted pioneering research on radioactivity. She was the first woman to win a Nobel Prize, the first person and only woman to win twice, the only person to win a Nobel Prize in two different sciences, and was part of the Curie family legacy of five Nobel Prizes. She was also the first woman to become a professor at the University of Paris, and in 1995 became the first woman to be entombed on her own merits in the Panthéon in Paris.

In 1903, Marie Curie and Pierre Curie (Fig. 13.2), along with Henri Becquerel, were awarded the Nobel Prize in physics for their contributions to understanding radioactivity, including the properties of uranium. To this day, the "curie" and the "becquerel" are used as units of measure in radiation studies.

13.3 TYPES OF RADIATION

Q. Describe different types of radiation.

These electromagnetic radiations are broadly of two types. The range of electromagnetic spectrum is summarized below (Fig. 13.3).

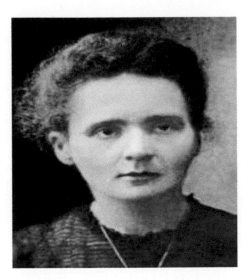

FIGURE 13.2

Marie Curie (1867–1934).

https://encrypted-tbn0.gstatic.com/images?q=tbn:ANd9GcR5o-LaoYDfwsplx8wS7iD8XEXkKY3_Zvf8vg3mR2D9Rsa-qje-

Non-ionising
ionising
Infrared
Radio
Ultraviolet
Extremely low frequency
Microwave
X-ray
Visble Light
Gamma Rays
Non-thermal
Thermal
Optical
Broken Bonds
Induces Low Currents
Induces High Currents
Exites Electrons
Damages DNA
Photo Chemical Effects
???
Heating
Static Field
Power Line
AM Radio
FM Radio
Wifi
Tanning Booth
Medical X-ray

FIGURE 13.3

Electromagnetic spectrum.

https://upload.wikimedia.org/wikipedia/commons/thumb/4/48/EM-spectrum.svg/400px-EM-spectrum.svg.png.

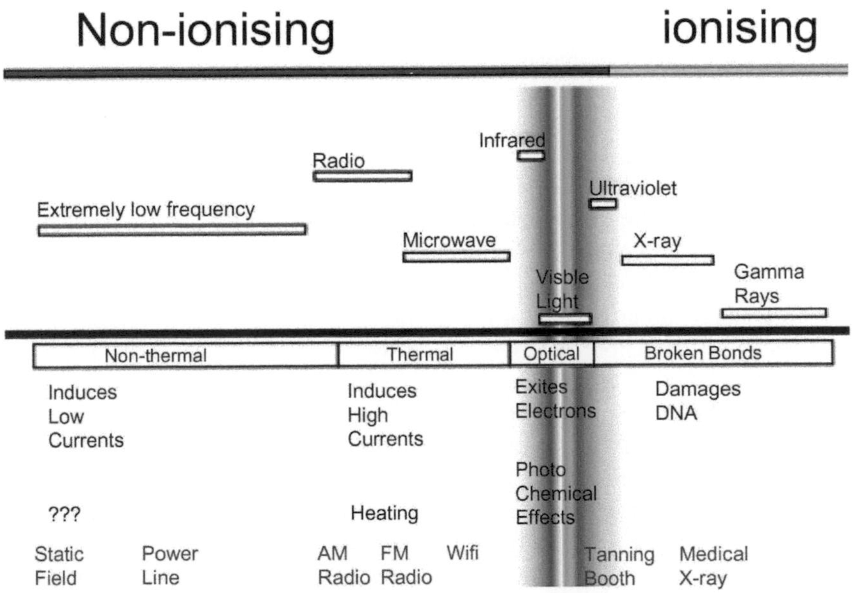

1. Nonionizing radiation: Nonionizing radiation includes ultraviolet, visible, infrared, radio and TV, and power transmission. We depend on the sun's radiation for photosynthesis and heat.

2. Ionizing radiation: Ionizing radiation includes high-energy radiation such as cosmic rays, x-rays, or gamma rays generated by nuclear decay. Ionizing radiation also includes several types of subatomic particles such as beta radiation (high-energy electrons) and alpha radiation (helium ions). Medical x-rays are an example of a common beneficial exposure to ionizing radiation. Nuclear radiation is not only used to generate electricity and cure disease but also an important element in military weapons. Uses of nuclear radiation pose serious problems of human exposure and environmental contamination.

13.3.1 NONIONIZING RADIATION

Q. What are the uses of nonionizing radiation?

Uses of nonionizing radiation include power transmission, TV, radio, and satellite transmissions, radar, light bulbs, heating, cooking, microwave ovens, lasers, photosynthesis (sunlight), mobile phones, and WiFi networks.

Q. What are the sources of nonionizing radiation?

Source of nonionizing radiation include ultraviolet light, visible light, infrared radiation, microwaves, radio and TV, mobile phones, and power transmission.

Q. Who are sensitive to nonionizing radiation?

Sensitive individuals: variable, e.g., fair-skinned children (sunburn).

Q. What are the biological effects of nonionizing radiations?

Nonionizing radiation is harmless; however, at higher levels and longer durations of exposure, it can be harmful. The classic example is sunlight or solar radiation. Ultraviolet radiation from the sun, part of the electromagnetic spectrum with wavelengths less than 400 nm, can damage the skin. Sunburn (erythema) is the result of excessive exposure of our skin to UV radiation when we lack the protection of UV-absorbing melanin. Acute cellular damage causes an inflammatory-type response and increased vascular circulation (vasodilation) close to the skin. The increased circulation cause the redness and hot feeling to the skin. Lightly pressing on the skin pushes the blood away and the spot appears white. Darker skinned people have an ongoing production of melanin, which protects them to some extent from UV radiation. In lighter skinned people, UV radiation stimulates the production of melanin, producing a tan and protection against UV radiation. Extreme exposure can result in blistering and severe skin damage. UV radiation can also damage cellular DNA, and repeated damage can overwhelm the DNA repair mechanism, resulting in skin cancer. Skin cancer accounts for approximately one-third of all cancers diagnosed each year. Thinning of the atmospheric ozone layer, which filters UV radiation, is suspected as being one cause of the increased incidence of skin cancer.

13.3.2 IONIZING RADIATION

Q. Describe ionizing radiation.

Ionizing radiation is higher energy radiation, with enough energy to remove an electron from an atom and damage biological material.

Q. What are the uses of ionizing radiation?

The uses are nuclear power, medical x-rays, medical diagnostics, scientific research, cancer treatment, and cathode ray tube displays.

Q. What is the source of ionizing radiation?

The source is radon, x-rays, radioactive material producing alpha, beta, and gamma radiation, and cosmic rays from the sun and space.

Q. What is the recommended daily dose of ionizing radiation?

Recommended daily intake is none (not essential).

Q. How ionizing radiation is absorbed in the body?

Absorption is done through interaction with atoms of tissue.

Q. What are the main types of ionizing radiation?

The four main types of ionizing radiation are:

1. alpha particles,
2. beta particles (electrons),
3. gamma rays, and
4. x-rays.

Q. What is the mechanism of action ionizing radiation?

Ionizing radiation has sufficient energy to produce ion pairs as it passes through matter, freeing electrons and leaving the rest of the atoms positively charged. In other words, there is enough energy to remove an electron from an atom. The energy released is also enough to break bonds in DNA, which can lead to significant cellular damage and cancer.

Q. Which radiation is more harmful?

Ionizing radiation is more harmful than nonionizing radiation because it has enough energy to remove an electron from an atom and thus directly damage biological material. The energy is enough to damage DNA, which can result in cell death or cancer.

Q. Describe the nature of alpha particles.

Alpha particles are heavyweight and relatively low-energy emissions from the nucleus of radioactive material. The transfer of energy occurs over a very short distance of about 10 cm in air. A piece of paper or layer of skin will stop an alpha particle. The primary hazard occurs in the case of internal exposure to an alpha-emitting material: cells close to the particle-emitting material will be damaged. Typical sites of accumulation include bone, kidney, liver, lung, and spleen. Radium is an alpha-particle emitter that accumulates in the bone after ingestion, causing a bone sarcoma. Airplane travel increases our exposure to cosmic and solar radiation that is normally blocked by the atmosphere. Radiation intensity is greater across the poles and at higher altitudes, thus individual exposure varies depending on the route of travel.

Storms on the sun can produce solar flares that release larger amounts of radiation than normal. For the occasional traveler, this radiation exposure is well below recommended limits established by regulatory authorities.

Q. Who are the sensitive individuals to ionizing radiation?

Children and developing organisms are sensitive to ionizing radiation.

13.4 HIROSHIMA AND NAGASAKI INCIDENCES

Q. What do you know about Hiroshima and Nagasaki incidences?

The US military dropped the first atomic bomb on Hiroshima, Japan, on August 6, 1945, and a second on Nagasaki, Japan, 3 days later. The bombs used two different types of radioactive material—235 U in the first bomb (Uranium-235 (^{235}U)) and 239 Pu (Plutonium-239) in the second. It is estimated that 64,000 people died from the initial blasts and radiation exposure. Approximately 100,000 survivors were enrolled in follow-up studies.

Q. What are the lessons learned from Hiroshima and Nagasaki incidences?

These incidences indicated that the greater the dose, the greater the likelihood of developing cancer. The second lesson was that there could be a very long delay in the onset of the cancer, from 10 to 40 years. This confirmed an increased incidence of cancer. It is estimated that 1 in 100 cancers are the result of this background exposure.

13.5 HEALTH EFFECTS OF RADIATION

Q. What are the health benefits from radiation?

All life is dependent on small doses of electromagnetic radiation. Radiations are produced by disintegration of unstable naturally occurring or man-made elements. Radiations have been utilized for many beneficial effects. For example, radiation-emitting devices help us to use many devices such as cell phones and radios, from medical x-rays to the electricity that powers our homes. X-rays were also used to treat disease such as ringworm in children. Subsequently during 1950s x-rays were used to treat a degenerative bone disease called ankylosing spondylitis.

Q. What are the adverse health effects/hazards of electromagnetic radiation?

Direct or indirect exposure to ionizing radiations produces number of deleterious effects on health of human beings as well as on animals. Ionizing radiations can cause different types of damages in mammalian systems including effects on both proliferative and nonproliferative tissues. A few of them are summarized in Table 13.2.

Table 13.2 Biological Effects of Electromagnetic Frequency Radiation

• Genetic effects	• Cardiovascular effects
• Cancer	• Sleeping disorders
• Cellular/molecular	• Hormonal disturbances
• Behavior changes	• Immune system
• Nervous system/brain	• Metabolic effects
• Blood brain barrier permeability	• Brittle diabetes
• Calcium efflux	• Autoimmunity
• Impaired learning	• Fertility impairment
	• Interpersonal effects

13.6 QUESTION AND ANSWER EXERCISES

13.6.1 SHORT QUESTIONS AND ANSWERS

Exercise 1

Q.1 What is the difference between radiation exposure and irradiation?

In both radiation exposure and irradiation, exposure to radiation occurs. However, in irradiation, contamination with radioactive material does not occur, which prevents postexposure radiation (e.g., γ-irradiation of syringes, irradiation used for treating cancers, etc.).

Q.2 Name the two elements that are responsible for natural background radiation in earth?

Radon (from uranium) and Thoron (from thorium) are responsible for 54% of the natural background radiation in earth.

Q.3 Why in the presence of heavy metals, more free radicals are generated?

Heavy metals (such as Fe, Pb, and Cd) have more number of electrons in outer shell. Hence, when a free radical attacks a heavy metal, there will be shower of electrons, which in turn produces more free radicals.

Q.4 Why are there so many different terms when it comes to radiation? Rem, rad, curie, gray, and so on. What are they all for?

One reason for so many different terms is that the United States uses traditional radiation units, whereas the rest of the world uses an international system of units (very similar to the United States using inches and other countries using centimeters). In the international system, sievert, gray, becquerel, and coulombs/kilogram are used, whereas traditional units are rem ($=0.01$ Sv), rad ($=0.01$ Gy), curie ($=3.7 \times 10^{10}$ Bq), and roentgen ($=2.5 \times 10^{-4}$ Coul/kg).

Another reason for all the different types of units is our need, as scientists, to be precise and accurate when we are describing radiation interactions and energy left behind.

Q.5 Can radioactive material affect the body? Explain how.

YES. Radiation is a "potentially harmful" agent. When radiation interacts with the tissue of our bodies, whether it is from radioactive atoms inside the body or from an external source such as an x-ray machine, it can cause damage to cells. This damage stems from the process of ionization. The radiation from radioactive atoms is called "ionizing radiation" because it causes ionization. Ionization is simply the "knocking off" of electrons from the atoms; they are normally said to "orbit." These electrons act as the "glue" that holds atoms together in chemical bonds. So, if some of the electrons get knocked loose by ionizing radiation, some of the chemical bonds get broken. This can result in damage to the cells. Because there is radioactive material in our bodies, this process goes on all the time.

Q.6 What is uranium?

Uranium is the heaviest metal that occurs in nature. It is an unstable material that gradually breaks apart or "decays" at the atomic level. Any such material is said to be "radioactive." As uranium slowly decays, it gives off invisible bursts of penetrating energy called "atomic radiation." It also produces more than a dozen other radioactive substances as by-products.

Q.7 What is radon?

These unstable by-products, having little or no commercial value, are called "uranium decay products." They are discarded as waste when uranium is mined. One of them is a toxic radioactive gas called radon. The others are radioactive solids.

Q.8 What is radioactivity?

Everything is made of tiny little particles called atoms. They are too small to be seen even under a powerful microscope. When a substance is radioactive, it means that its atoms are exploding (submicroscopically) and throwing off pieces of themselves with great force. This process is called "radioactive decay."

During radioactive decay, two types of tiny electrically charged particles are given off, traveling very fast. They are called alpha and beta particles. Some radioactive materials are alpha emitters, and others are beta emitters. In addition, highly energetic rays called gamma rays are often emitted. Gamma rays are not material particles at all, but a form of pure energy very similar to x-rays, traveling at the speed of light.

Q.9 How far can atomic radiation penetrate?

Gamma rays penetrate through soft tissue just as light shines through a window. Beta particles have less penetrating power, traveling less than 2 cm in soft tissue. Alpha particles have the least penetrating power, traveling just a few micrometers in soft tissue, equivalent to a few cell diameters.

Q.10 Is radioactivity dangerous?

Alpha particles, beta particles, and gamma rays can do great harm to a living cell by breaking its chemical bonds at random and disrupting the cell's genetic instructions.

Massive exposure to atomic radiation can cause death within a few days or weeks. Smaller doses can cause burns, loss of hair, nausea, loss of fertility, and pronounced changes in the blood. Still smaller doses, too small to cause any immediate visible damage, can result in cancer or leukemia in the person exposed, congenital abnormalities in his or her children (including physical deformities, diseases, and mental retardation), and possible genetic defects in future generations.

Outside the body, alpha emitters are the least harmful, and gamma emitters are more dangerous than beta emitters.

Inside the body, however, alpha emitters are the most dangerous. They are about 20 times more damaging than beta emitters or gamma emitters. Thus, although alpha radiation cannot penetrate through a sheet of paper or a dead layer of skin, alpha emitters are extremely hazardous when taken into the body by inhalation or ingestion, or through a cut or open sore.

Exercise 2

Q.1 How do radioactive elements produce other radioactive elements?

When atoms undergo radioactive decay, they change into new substances, because they have lost something of themselves. These by-products of radioactive decay are called "decay products" or "progeny." In many cases, the decay products are also radioactive. If so, they too will disintegrate, producing even more decay products and giving off even more atomic radiation.

Q.2 What is the difference between ionizing radiation and radioactivity?

A radioactive atom is unstable because its nucleus contains extra energy. When this atom decays to a more stable atom, it releases this extra energy as ionizing radiation.

Q.3 Is there more than one kind of radiation?

Yes, in addition to x-rays, three are common: the alpha, beta, and gamma radiations. Alpha rays (the nuclei of helium atom) may be stopped by paper, beta rays (high-speed electrons) are stopped less easily, and gamma rays (such as x-rays) may need lead or concrete to stop them.

Q.4 Will these ionizing radiations make me radioactive?

No, just as light will not make you glow in the dark, a chest x-ray will not make you radioactive.

Q.5 If ionizing radiation does not make a thing radioactive, how do items become radioactive in a nuclear reactor?

In a nuclear reactor there are billions of free nuclear projectiles called neutrons. When absorbed in a material, they make it radioactive, i.e., it emits its own radiation. This is how radioisotopes are made. There are very few free neutrons in the environment.

Q.6 Will radiation build up in the body until it gets to a point where it kills you?

No, ionizing radiation does not build up in the body. All radiation will eventually disperse. However, radiation effect may appear, after exposure to a high intensity of radiation, just as you may get sunburn from overexposure to sunlight.

Q.7 When radiation does not build up in the body, how does it harm a person?

All radiation carries energy that may damage living cells. This damage may cause cells either to die or to change their structure and function.

Q.8 If anyone gets a dose of radiation, will he die?

Very unlikely, because it would take a very large dose to kill sufficient numbers of your cells to cause death.

Q.9 Where does natural radiation dose come from?

The major part derives from the decay of natural radioactivity in the earth, most of it from uranium and thorium: they give rise to a radioactive gas called radon in the air we breathe. Radon is present in all buildings. Smaller, and roughly equal, parts of everyday radiation come from cosmic rays and from the natural radioactivity of our food and drink. Some other radiations are man-made.

Q.10 What are the man-made sources of radiation?

Medical uses of ionizing radiation are the major sources. These include the use of x-rays for radiography and computer tomography, and radiopharmaceuticals in nuclear medicine.

13.6.2 MULTIPLE CHOICE QUESTIONS (CHOOSE THE BEST STATEMENT, IT CAN BE ONE, TWO OR ALL OR NONE)

Exercise 3

Q.1 Which of the following ionizing radiations has the shortest range (i.e., travels the shortest distance in tissue) for the same initial energy?
 a. alpha particle
 b. beta particle
 c. gamma ray
 d. x ray
 e. cosmic ray

Q.2 An individual exposed to 10 rads (0.1 Gy) of whole body x-irradiation would be expected to _____
 a. have a severe bone marrow depression
 b. die
 c. be permanently sterilized
 d. exhibit no symptoms
 e. vomit

Q.3 The cellular component, which is affected during radiation damage is ____
 a. lipid
 b. DNA
 c. RNA
 d. sugar

Q.4 Molecules with unpaired electrons in the outer shells are known as _____
 a. free radicals
 b. sulfur

c. nitrogen
d. carbon

Q.5 Cells are more susceptible for radiation in the following stage(s) of cell cycle:
  a. M-Phase (mitosis)
  b. early G-phase
  c. late G-phase
  d. S-phase

Q.6 The following organ is resistant to radiation:
  a. Endocrine glands
  b. Kidney
  c. Bone marrow
  d. Germinal cells.

Q.7 More than 99% of the energy from the sun is within the spectral range of _____ nanometers.
  a. 150–4000
  b. 700–4000
  c. 140–400
  d. 400–700

Q.8 Which of the following inversions is short-lived?
  a. Radiation
  b. Subsidence

Q.9 The most common type of free radicals produced in the body are _____
  a. NO
  b. O_2
  c. SO_2
  d. reactive oxygen species (ROS)

Q.10 The part of the head, which can be affected by the heating effects of mobile phone, is _____.
  a. ears
  b. nose
  c. tongue
  d. cornea

Answers

1. a; 2. d; 3. b; 4. a; 5. a and b; 6. a. (Because the proliferation rate of endocrine glands is very low, the other organs are very sensitive due to high proliferative rate); 7. a; 8. a; 9. d (ROS include Hydroxyl (OH^-), Superoxide (O^{-2}), Singlet oxygen (O^-), Hydrogen peroxide (H_2O_2), etc.; the other types are reactive nitrogen species (RNS)—Nitric oxide (NO), peroxynitrate, etc.; 10. d (cornea of the eye lacks temperature regulating mechanism and hence could be affected by dielectric heating from mobile phones during usage).

13.6.3 FILL IN THE BLANKS

Exercise 4

Q.1 The process of transmission of electromagnetic waves through a medium or vacuum is known as _____.

Q.2 Ionizing radiations produce ions by knocking out _____ from atoms.

Q.3 The most sensitive hematological test for detecting radiation damage is _____.

Q.4 The ionizing radiation that has the least penetrating capacity is _____.

Q.5 The ionizing radiation that has the highest penetrating capacity is _____.

Q.6 The type of UV rays, which can only reach the earth, is _____.

Q.7 Nonionizing radiations include _____, _____, _____, and _____.

Q.8 The SI unit of radiation is _____ and depreciated unit in CGS system is _____.

Q.9 One _____ is equal to 100 rad (or 1 rad = 0.01 Gy).

Q.10 The instrument that is used to measure radiation is called _____.

Q.11 The most potent among the free radical is _____.

Q.12 The damaging effect of free radicals on protein is _____ and on DNA is _____.

Answers

1. RADIATION; 2. ELECTRONS; 3. ABSOLUTE LYMPHOCYTE COUNT (lymphocyte count (LC) <1000 cells/cc within 24 h or <500 cells/cc within 48 h indicates severe exposure. If LC is >1500/cc after 48 h postexposure, it rules out radiation); 4. ALPHA (α)-PARTICLES (α-particles are large in size (two protons + two neutrons = α-particle). Hence, they have the least penetration ability. However, due to their high mass, they have high linear energy transfer (LET) ability; 5. GAMMA (γ) RAYS (because γ-rays are nonparticulate electromagnetic radiation, they have the highest penetration ability. However, as the mass is least, LET is very low); 6. UV-A TYPE (UV-B and C are more powerful than UV-A rays; however, they are filtered by ozone layer (up to 99%). A sunscreen with both UV-A and B sun protection factor (SPF) of at least 25 is recommended in Indian conditions; 7. visible light, infrared rays, microwaves, radio waves; 8. GRAY (Gy) and RAD (rad); 9. Gray; 10. GEIGER-MULLER COUNTER; 11. HYDROXYL (OH−), (OH− is produced through Fenton's reaction in the body when hydrogen peroxide acts on iron); 12. PROTEIN OXIDATION and DNA FRAGMENTATION.

Exercise 5

Q.1 During nuclear explosion, the ascent and subsequent descent of radioactive material either in the vicinity or away from site of explosion is known as _____.

Q.2 Among the radioactive material produced by nuclear explosions, the elements with biological significance are _____ and _____.

Q.3 The environmental hazard from nuclear power plants is due to the release of radioactive _____.

Q.4 The group of symptoms that appear within 48 h of exposure to radiation are known as _____.

Q.5 The most common type of cancer induced by radiation is _____.

Q.6 In case of grazing animals on fall-out pastures, the system that is primarily affected is _____.

Q.7 The amount of radio frequency radiation absorbed by human body while using mobile phone is measured by _____.

Q.8 The sensitivity of rapidly proliferating cells to radiation is _____.

Q.9 The system in the body, which is more susceptible to radiation exposure is_____.

Q.10 The lethal dose of radiation in humans is expressed as _____.

Answers

1. FALL OUT (Fall out can occur within few minutes to months and either in the vicinity or very far away); 2. STRONTIUM (ST90) and CESIUM (CS137) (due to long half-lives); 3. COOLANT (light water, heavy water, liquid sodium, etc., are used as coolants); 4. PRODROMAL SYNDROME (the symptoms include nausea, vomiting, anorexia, fatigue, diarrhea, and sweating); 5. LEUKEMIA; 6. GASTROINTESTINAL SYSTEM; 7. SPECIFIC ABSORPTION RATE (SAR) (In the United States, permissible SAR is set at 1.6 W/kg user mass; In Europe, SAR is set at 2.0 W/kg); 8. MORE; 9. HEMOPOETIC SYSTEM; 10. LD50/60 (lethal dose required to causes 50% mortality in 30 days; in animals it is LD50/30).

FURTHER READING

Gupta, P.K., 1988. Veterinary Toxicology. Cosmo Publications, New Delhi, India (Chapter 10).

Gupta, P.K., 2014. Essential Concepts in Toxicology. BSP Pvt Ltd, Hyderabad, India (Chapter 30).

Gupta, P.K., 2016. Fundamental in Toxicology: Essential Concepts and Applications in Toxicology. Elsevier/BSP, San Diego, USA (Chapters 30).

Henriksen, T., Maillie, D.H., 2003. Radiation and Health. Taylor and Francis, USA.

Hoel, D.G., 2013. Toxic effects of radiation and radioactive materials. In: Klaassen, C.D. (Ed.), Casarett and Doull's Toxicology: The Basic Science of Poisons, eighth ed. McGraw-Hill, New York, NY, pp. 1113–1130.

Murphy, L., 2018. Ionizing radiation and radioactive materials in health and disease. In: Gupta, R.C. (Ed.), Veterinary Toxicology: Basic and Clinical Principles, second ed. Academic Press/Elsevier, San Diego, USA, pp. 327–338.

Environmental and ecotoxicology

14

CHAPTER OUTLINE

14.1 ENVIRONMENTAL TOXICOLOGY

Q. Define environmental toxicology.

Environmental toxicology deals with the effects of environmental toxicants on health and the environment.

Q. How do environmental toxicants affect health?

Environmental toxicants are agents released into the general environment that can cause adverse effects on health. Links between the natural environment and human health have been recognized for centuries. The word "health" here refers to not only the human health but also the health of animals and plants. Therefore, the study of environmental toxicology stems from the recognition that:

1. human survival depends upon the well-being of other species and upon the availability of clean air, water, and food;
2. anthropogenic and naturally occurring chemicals can have detrimental effects on living organisms and ecological processes.

Environmental toxicology is thus concerned with how environmental toxicants, through their interaction with humans, animals, and plants, influence the health and welfare of these organisms.

Illustrated Toxicology. DOI: http://dx.doi.org/10.1016/B978-0-12-813213-5.00014-6

Q. What is photodegradation?

Photodegradation is the alteration of materials by light. Typically, the term refers to the combined action of sunlight and air. Photodegradation is usually oxidation and hydrolysis.

Explanation: Photodegradation implies reduction in toxicity and, in the case of many complex molecules containing chlorine, bromine, or fluorine, can result from ultraviolet (UV)-induced dehalogenation. Although many man-made chemicals are rapidly photodegraded by sunlight, some chemicals become more toxic to organisms through photoactivation. For example, dechlorination of hexachlordibenzo-p-dioxin may produce lower chlorinated but more toxic dioxin congeners.

Q. How photosynthesis takes place?

Photosynthesis is the process used by plants, algae, and certain bacteria to harness energy from sunlight into chemical energy (Fig. 14.1).

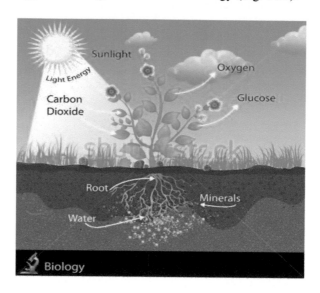

FIGURE 14.1

Photosynthesis in plants.

https://thumb9.shutterstock.com/display_pic_with_logo/1120544/139536956/stock-vector-easy-to-edit-vector-illustration-of-photosynthesis-in-plant-139536956.jpg.

Q. What is sunburn?

Sunburn is a form of radiation burn that affects living tissue, such as skin, that results from an overexposure to ultraviolet (UV) radiation, commonly from the sun.

Q. Describe in brief signs and symptoms of sunburn.

Typically, there is initial redness (erythema), followed by varying degrees of pain, proportional in severity to both the duration and intensity of exposure (Fig. 14.2).

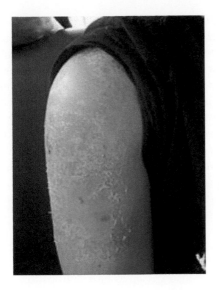

FIGURE 14.2

Sunburn peeling. The destruction of lower layers of the epidermis causes rapid loss of the top layers.

https://upload.wikimedia.org/wikipedia/commons/thumb/c/c8/Sun_burn.JPG/255px-Sun_burn.jpg.

Other symptoms can include edema, itching, peeling skin, rash, nausea, fever, chills, and syncope. Also, a small amount of heat is given off from the burn, caused by the concentration of blood in the healing process, giving a warm feeling to the affected area. Sunburns may be classified as superficial or partial thickness burns.

Q. What is biotransformation?

Biotransformation is the chemical modification (or modifications) made by an organism on a chemical compound. If this modification ends in mineral compounds such as CO_2, NH_4^+, or H_2O, the biotransformation is called mineralization. Biotransformation occurs not only in animals and plants but also in soil microbes such as fungi and bacteria under aerobic or anaerobic conditions. In vertebrates, microbes within digestive tracts can also greatly influence the biotransformation of environmental contaminants. Metabolism and conjugation of xenobiotics often reduces toxicity and enhances the ability of the animal to eliminate the agent from the body.

Q. What is bioactivation?

Bioactivation is the process where enzymes or other biologically active molecules acquire the ability to perform their biological function, such as inactive proenzymes being converted into active enzymes that are able to catalyze their substrates into products to produce (by definition) metabolites that are more toxic than their parent compounds.

Explanation: The organochlorine pesticide DDT is not itself highly toxic to birds, but its metabolite p, p'-DDE can cause thinning of eggshells due to disruption of calcium metabolism. Also, microbial metabolism in anaerobic sediments converts inorganic mercury to methylmercury, which is responsible for cognitive, motor, and visual–spatial disabilities, especially in the developing young of a wide array of animals including human beings. Efforts by organisms to detoxify exogenous compounds can sometimes produce temporary bioactivation manifested in reactive species such as singlet oxygen or hydroxy radicals. These free radicals or oxidants, as well as their depletion of natural antioxidants in the body (e.g., glutathione, ascorbic acid, and carotenoids), can lead to oxidative stress, damaging macromolecules, cells, and tissues. Such processes can culminate in overt tissue injury and also DNA damage leading to degenerative diseases, mutagenesis, carcinogenesis, and hereditary defects, as well as their metabolites, and their environmental degradation products.

Q. What is biomagnification?

Biomagnification, also known as bioamplification or biological magnification, is the increasing concentration of a substance, such as a toxic chemical, in the tissues of organisms at successively higher levels in a food chain (Fig. 14.3).

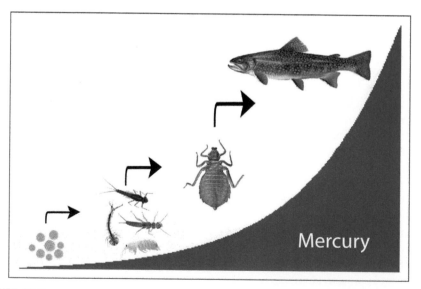

FIGURE 14.3

Biological magnification of mercury.

14.1.1 EXPOSURE OF TOXICANTS

Q. What are the different steps involved from exposure to toxic substance at concentration that are harmful?

1. Release of pollutant into the environment
2. Transport and fate into biota (with/out chemical transformation)
3. Exposure to biological and ecological system
4. Understanding responses and/or effects (molecular to ecological systems)
5. Design remediation, minimization, conservation, and risk assessment plans to eliminate, prevent or predict environmental and human health pollutions situations

   It is therefore the study that involves air pollution that includes the earth, air, water, living environments, and social components, and on ecotoxicology (ecology + toxicology) that want to protect many individuals, populations, communities, and ecosystems from exposure to toxic substance at concentrations that are harmful.

Q. Describe health effects of indoor air pollution.

   Many of the health problems associated with indoor air pollution generally involve nonspecific symptomatology and appear to involve a wide range of potential toxicants and sources. Two broadly defined illnesses that are largely unique to the indoor environment are Sick-Building Syndromes. Frequently, but not always, this syndrome occurs in new, poorly ventilated, or recently refurbished office buildings. The suspected causes include combustion products, household chemicals, biological materials and vapors, and emissions from furnishings; they are exacerbated by the effect of poor ventilation on comfort factors. The perception of irritancy to the eyes, nose, and throat ranks among the predominant symptoms that can become intolerable with repeated exposures (Table 14.1).

Table 14.1 Symptoms Commonly Associated With the Sick-Building Syndromes

Eyes, nose, and throat irritation
Headaches
Fatigue
Reduced attention span
Irritability
Nasal congestion
Difficulty in breathing
Nosebleeds
Dry skin
Nausea

Q. Describe some major incidences of outdoor air pollution.

1. A single chemical has been accidentally released (e.g., methyl isocyanate in Bhopal, India), establishing the relationship between cause and ill effect is straightforward.

2. Three acute episodes of community air pollution are considered classic (Meuse Valley, Belgium; Donora, Pennsylvania; and London, United Kingdom). In each event, community inhabitants were clearly affected adversely; hospitalizations were concomitant with an elevated mortality rate. The famous "London smog" of 1952 is estimated to have resulted in 4000 excess deaths during the event itself.

3. Episodes in the more recent past include New York City, Steubenville, Ohio; Pittsburgh, Pennsylvania; Athens, Greece, and entire regions of Western Europe from the Netherlands to the Ruhr Valley of Germany have all had air pollution episodes of note between 1970 and 1995.

Q. What is the source of environmental contamination?

Environmental contamination can emanate from:

1. industries
2. mines
3. refineries
4. coal-burning power plants
5. sewage treatment plants.

Nonpoint sources, such as pesticides washed from large areas of land after precipitation, effluents from the tailpipes of myriad motor vehicles, or semivolatile pollutants that circle the globe after evaporation from the soils of agricultural and urban environments.

Q. What are the possible adverse effects of dust inhalation of different particles size on lung?

Possible health issues arising from dust inhalation of different particles sizes are summarized in Fig. 14.4.

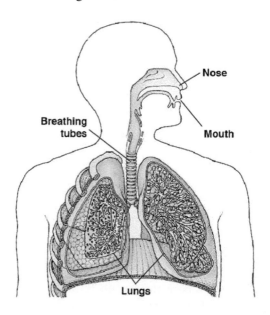

FIGURE 14.4

Possible health issues arising from dust inhalation.

Reproduced from Health and Safety Executive.

Q. What are main health hazards of pollution?

The main health hazards due to air and water pollution and due to soil contamination are shown in Fig. 14.5.

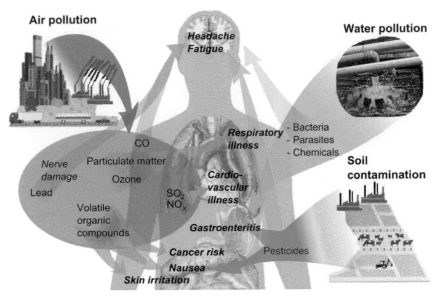

FIGURE 14.5

Health effects of pollution.

https://encrypted-tbn3.gstatic.com/images?q=tbn:ANd9GcQEdcFNcowki8-uFx6mj9pSKvTz_5fwVm-
BAvehcbZNUMbmKYuNFWZufFvz.

Q. What is nitrogen cycle?

The nitrogen cycle is a model that explains how nitrogen is recycled. It includes a series of processes by which nitrogen and its compounds are interconverted in the environment and in living organisms, including nitrogen fixation and decomposition.

Q. Describe in brief nitrogen cycle.

Nitrogen is essential for the formation of amino acids in proteins.

There is lot of nitrogen in air—about 78% of the air is nitrogen. Because nitrogen is so unreactive, it cannot be used directly by plants to make protein. Only nitrates are useful to plants, so we are dependent on other processes to convert nitrogen to nitrates in the soil (Fig. 14.6).

1. Nitrogen gas is converted to nitrate compounds by nitrogen-fixing bacteria in soil or root nodules. Lightning also converts nitrogen gas to nitrate compounds. The Haber process converts nitrogen gas into ammonia used in fertilizers. Ammonia is converted to nitrates by nitrifying bacteria in the soil.

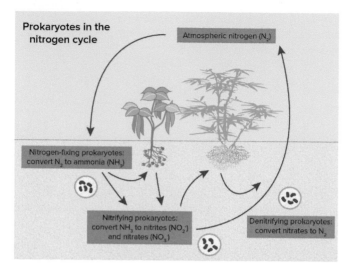

FIGURE 14.6

Nitrogen cycle.

Reproduced with permission from Khan Academy: Modified from Nitrogen cycle by Johann Dréo.

2. Plants absorb nitrates from the soil and use these to build up proteins. The plant may be eaten by an animal, and its biomass is used to produce animal protein.

3. Urea and egested material is broken down by decomposers. This results in nitrogen being returned to the soil as ammonia.

4. Decomposers also break down the bodies of dead organisms resulting in nitrogen being returned to the soil as ammonia.

5. Higher only: In some conditions denitrifying bacteria in the soil break down nitrates and return nitrogen to the air. This is usually in waterlogged soil. Improving drainage reduces this effect, making the soil more fertile.

Q. What is oxygen cycle?

The oxygen cycle is the biogeochemical cycle of oxygen within its three main reservoirs: the atmosphere (air), the total content of biological matter within the biosphere (the global sum of all ecosystems), and the Earth's crust (Fig. 14.7).

Q. What is carbon dioxide cycle?

1. Carbon enters the atmosphere as carbon dioxide from respiration and combustion.

2. Carbon dioxide is absorbed by producers to make carbohydrates in photosynthesis.

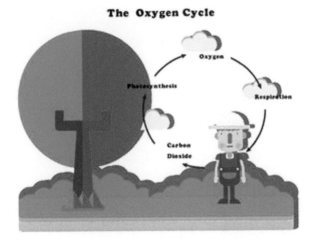

FIGURE 14.7

Oxygen cycle.

3. Animals feed on the plant passing the carbon compounds along the food chain. Most of the carbon they consume is exhaled as carbon dioxide formed during respiration. The animals and plants eventually die.

4. The dead organisms are eaten by decomposers and the carbon in their bodies is returned to the atmosphere as carbon dioxide. In some conditions decomposition is blocked. The plant and animal material may then be available as fossil fuel in the future for combustion (Fig. 14.8).

Q. Describe carbon cycle in the sea.

In the sea, marine animals may convert some of the carbon in their diet to calcium carbonate that is used to make their shells. Over time, the shells of dead organisms collect on the seabed and form limestone. Due to earth movements, this limestone may eventually become exposed to the air where it is weathered and the carbon is released back into the atmosphere as carbon dioxide. Volcanic action may also release carbon dioxide (Fig. 14.9).

YOU WILL DIE BUT THE CARBON WILL NOT; ITS CAREER DOES NOT END WITH YOU. IT WILL RETURN TO THE SOIL, AND THERE A PLANT MAY TAKE IT UP AGAIN IN TIME, SENDING IT ONCE MORE ON A CYCLE OF PLANT AND ANIMAL LIFE.

JACOB BRONOWSKI

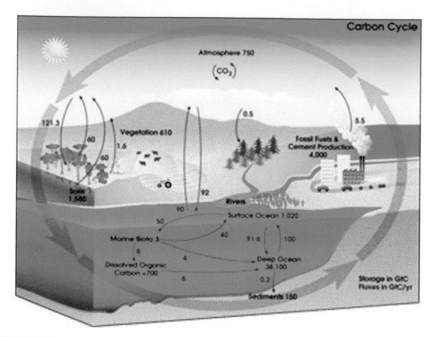

FIGURE 14.8

Carbon dioxide cycle.

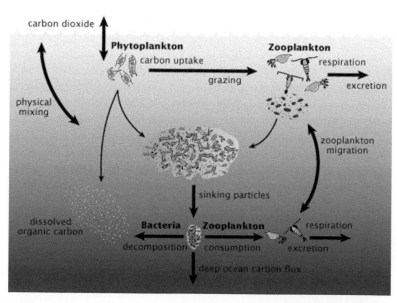

FIGURE 14.9

Global carbon cycle.

14.1.2 MAJOR POLLUTANTS

Q. What are major pollutants in the air?

1. ozone (O_3)
2. sulfur dioxide (SO_2)
3. oxides of nitrogen (NO_2)
4. carbon monoxide (CO)
5. particulate matter (PM)
6. lead (Pb)

Six major air pollutants account for 98% of pollution.

Others include volatile organic compounds and a myriad of other compounds considered under the category of hazardous air pollutants (HAPs).

14.1.2.1 Ozone (O_3)

Q. What is the effect of stratosphere ozone depletion?

Ozone in the stratosphere protects us from the harmful effects of excess ultraviolet radiation from the sun that, among other things, causes skin cancer. CFCs—chlorofluorocarbons (formerly used extensively as refrigerants and solvents), after entering the stratosphere, catalytically reacts with the ozone, thereby reducing the ozone layer leading to harmful effects of excess ultraviolet radiation from the sun that, among other things, causes skin cancer.

14.1.2.2 Sulfur dioxide (SO_2)

Q. What is sulfate aerosis?

The term sulfate aerosis is used for a suspension of fine solid particles of a sulfate or tiny droplets of a solution of a sulfate or of sulfuric acid (which is not technically a sulfate). They are produced by chemical reactions in the atmosphere from gaseous precursors (with the exception of sea salt sulfate and gypsum dust particles). The two main sulfuric acid precursors are sulfur dioxide (SO_2) from anthropogenic sources and volcanoes, and dimethyl sulfide from biogenic sources, especially marine plankton. These aerosols can cause a cooling effect on earth.

Q. What are health hazards of sulfuric acid and related sulfates?

Sulfuric acid increases the irritant response to ozone in the lung. These changes resemble those produced by cigarette smoke and could well lead to chronic bronchitis including functional, morphological, and biochemical pulmonary effects. Sulfur dioxide is a water-soluble irritant gas and can stimulate bronchoconstriction and mucus secretion in a number of species, including humans. Once deposited along the airway, SO_2 dissolves into surface lining fluid as sulfite or bisulfite and is readily distributed throughout the body. Concurrent exposures to sulfur dioxide, smoke, and particulates have been associated with symptoms including increased respiratory effects, increased frequencies of respiratory illness, excess mortality, and worsening of existing respiratory disease. Health effects of sulfur dioxide exposure in humans are summarized in Table 14.2.

Table 14.2 Health Effects of Sulfur Dioxide Exposure

Sulfur Dioxide Concentration (ppm)	Effects
0.01	Increased respiratory symptoms among the general population and increased frequencies of respiratory illness among children
0.04	Excess mortality among the elderly or the chronically sick
0.04	Worsening of the condition of patients with existing respiratory disease

Explanation: The conversion of SO_2 to sulfate is favored in the environment with subsequent ammonia neutralization to ammonium sulfate [$(NH_4)2SO_4$] or as ammonium bisulfate [NH_4HSO_4]. During oil and coal combustion or the smelting of metal ores, sulfuric acid condenses downstream of the combustion processes with available metal ions and water vapor to form submicron sulfuric acid fume and sulfated fly ash. Sulfur dioxide continues to oxidize to sulfate within dispersing smokestack plumes, which can be augmented by the presence of free soluble or partially coordinated transition metals such as iron, manganese, and vanadium within the effluent ash. Sulfuric acid irritates by virtue of its ability to protonate ($H+$) receptor ligands and other biomolecules. This action can either directly damage membranes or activate sensory reflexes that initiate inflammation. Interestingly, there is considerable species variability in sensitivity to sulfuric acid, with guinea pigs being quite responsive to acid sulfates, in contrast to rats, which seem generally resistant. Asthmatics appear to be somewhat more sensitive to the bronchoconstrictive effects of sulfuric acid than are healthy individuals,

14.1.2.3 Oxides of nitrogen (NO_2)

Q. What are health effects of oxides of NO_2?

NO_2 irritates lungs and promotes respiratory infections. Short-term NO_2 exposures, ranging from 30 minutes to 24 hours, have adverse respiratory effects including airway inflammation. Nitrogen dioxide, like O_3, is a deep lung irritant that can produce pulmonary edema if it is inhaled at high concentrations. It is a much less potent irritant and oxidant than O_3, but NO_2 can pose clear toxicological problems. Exposure to nitrogen oxides to farmers lead to "silo-filler disease" (a toxic gas-induced pneumonitis and bronchiolitis caused by inhalation of nitrogen oxides in freshly filled grain silos, often coupled with asphyxia.

Explanation: Lethal high levels of NO_2 can be liberated from fermenting fresh silage. Being heavier than air, the generated NO_2 and CO_2 displace air and oxygen at the base of silo and diffuse into closed spaces where workers can inadvertently get exposed to very high concentrations perhaps with depleted oxygen. Typically, shortness of breath rapidly ensues with exposures nearing $75-100$ ppm NO_2, with delayed edema and symptoms of pulmonary damage. Not surprisingly, the symptoms are collectively termed "silo-filler's disease." Nitrogen dioxide is also an important indoor pollutant, especially in *homes with unventilated gas stoves or kerosene heaters. Unlike O_3, NO_2 does not induce significant neutrophilic inflammation in humans at exposure concentrations encountered in the ambient outdoor environment. However, there is some evidence for bronchial inflammation. Typical symptoms of "silo-filler's disease" include cough, light headedness, dyspnea, cyanosis, hemoptysis, and choking.*

14.1.2.4 Carbon monoxide (CO)

Q. What are the harmful effects of CO?

CO is ubiquitous and most commonly produced by incomplete hydrocarbon combustion. A component of CO poisoning is almost always present in cases of smoke inhalation injury. It is a chemical asphyxiant because its toxic action stems from its formation of carboxyhemoglobin (COHb), preventing oxygenation of the blood for systemic transport. The normal concentration of COHb in the blood of nonsmokers is about 0.5%. This is attributed to endogenous production of CO from heme catabolism. No overt human health effects have been demonstrated for COHb levels below 2%, whereas levels above 40% cause fatal asphyxiation. Fig. 14.10 summarizes difference in CO and cyanide toxicity.

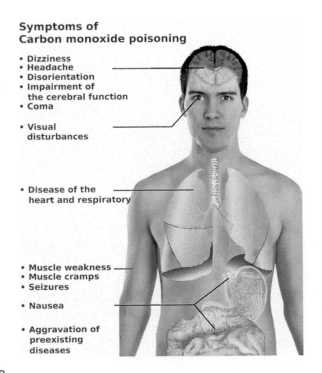

FIGURE 14.10

Symptoms of Carbon monoxide poisoning.

Reproduced from https://commons.wikimedia.org/wiki/File:CO_toxicity_symptoms_(en).jpg.

14.1.2.5 Particulate matter

Q. What do you mean by PM?

Atmospheric PM—also known as PM or particulates—are microscopic solid or liquid matter suspended in the earth's atmosphere.

Q. What is aerosol?

The term aerosol commonly refers to the particulate/air mixture, as opposed to the PM alone.

Q. What are the sources of PM?

Sources of PM can be man-made or natural. They have impacts on climate and precipitation that adversely affect human health.

Q. What are the subtypes of PM?

Subtypes of atmospheric PM include:
- suspended particulate matter,
- thoracic and respirable particles,
- inhalable coarse particles, which are [coarse] particles with a diameter between 2.5 and 10 μm,
- fine particles with a diameter of 2.5 μm or less,
- $PM_{2.5}$,
- PM_{10},
- ultrafine particles, and
- Soot.

PM are completely burned carbonaceous materials such as
1. acid sulfates,
2. various metals,
3. silicates associated with the solid nature of the fuel, and
4. metals with a considerable amount of zinc in the form of zinc sulfate—as reported from postepisode analyses of the Donora PM.

Q. How soot differ from PM?

Soot is indicative of poorly (inefficiently) combusted fuel. PM in the atmosphere can be solid, liquid, or a combination of both with a melange of organic, inorganic, and biological compounds. The compositional matrix of PM can vary significantly depending on the emission source and secondary transformations, many of which involve gas to particle conversions.

Q. How does PM contribute to environmental effects?

PM includes several organic constituents, as well as other constituents, which can induce toxicity either directly or via metabolism product—some of which are genotoxic. Studies focusing on very small, ultrafine particles suggest that although these particles are low in mass, they are high in number and thus provide substantial reactive particle surface to interact with biological substances. Particle type contributes to soil-reduced visibility; organic carbon compounds: ozone-reduced visibility; sulfates: acid deposition—reduced visibility, and nitrates: acid deposition ozone (Table 14.3).

Table 14.3 Contributions of PM$_{2.5}$ Particles to Environmental Effects

Particle Type	Contributes To
Soil	Reduced visibility
Organic carbon compounds	Ozone-reduced visibility
Sulfates	Acid deposition–reduced visibility
Nitrates	Acid deposition ozone

Q. What does PM$_{2.5}$ means?

Particles less than 2.5 μm in diameter (PM$_{2.5}$) are referred to as "fine" particles and are believed to pose the greatest health risks. Because of their small size (approximately 1/30th the average width of a human hair), fine particles can lodge deeply into the lungs.

14.1.2.6 Lead

Q. How does lead get in the air?

Sources of lead emissions vary from one area to another. At the national level, major sources of lead in the air are ore and metals processing and piston-engine aircraft operating on leaded aviation fuel. Other sources are waste incinerators, utilities, and lead-acid battery manufacturers. The highest air concentrations of lead are usually found near lead smelters.

As a result of EPA's regulatory efforts including the removal of lead from motor vehicle gasoline, levels of lead in the air decreased by 98% between 1980 and 2014.

Q. What are the effects of lead on human health?

Once taken into the body, lead distributes throughout the body in the blood and is accumulated in the bones. Depending on the level of exposure, lead can adversely affect the nervous system, kidney function, immune system, reproductive and developmental systems, and the cardiovascular system. Lead exposure also affects the oxygen-carrying capacity of the blood. The lead effects most commonly encountered in current populations are neurological effects in children and cardiovascular effects (e.g., high blood pressure and heart disease) in adults. Infants and young children are especially sensitive to even low levels of lead, which may contribute to behavioral problems, learning deficits, and lowered IQ.

14.1.2.7 Other air pollutants

Q. What are HAPs?

HAPs are also known as toxic air pollutants or air toxics. Examples of toxic air pollutants include benzene, which is found in gasoline; perchloroethylene, which is emitted from some dry cleaning facilities, and methylene chloride, which is used as a solvent and paint stripper by a number of industries. Examples of other listed air toxics include dioxin, asbestos, toluene, pesticides, and metals such as cadmium, mercury, chromium, and lead compounds.

Q. What are health and environmental effects of HAPs?

People exposed to toxic air pollutants at sufficient concentrations and durations may have an increased chance of getting cancer or experiencing other serious health effects. These health effects can include damage to the immune system, as well as neurological, reproductive (e.g., reduced fertility), developmental, respiratory, and other health problems. In addition to exposure from breathing air toxics, some toxic air pollutants such as mercury can deposit onto soils or surface waters, where they are taken up by plants and ingested by animals and are eventually magnified up through the food chain. Like humans, animals may experience health problems if exposed to sufficient quantities of air toxics over time.

Q. What is photochemical air pollution?

Photochemical air pollutants (notably O_3) arise secondarily from a series of complex reactions in the troposphere activated by the ultraviolet (UV) spectrum of sunlight. In addition to O_3, it comprises a mixture of nitric oxides (NOx), aldehydes, peroxyacetyl nitrates (PAN), and a myriad of aromatics and alkenes along with analog reactive radicals. If SO_2 is present, sulfates may also be formed and, collectively, they yield "summer haze." Likewise, the complex chemistry can generate organic PM, nitric acid vapor, and various condensates. O_3 is by far the toxicant of greatest concern that can lead to pulmonary dysfunction. It is highly reactive and more toxic than NOx, and because its generation is fueled through cyclic hydrocarbon radicals, it reaches greater concentrations than the hydrocarbon radical intermediates.

Q. Describe gas—particle interactions.

These interactions can be extremely complex involving multiple components of the particles, gases/vapors, and sunlight. In view of several components together with those focusing on irritancy and infectivity, raise the question of realistic exposure scenarios of gaseous and particulate pollutants that can interact through either chemical or physiologic mechanisms to enhance health risks of complex polluted atmospheres.

Q. What is ultrafine carbonaceous matter?

Particles that are less than 100 nm in diameter are commonly defined as ultrafine. This matter typically results from high temperature oxidation or as the product the atmospheric transformation involving organic vapors and sunlight. The size of these particles allows them to slip between gas molecules moving primarily by diffusion and principles of Brownian motion. When concentrations exceed approximately million per cubic centimeter, they rapidly agglomerate with each other to form larger clumps or chains of ultrafine particles. The diesel particulate emissions are largely ultrafine; there has been growing interest in ultrafine ambient particles. Diesel particles vary widely in the ratio of organic and elemental carbonaceous materials that have shown to influence toxic outcomes such as inflammatory and carcinogenic potential.

14.1.2.8 E-wastes

Q. Define contaminants from electronic wastes (e-wastes).

"Electronic waste" may be defined as discarded computers, office electronic equipment, entertainment device electronics, mobile phones, television sets, and refrigerators. This includes used electronics that are destined for reuse, resale, salvage, recycling, or disposal.

Q. How do e-wastes enter the environment?

Burning of e-components, circuit boards, and other plastic components releases plasticizers including bisphenol A, triphenyl phosphate, palmitic and stearic acids, brominated flame retardants, and the highly chlorinated flame retardant Dechlorane Plus (Dechlorane A) into the air, soils, and tissues of resident people and animals near the recycling facilities.

14.1.2.9 Smog

Q. What is smog?

The term "smog" was first used in London during the early 1900s to describe the combination of smoke and fog. What we typically call "smog" today is a mixture of pollutants that is primarily made up of ground-level ozone. In other words, we can say combination of smoke and fog is SMOG which considerably reduces visibility (Fig. 14.11).

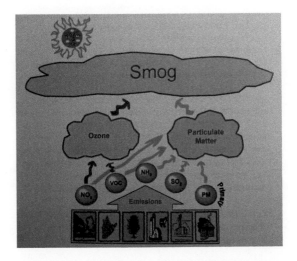

FIGURE 14.11

Smog.

Q. What are the adverse effects of smog?

Smog is made up of a combination of air pollutants that can injure health, harm the environment, and cause property damage. Smog causes health problems such as difficulty in breathing, asthma, reduced resistance to lung infections and colds, and eye irritation. The ozone in smog also inhibits plants growth and can cause widespread damage to crops and forest, and the haze reduces visibility. The smog or haze is particularly noticeable from mountains and other beautiful vistas, such as those in National Parks.

Q. What is photochemical smog?

Haze in the atmosphere accompanied by high levels of ozone and nitrogen oxides, caused by the action of sunlight on pollutants, is called photochemical smog (Fig. 14.12). It is short-lived because of their reaction with co-pollutants. PAN is believed to be responsible for much of the eye-stinging activity of smog. It is more soluble and reactive than O_3, and hence rapidly decomposes in mucous membranes before it can penetrate into the respiratory tract. The cornea is a sensitive target and is prominent in the burning/stinging discomfort often associated with oxidant smog.

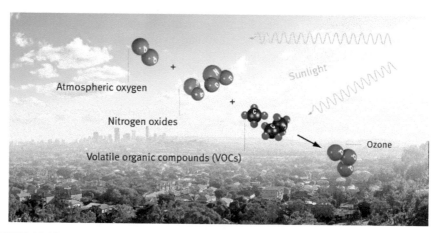

Atmospheric oxygen

Sunlight

Nitrogen oxides

Ozone

Volatile organic compounds (VOCs)

FIGURE 14.12

Photochemical smog.

Reproduced from The State of Queensland (https://www.qld.gov.au/environment/assets/images/pollution/monitoring/air/ozone-formation-large.jpg).

Q. What is the difference between photochemical smog and London-type smog?

London-type smog is caused mainly by air pollution due to combustion of coal and emission of sulfur dioxide and dust.

Photochemical smog is a type of air pollution produced when sunlight acts upon motor vehicle exhaust gases to form harmful substances.

Explanation: Carbonyl compounds, notably short-chained (2–4C) aldehydes, are common photooxidation products of unsaturated hydrocarbons. Two aldehydes are of major interest by virtue of their concentrations and irritancy: formaldehyde (HCHO) and acrolein ($H_2C = CHCHO$).

*They contribute to the odor as well as eye and sensory effects of smog.
Formaldehyde is a primary sensory irritant. Because it is very soluble in water,
it is absorbed in mucous membranes in the nose, upper respiratory tract, and
eyes. Acrolein is an unsaturated aldehyde, and it is more reactive than
formaldehyde. It penetrates a bit deeper into the airways and may not have the
same degree of sensory irritancy but it may cause more damage. Thus, as a
class the aldehydes can be very irritating and may constitute a significant
fraction of the discomfort and sensation experienced during an oxidant
pollution episode, especially in mixed atmospheres containing particles.*

Q. What are adverse effects of smog on human health?

Due to ozone, smog exposure may lead to several different types of
short-term health problems:

1. coughing and throat/chest irritation

2. high levels of ozone can irritate respiratory system

General adverse effects of smog on human heath are summarized in Fig. 14.13.

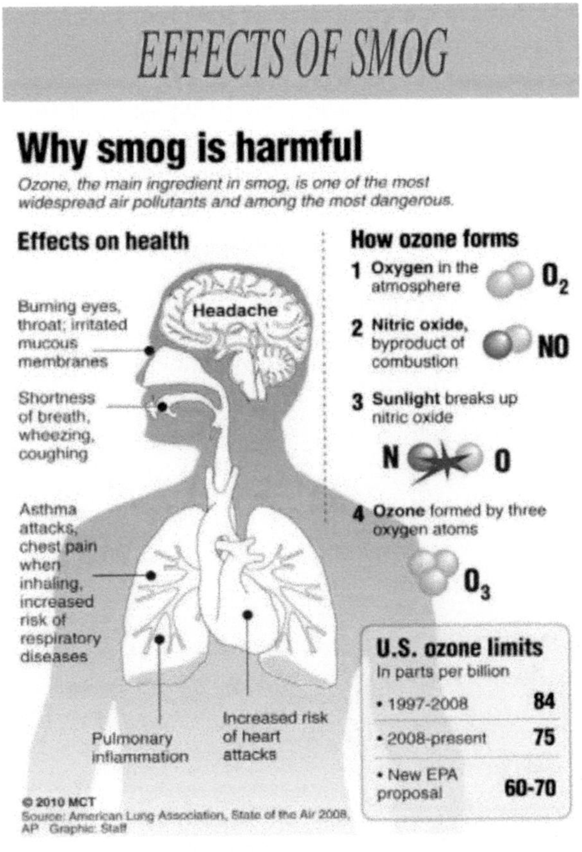

FIGURE 14.13

Adverse effects of smog on human health.

https://s-media-cache-ak0.pinimg.com/736x/c3/e4/6a/c3e46a0fa1f6a60202a297926d41feb9.jpg.

14.2 ECOTOXICOLOGY

Q. Define ecotoxicology.

Ecotoxicology is defined as the branch of science that deals with the nature, effects, and interactions of substances that are harmful to the environment.

Q. What is the difference between ecotoxicology and environmental toxicology?

Ecotoxicology differs from environmental toxicology in that it integrates the effects of stressors across all levels of biological organization from the molecular to whole communities and ecosystems, whereas environmental toxicology focuses upon effects at the level of the individual and below.

Q. How do nutrients enter our ecosystem?

Nutrients, primarily N and phosphorus (P), enter environments from chemical fertilizers, manure, urine, sewage effluents, burning fossil fuels, fires, decay of plants and animals, and industrial processes such as pulp/paper milling and nitric acid production. Free nutrients are washed into water bodies and enter groundwater and aquifers, some of which feed streams, ponds, lakes, estuaries, bays, and oceans. Agricultural production of plants and animals is the primary source of excess nutrients in the environment.

Q. How do petroleum products enter our ecosystem?

Petroleum products include a wide array of aliphatic and aromatic hydrocarbons. Aromatic hydrocarbons are also present at high concentrations in coal tar and are formed during incomplete combustion of coal, oil, gas, garbage, and other materials. Among the best-known polycyclic aromatic hydrocarbons (PAHs) is benzo (*a*) pyrene, which is a component of cigarette smoke.

Q. What is the impact of nutrient pollution on ecosystem?

Nutrient pollution is the process where too many nutrients, mainly nitrogen and phosphorus, are added to bodies of water and can act like fertilizer, causing excessive growth of algae (Fig. 14.14). Nutrients can run off

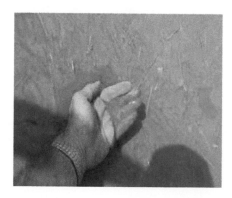

FIGURE 14.14

Harmful Lake Erie algal blooms worsened by power plant pollution.

of land in urban areas where lawn fertilizers are used. Too much nitrogen and phosphorus in the water can have diverse and far-reaching impacts on public health, the environment, and the ecosystem.

Q. What is the impact of wastes on ecosystem?

Introduction of vast amounts of cast-off food, chemicals, and other wastes alter the relationship between predators and prey in various environments and ecosystem leading to death of wildlife, birds, fishes, and other species of plants (Fig. 14.15).

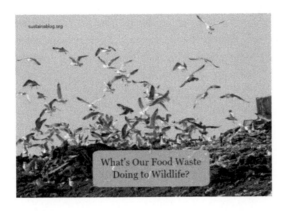

FIGURE 14.15

Impact of wastes on ecosystem.

http://sustainablog.org/wp-content/uploads/2016/01/wildlife-and-waste.jpg.

For example, the Pasión River in Guatemala was declared an ecological disaster after thousands of dead fish surfaced in June as a result of agrochemicals pollution from a nearby palm oil production site (Fig. 14.16).

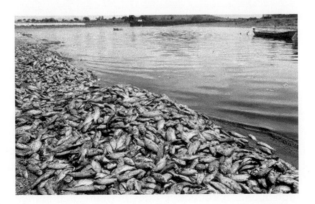

FIGURE 14.16

Dead fish on the banks of Guatemala's "Pasión River." I Photo: De Guate.

Reproduced from http://www.telesurtv.net/export/sites/telesur/img/news/2015/12/01/rio-pasion-dead-fish-palm-pollution.jpg_215828346.jpg.

Explanation: Persistent organic pollutants and semivolatile chemicals, such as organochlorine insecticides, the fungicide hexachlorobenzene, and polychlorinated dibenzodioxins and polychlorinated dibenzofurans, which are toxic byproducts of organochlorine, synthesis, manufacturing processes, such as the Kraft paper, bleaching process can have serious effects on the immune, nervous, and reproductive systems, especially those of developing organisms. Such compounds can also reduce control of impulsive behaviors, impair learning, cause liver damage, and disrupt reproductive and thyroid hormone functions. Likewise leakage of acids from coal mines and drainage of hazardous substances, pollutants, or contaminants into the environment lead harm to fish and other aquatic life: If mine waste is acid-generating, the impacts to fish, animals, and plants can be severe (Fig. 14.17).

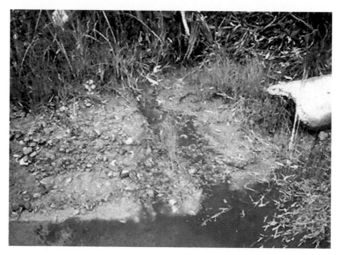

FIGURE 14.17

Acid rock drainage (Andalusia coal mines, Spain).

Reproduced from US Fish and Wildlife Service.

Q. What are the effects of lead on ecosystems?

Lead is persistent in the environment and can be added to soils and sediments through deposition from sources of lead air pollution. Other sources of lead to ecosystems include direct discharge of waste streams to water bodies and mining. Elevated lead in the environment can result in decreased growth and reproductive rates in plants and animals, and neurological effects in vertebrates.

14.3 QUESTION AND ANSWER EXERCISES

14.3.1 SHORT QUESTIONS AND ANSWERS

Exercise 1

Q.1 Describe briefly the greenhouse effect.

Heat energy (infrared) reflected from the earth may be absorbed by infrared-absorbing gases such as carbon dioxide, CFCs, methane, and water vapors. Such gases then trap the warmth and reflect it back to the Earth's atmosphere in a process known as the greenhouse effect. If the greenhouse gases increase in concentration, it is logical that more heat energy will be absorbed and the average annual global temperature may rise causing a global warming trend.

Q.2 Describe what happens during an asthma attack.

The beginning signs of an attack include wheezing, coughing, and difficulty breathing. As the problem persists, the airways begin to spasm. During a spasm, the muscles in the bronchi and bronchioles contract and membranes swell. Mucus forms in the airways, and this narrowing of the airway makes it difficult to breathe. With an extended attack, the person sweats, the pulse becomes rapid, the skin turns blue, and the arms and legs become chilled or cold.

Q.3 Describe the nature of a subsidence inversion.

Subsidence refers to the descent of air masses. Cool air masses (anticyclones) associated with Hadley cells descend causing air molecules to compress in a layer above the ground. This layer becomes warmed by compression, whereas the air at ground level remains unchanged and often cooler than the air above, producing an inversion layer at distances of 500−1000 m above the ground. Such inversions may occur frequently along coastal areas such as California that has documented inversions more than 300 days of the year. Such subsidence inversions occur most often during the fall and winter months and are particularly troublesome because they may persist for days.

Q.4 Discuss the impact of acid rain on plant life.

Acidic deposition at levels of pH 4.0−5.0 are most common and do not appear to cause widespread adverse effects on forest ecosystems. However, acid clouds (as low as pH 2.2) can have the following adverse effects:

1. damage leaves,
2. mobilize toxic metals in soil, such as aluminum, which adversely effects roots,
3. leach nutrients from soil, and
4. overstimulate plants from excess nitrates that aggravate deficiencies of other nutrients.

These factors may combine to increase forest susceptibility to insect and fungal pathogens.

Q.5 List some of the indicators of indoor air pollution.

Signs of indoor air pollution may include physical or health signs or both.

1. Physical symptoms may include:
   a. heating or cooling equipment that is dirty and/or moldy;
   b. moisture condensation on walls and windows;
   c. air that has a stuffy or has an unpleasant odor; and
   d. signs of water leakage anywhere in the building with the growth of molds.
2. Health indicators of indoor air pollution may include immediate or acute effects such as eye irritation, dry throat, headaches, fatigue, sinus congestion, shortness of breath, cough dizziness, nausea, sneezing, and nose irritation.

Q.6 What are the possible toxic mechanisms for chemicals?
1. Produce reversible or irreversible bodily injury
2. Have the capacity to cause tumors, neoplastic effects, or cancer
3. Cause reproductive errors including mutations and teratogenic effects
4. Produce irritation and sensitization of mucous membranes
5. Cause a reduction in motivation, mental alertness, or capability
6. Alter behavior or cause death of the organism

Q.7 List the variety of processes of absorption including their characteristics.
1. Diffusion: Molecules move from areas of high concentration to low concentration.
2. Facilitated Diffusion: Require specialized carrier proteins, no-high energy phosphate bonds are required.
3. Active Transport: ATP is required in conjunction with special carrier proteins to move molecules through a membrane against a concentration gradient.
4. Endocytosis: Particles and large molecules that might otherwise be restricted from crossing a plasma membrane can be brought in or removed by this process.

Q.8 How do toxic substances enter the body?

There are several ways in which toxic substances can enter the body. They may enter through:
1. lungs by inhalation,
2. skin,
3. oral, and
4. mucous membranes or eyes by absorption

Q.9 What are the major functions of the skin?

The skin can help to:
1. regulate body temperature through sweat glands;
2. provide a physical barrier to dehydration, microbial invasion, and some chemical insults;
3. excrete salts, water, and organic compounds;

    4. serve as a sensory organ for touch, temperature, pressure, and pain; and

    5. provide some important components of immunity.

Q.10 What are the three major mechanisms for the harmful effects of environmental toxins?

    1. The toxins influence on enzymes

    2. Direct chemical combination of the toxin with a cell constituent

    3. Secondary action as a result of the toxins presence in the system

Exercise 2

Q.1 List the four major types of hypersensitivity reactions

    1. Cytotoxic

    2. Cell-mediated

    3. Immune complex

    4. Anaphylactic

Q.2 What are the messages given through the public media about toxic chemicals?

    1. Exposure to toxic chemicals has dramatically increased the risk of cancer.

    2. Common household and agricultural chemicals are causing many human diseases and death.

    3. Polluted air and water are major sources of disease risk.

    4. Environmental chemicals are interfering with the reproductive process in humans and producing harmful effects in the fetus and young children.

Q.3 What are the major mechanisms for chemical injury?

    1. interfere with enzyme activity;

    2. directly combine with some cell component other than enzymes; and

    3. produce a secondary action in which a chemical causes the release or formation of a more harmful substance.

Q.4 What is environmental disease and what are its external causal factors?

    Environmental disease refers to any pathologic process having a characteristic set of signs and symptoms that are detrimental to the well-being of the individual and are the consequence of external factors, including exposure to physical or chemical agents, poor nutrition, and social or cultural behaviors.

Q.5 What are the differences between DNA and messenger RNA?

    Messenger RNA is quite similar to its DNA counterpart except the fact that it is single stranded, contains the nucleotide base uracil instead of thymine and the sugar D-ribose instead of 2-deoxyribose in the four mononucleotides.

Q.6 What are the health consequences of air pollution?

    Air pollution increases the risk of respiratory and heart disease in the population. Both short- and long-term exposure to air pollutants have been associated to health impacts. More severe impacts affect people who are already ill. Children, the elderly, and poor people are more susceptible.

Q.7 How bad is air pollution?

Air pollution is a major environmental health problem affecting everyone. It is a problem from exhaust fumes from cars, domestic combustion, or factory smoke. Worldwide there are risks to health from exposure to PM and ozone (O3) in many cities of developed and developing countries alike.

Q.8 What are the most polluted cities in the world?

Unfortunately, there is no comprehensive, worldwide database allowing precise answer to this question. Nevertheless, the available data indicate that air pollution is very high in a number of Asian cities (Karachi, New Delhi, Katmandu, and Beijing), in Latin American cities (Lima and Arequipa), and in Africa (Cairo).

Q.9 In which regions of the world/countries and cities are PM concentrations particularly high?

As often is the case, the biggest air pollution—related burden to health is observed in developing countries. The lack of knowledge of the health impacts from pollution is a big obstacle in defining the actions and mobilizing local and international resources.

Q.10 Have there been any new guidelines or other significant, relevant documents since 2005 about the health impact of air pollution?

The 2005 global guidelines are the most up to date providing the latest scientific evidence. They set targets for air quality that would protect the large majority of individuals from the effects of air pollution on health.

Exercise 3

Q.1 Which effects can be expected of long-term exposure to levels of PM observed currently in Europe (include both clinical and preclinical effects, e.g., development of respiratory system)?

Long-term exposure to current ambient PM concentrations may lead to a marked reduction in life expectancy. The reduction in life expectancy is primarily due to the increased cardiopulmonary and lung cancer mortality. Increases are likely in lower respiratory symptoms and reduced lung function in children, and chronic obstructive pulmonary disease and reduced lung function in adults.

Q.2 Is there a threshold below which no effects on health of PM are expected to occur in all people?

Epidemiological studies on large populations have been unable to identify a threshold concentration below which ambient PM has no effect on health. It is likely that within any large human population, there is such a wide range in susceptibility that some subjects are at risk even at the lowest end of the concentration range.

Q.3 Are effects of the pollutant dependent upon the subjects' characteristics such as age, gender, underlying disease, smoking status, atopy, and education? What are the critical characteristics?

In short-term studies, elderly subjects and subjects with preexisting heart and lung disease were found to be more susceptible to effects of ambient PM on mortality and morbidity. In panel studies, asthmatics have also been shown to respond to ambient PM with more symptoms, larger lung function changes, and with increased medication use than non-asthmatics. In long-term studies, it has been suggested that socially disadvantaged and poorly educated populations respond more strongly in terms of mortality. PM also is related to reduced lung growth in children. No consistent differences have been found between men and women, and between smokers and nonsmokers in PM responses in the cohort studies.

Q.4 To what extent is mortality being accelerated by long- and short-term exposure to the pollutant (harvesting)?

Cohort studies have suggested that life expectancy is decreased by long-term exposure to PM. This is supported by new analyses of time-series studies that have shown death being advanced by periods of at least a few months, for causes of death such as cardiovascular and chronic pulmonary disease.

Q.5 For PM, which of the physical and chemical characteristics of particulate air pollution are responsible for health effects?

There is strong evidence to conclude that fine particles (<2.5 μm, PM2.5) are more hazardous than larger ones (coarse particles) in terms of mortality and cardiovascular and respiratory endpoints in panel studies. This does not imply that the coarse fraction of PM10 is innocuous. In toxicological and controlled human exposure studies, several physical, biological, and chemical characteristics of particles have been found to elicit cardiopulmonary responses. Among the characteristics found to be contributing to toxicity in epidemiological and controlled exposure studies are metal content, the presence of PAHs, other organic components, endotoxin, and both small (<2.5 μm) and extremely small size (<100 nm).

Q.6 What is the evidence of synergy/interaction of the pollutant with other air pollutants?

Few epidemiological studies have addressed interactions of PM with other pollutants. Toxicological and controlled human exposure studies have shown additive and, in some cases, more than additive effects, especially for combinations of PM and ozone, and of PM (especially diesel particles) and allergens. Finally, studies of atmospheric chemistry demonstrate that PM interacts with gases to alter its composition and hence its toxicity.

Q.7 What is the relationship between ambient levels and personal exposure to the pollutant over short and long term (including exposures indoors)? Can the differences influence the results of studies?

Although personal exposure to PM and its components is influenced by indoor sources (such as smoking) in addition to outdoor sources, there is a clear relationship on population level between ambient PM and personal PM of ambient origin over time, especially for fine combustion particles. On a population level, personal PM of ambient origin "tracks" ambient PM over time, thus measurements of PM in ambient air can serve as a reasonable "proxy" for personal exposure in time-series studies. The relationship between long-term average ambient PM concentrations and long-term average personal PM exposure has been studied less. Contributions to personal PM exposure from smoking and occupation need to be taken into account. However, the available data suggest that imperfect relationship between ambient and personal PM does not invalidate the results of the long-term studies.

Q.8 Which effects can be expected of long-term exposure to levels of O3 observed currently in Europe (both clinical and preclinical effects)?

There are few epidemiological studies on the chronic effects of ozone on human health. Incidence of asthma, a decreased lung function growth, lung cancer, and total mortality are the main outcomes studied. At levels currently observed in Europe, the evidence linking O3 exposure to asthma incidence and prevalence in children and adults is not consistent. Available evidence suggests that long-term O3 exposure reduces lung function growth in children. There is little evidence for an independent long-term O3 effect on lung cancer or total mortality. The plausibility of chronic damage to the human lung from prolonged O3 exposure is supported by the results of a series of chronic animal exposure studies.

Q.9 Is there a threshold below which ozone have no effects on health are expected to occur in all people?

There may be different concentration−response curves for individuals in the population response to O3 exposure. There is evidence for a threshold for lung damage and inflammation at about 60−80 ppb ($120-160 \,\mu g/m^3$) for short-term exposure (6.6 hours) with intermittent moderate exercise. Where there are thresholds, they depend on the individual exercise levels.

Q.10 What is the evidence of synergy/interaction of O3 with other air pollutants?

Epidemiological studies show that short-term effects of O3 can be enhanced by PM and vice versa. Experimental evidence from studies at higher O3 concentrations shows synergistic, additive, or antagonistic effects, depending on the experimental design, but their relevance for ambient exposures is unclear. O3 may act as a primer for allergen response.

Exercise 4

Q.1 Are effects of NO2 dependent upon the subjects' characteristics such as age, gender, underlying disease, smoking status, atopy, and education? What are the critical characteristics?

In general, individuals with asthma are expected to be more responsive to short-term exposure to inhaled agents, when compared to individuals without asthma. Controlled human exposure studies of short-term responses of persons with and without asthma to NO2 have not been carried out. There is limited evidence from epidemiological studies that individuals with asthma show steeper concentration—response relationships. Small-scale human exposure studies have not shown consistent effects of NO2 exposure on airways reactivity in persons with asthma, even at exposure levels higher than typical ambient concentrations. As for other pollutants, children can reasonably be considered to be at an increased risk. There is limited evidence for influence of the other listed factors on the effects of NO2.

Q.2 Is the considered pollutant NO2 per se responsible for effects on health?

The evidence for acute effects of NO2 comes from controlled human exposure studies to NO2 alone. For the effects observed in epidemiological studies, a clear answer to the question cannot be given. Effects estimated for NO2 exposure in epidemiological studies may reflect other traffic-related pollutants, for which NO2 is a surrogate. Additionally, there are complex interrelationships among the concentrations of NO2, PM, and O3 in ambient air.

Q.3 What is the evidence of synergy/interaction of the pollutant NO2 with other air pollutants?

There have been few controlled human exposure studies on interactions with other chemical pollutants, although several studies show that NO2 exposure enhances responses to inhaled pollens. Some epidemiological studies have explored statistical interactions of NO2 with other pollutants, including particles, but the findings are not readily interpretable.

Q.4 Which are the critical sources of the pollutant NO2 responsible for health effects?

In most urban environments in Europe, the principal source of NO2 is NOx from motor vehicles of all types and energy production in some places.

Q.5 How is ozone produced and destroyed?

The ozone molecule (O3) contains three atoms of oxygen and is mainly formed by the action of the UV rays of the sun on oxygen molecules (diatomic oxygen, O2) in the upper part of Earth's atmosphere (called the stratosphere). Ozone is also produced locally near Earth's surface from the action of UV radiation on some air pollutants.

Q.6 What is the relationship between ozone and solar UV radiation?

There is an inverse relationship between the concentration of ozone and the amount of harmful UV radiation transmitted through the atmosphere since ozone absorbs some of the UV radiation.

Q.7 How and why has the situation regarding the ozone layer changed over the past 35 years?

Stratospheric ozone has decreased over the globe since the 1980s. Averaged over the globe, ozone in the period 1996—2009 is about 4%

lower than before 1980. Much larger depletion, up to 40%, occurs over the high latitudes of the Southern Hemisphere in October.

Q.8 What determines the level of solar UV-B radiation at a specific place?

The Sun is the source of the UV radiation reaching Earth. UV radiation is partly absorbed by the components of Earth's atmosphere. The amount of UV radiation that is absorbed depends mainly on the length of the path of the sunlight through the atmosphere.

Q.9 What is the solar UV Index (UVI)?

The solar UVI describes the level of solar UV radiation relevant to human sunburn (erythema).

Q.10 How does the UVI vary with location and time?

The combination of total ozone, aerosols, clouds, air pollution, altitude, surface reflectivity, and solar zenith angle (that is determined by the geographical position, season, and time of the day) are the main factors resulting in variation in the UVI.

Exercise 5

Q.1 What is the effect of the interaction between UV-B radiation, climate change, and human activity on air pollution?

Pollutants emitted by human activities can reduce UV-B radiation near the surface, whereas particles may lead to enhancement by scattering. These processes decrease some exposures to UV while enhancing others. Interactions between UV radiation and pollutants resulting from changes in climate and burning of fossil and plant fuels will worsen the effects of ozone on humans and plants in the lower atmosphere.

Q.2 What are the effects of exposure to solar UV radiation on the human eye and how can the eye be protected?

The effects of UV radiation on the eye can be almost immediate (acute) occurring several hours after a short, intense exposure. They can also be long-term (chronic), following exposure of the eye to levels of UV radiation below those required for the acute effects but occurring repeatedly over a long period of time. The commonest acute effect, photokeratitis (snow blindness), leaves few or no permanent effects, whereas cataract due to chronic exposure is irreversible and ultimately leads to severe loss of vision requiring surgery.

Q.3 What are the adverse effects of exposure to solar UV-B on human skin?

Acute overexposure of the skin to solar UV radiation causes sunburn; chronic sunlight exposure can lead to the development of skin cancers.

Q.4 Do ozone-depleting gases and their substitutes have an effect on climate?

Stratospheric ozone depletion has an influence on climate change because both ozone and the compounds responsible for its depletion are active greenhouse gases.

Q.5 Is ozone depletion affected by climate change?

Climate change affects ozone depletion through changes in atmospheric conditions that affect the chemical production and loss of stratospheric ozone. The interactions are complex. Climate change is expected to decrease temperatures and water vapor abundances in the stratosphere. This will tend to speed up ozone recovery outside Polar Regions but slow down the recovery in Polar Regions.

Q.6 Name at least three things the word climate takes into consideration.

Temperature, precipitation, humidity, wind velocity and direction, and cloud cover and solar radiation.

Q.7 Name different phenomena associated with climatic change.

1. Changes in ocean temperature
2. Changes in Earth's orbital geometry
3. Volcanic activity with increased atmosphere dust and reduced sunlight penetration
4. Variations in solar radiation
5. Increases in atmospheric gases that absorb hear energy

Q.8 Which is the most important factor(s) that affect the climate?

Temperature or the sun.

Q.9 Give two examples of ecosystem.

The planet, an ant farm, tidal pool, pond, river valley, and garbage can.

Q.10 Give two examples of physical or abiotic components of an ecosystem.

Water, air, sunlight, and minerals.

Exercise 6

Q.1 By which process green plants and some other organisms use sunlight to synthesize nutrients from carbon dioxide and water.

Photosynthesis.

Q.2 What is the term associated with the accumulation of organic material in an ecosystem?

Biomass.

Q.3 What term describes the amount of energy stored by a plant to be used as chemical energy?

Kilocalories.

Q.4 Give an example of an organism in the first trophic level.

Plant.

Q.5 Give examples of primary consumers.

Caterpillar, grasshopper, cattle, and elephants.

Q.6 Name macronutrients.

Sulfur, carbon, oxygen, phosphorus, nitrogen, and hydrogen.

Q.7 List three sources from which carbon dioxide is released into the atmosphere.

1. Respiratory process of plants and animals that consume oxygen and release carbon dioxide.

2. Combustion of fossil or organic fuels.

3. Decomposition of organic matter.

Q.8 What part of the carbon cycle do scientists think is contributing to the greenhouse effect?

The increase of carbon dioxide due to the burning of forests and fossil fuels.

Q.9 What macronutrient makes up the largest percent of the earth's air?

Nitrogen.

Q.10 Briefly describe the greenhouse effect.

Heat energy (infrared) reflected from the earth may be absorbed by infrared-absorbing gases such as carbon dioxide, CFCs, methane, and water vapor. Such gases then trap the warmth and reflect it back to the Earth's atmosphere in a process known as the greenhouse effect. If the greenhouse gases increase in concentration, it is logical that more heat energy will be absorbed and the average annual global temperature may rise causing a global warming trend. This is the focus of world attention.

Q.11 In which state carbon is found?

Carbon can be found in three different states:

1. gas,

2. liquid, and

3. solid.

Q.12 Discuss the impact of acid rain on plant life.

Acidic deposition at levels of pH 4.0−5.0, which are most common, do not appear to cause widespread adverse effects on forest ecosystems. However, conifer forests such as Red Spruce on mountaintops in New Hampshire, Vermont, and in the Appalachians have been more than 80% decimated at the cloud line. Severe damage is also evidenced in Central Europe in such places as the Czech Republic and Poland where 60%−70% of forests show evidence of damage associated with sulfur and nitrogen disposition. The mechanisms for such destruction are not immediately obvious but may be attributed to combinations of ozone and acid clouds (as low as pH 2.2) which (1) directly damage leaves; (2) mobilize toxic metals in soil such as aluminum, which adversely effects roots; (3) leach nutrients from soil; and (4) overstimulate plants from excess nitrates that aggravate deficiencies of other nutrients. These factors may combine to increase forest susceptibility to insect and fungal pathogens.

Q.13 What causes depletion of ozone?

Scientific evidence indicates that stratospheric ozone is being destroyed by a group of manufactured chemicals, containing chlorine and/or bromine. These chemicals are called "ozone-depleting substances".

Q.14 How do CFCs lead to ozone depletion?

Because of their relative stability, CFCs rise into the stratosphere where they are eventually broken down by UV rays from the Sun. This causes them to release free chlorine. The chlorine reacts with oxygen, which leads to the chemical process of destroying ozone molecules.

Q.15 What is causing the depletion of the ozone layer?

Ozone depletion occurs when CFCs—formerly found in aerosol spray cans and refrigerants—are released into the atmosphere. These gases, through several chemical reactions, cause the ozone molecules to break down, reducing ozone's UV radiation-absorbing capacity.

14.3.2 MULTIPLE CHOICE QUESTIONS (CHOOSE THE BEST STATEMENT, IT CAN BE ONE, TWO OR ALL OR NONE)

Exercise 7

Q.1 A threshold limit value-time weighted average for a chemical represents:
- **a.** an airborne concentration of a chemical that can never be exceeded.
- **b.** an airborne concentration of a chemical that is believed to cause no adverse health effect to a worker exposed for 8 hours a day, 40 hours a week.
- **c.** an airborne concentration of a chemical that cannot be exceeded for longer than 15 minutes a day.
- **d.** a value for an acceptable airborne concentration of a chemical established by the Occupational Safety and Health Administration.
- **e.** an airborne concentration that cannot be measured using available technology.

Q.2 Which of the following is the most significant contributor to air pollution by mass in suburban areas?
- **a.** Manufacturing
- **b.** Transportation
- **c.** Space heaters
- **d.** Electric power generation
- **e.** Waste disposal

Q.3 The major toxic effect of hydrogen cyanide exposure is
- **a.** lung damage
- **b.** hemoglobin alteration
- **c.** hemolysis of RBCs
- **d.** inhibition of mitochondrial respiration.
- **e.** lipid peroxidation

Q.4 Which of the following agents would NOT likely produce reactive airways dysfunction syndrome?
- **a.** Carbon monoxide
- **b.** Chlorine
- **c.** Ammonia
- **d.** Toluene di isocyanate
- **e.** Acetic acid

Q.5 Benzene is similar to toluene
- **a.** in its metabolism to redox active metabolites.
- **b.** regarding covalent binding of its metabolites to proteins.
- **c.** in its ability to produce CNS depression.

d. in its ability to produce acute myelogenous leukemia.

e. in its ability to be metabolized to benzoquinone.

Q.6 Which of the following is not a primary pollutant?

a. Carbon monoxide

b. Lead

c. Ozone

d. Nitrogen dioxide

Q.7 Most automobiles emit up to _____% less pollutants now than in 1960.

a. 80

b. 30

c. 99

d. 50

Q.8 Particulates may cause which of the following health hazards to humans.

a. Respiratory distress

b. Damage to nervous system

c. Blindness

d. Learning disabilities

Q.9 Carbon monoxide may produce _____ as one of the symptoms of exposure in humans.

a. excess urination

b. headache

c. throat irritation

d. hearing loss

Q.10 Tropospheric ozone may cause which of the following effects:

a. grime deposits

b. reduced visibility

c. retardation of plant growth

d. metal corrosion

Answers

1. b; 2. b; 3. d; 4. a; 5. c; 6. c; 7. a; 8. a; 9. b; 10. c.

Exercise 8

Q.1 Fine particulates from motor vehicles and power plants are reported to kill about _____ Americans annually.

a. 38,000

b. 2 million

c. 9100

d. 64,000

Q.2 _____ may be the primary health problem when a person's bronchial tubes respond to allergens, pollution, etc., resulting in hyperactive airways.

a. Cardiac arrest

b. Asthma

c. Laryngitis

d. Sneezing

Q.3 Signs of an extended asthma attack may include:
    a. sweating
    b. rapid pulse
    c. skin turns blue
    d. all of the above

Q.4 Most adult people spend an average of _____% of their time indoors.
    a. 50
    b. 25
    c. 90
    d. 10

Q.5 Which is a potential source of indoor air pollution?
    a. Moisture
    b. Room air fresheners
    c. Personal care products
    d. All of the above

Q.6 A smoker is exposed to nearly _____ compounds in mainstream cigarette smoke.
    a. 4700
    b. 320
    c. 9400
    d. 560

Q.7 Building-related illnesses refers to:
    a. well-defined illnesses occurring in a building that can be traced to specific building problems.
    b. the display of acute symptoms by a number of people in a building without a particular pattern and the varied symptoms cannot be associated with a particular pattern.
    c. well-defined illnesses occurring in a building that cannot be traced to specific building problems.
    d. the display of acute symptoms by a number of people in a building with a specific pattern of disease associated with a particular pattern.

Q.8 Biological contaminants are most likely aggravated by what problem?
    a. Auto exhaust
    b. Unvented gas stove
    c. Moisture
    d. Household chemicals

Q.9 Air that drawn into the home by cracks in the foundation is known as:
    a. natural ventilation
    b. infiltration
    c. mechanical filtration
    d. foundation suction

Q.10 When considering the contribution of all greenhouse gases, carbon monoxide contributes approximately _____% to global warming?
a. 24
b. 6
c. 55
d. 15

Answers

1. d; 2. b; 3. d; 4. c; 5. d; 6. a; 7. a; 8. c; 9. b; 10. c.

Exercise 9

Q.1 What event in 1978 was (one of) the first that raised public consciousness focusing attention on the hazards to the environment and human health of improperly disposed chemicals?
a. Love canal
b. 3 mile island
c. Chernobyl
d. Valdez oil spill
e. None of them

Q.2 _____ is the leading factor among those listed below, associated with cancer risk.
a. Occupation
b. Alcohol
c. Pollution
d. Medicines and medical procedures
e. Poor diet

Q.3 Which of the following diseases is an acute disease?
a. AIDS
b. Emphysema
c. Cancer
d. Flu
e. Heart disease

Q.4 The leading cause of injury-related death in the United States is _____.
a. shootings
b. falls
c. motor vehicles
d. stabbings
e. other forms of trauma to human body

Q.5 What is the major mechanism for chemical injury caused by allergens:
a. interference with enzyme activity
b. directly combing with some cell component other than enzymes
c. producing a secondary action in which a chemical causes the release or formation of a more harmful substance
d. none of above
e. all of above

Q.6 Which of the following chemicals is most associated with systemic disease involving the central nervous system, the gastrointestinal system, and the blood-forming tissues?
  a. Lead
  b. Pollen
  c. Animal dander
  d. CO
  e. None of the above
  f. All of the above

Q.7 Which of the following is not an exogenous factor of malignant tumors?
  a. Habits
  b. Ionizing radiation
  c. Chemical exposure
  d. Environment (socioeconomic, geographical, and occupational)
  e. Gender

Q.8 Which of the following is not an endogenous factor of malignant tumors?
  a. Oncogenic viruses
  b. Gender
  c. Age
  d. Hormonal imbalance
  e. Impaired immune system

Q.9 How many homologous pairs of chromosomes are there in human nucleus?
  a. 20
  b. 21
  c. 22
  d. 23
  e. 24

Q.10 Which of the following diseases is due to the point mutation on the codominant genes resulting in abnormal hemoglobin?
  a. Phenylketonuria
  b. Cystic fibrosis
  c. Sickle cell disease
  d. Huntington's disease
  e. Spherocytosis

Answers
1. a; 2. e; 3. d; 4. c; 5. c; 6. a; 7. e; 8. a; 9. d; 10. c.

Exercise 10

Q.1 How many synthetic chemicals are currently in commercial use in the United States, and whose toxicity is not widely known or understood?
  a. 70,000
  b. 6000
  c. 500
  d. 800,000
  e. 15,000

Q.2 _____is the most likely process of absorption for amino acids.
  a. Diffusion
  b. Facilitated diffusion
  c. Active transport
  d. Endocytosis
  e. None of the above

Q.3 Which of the following sites in the respiratory system is the most likely place for the carbon dioxide and oxygen to exchange in the blood?
  a. Nose
  b. Pharynx
  c. Larynx
  d. Trachea
  e. Alveoli

Q.4 Which of the following processes, when prolonged and severe, can be life threatening such as in asthmatic attacks?
  a. Mucociliary streaming
  b. Coughing
  c. Sneezing
  d. Bronchoconstriction
  e. None of the above

Q.5 What is the best estimate for the area of skin coverage in the average adult?
  a. 2500 in^2
  b. 3000 in^2
  c. 3500 in^2
  d. 4000 in^2
  e. 4500 in^2

Q.6 By what absorptive process does hexane pass through the skin?
  a. Passive diffusion
  b. Facilitated diffusion
  c. Active transport
  d. Endocytosis
  e. None of the above

Q.7 How long is the average adult human gastrointestinal tract?
  a. 20 ft
  b. 22 ft
  c. 30 ft
  d. 41 ft
  e. 52 ft

Q.8 Where is the most likely site for the absorption of toxic agents in the gastrointestinal tract?
  a. Between the stomach and the upper portion of the intestine
  b. Stomach

   c. Small intestine
   d. Large intestine
   e. The lower portion of large intestine
Q.9 What is the mechanism for the harmful effects of CO (carbon monoxide)?
   a. Interfere with or block the active sites of some important enzymes
   b. Direct chemical combination with a cell constituent
   c. Secondary action as a result of its presence in the system
   d. Compete with the cofactors for a site on an important enzyme
   e. None of the above
Q.10 What is the major organ responsible for detoxification in the body?
   a. Lung
   b. Intestines
   c. Kidney
   d. Liver
   e. Skin

Answers
1. a; 2. b; 3. e; 4. d; 5. b; 6. a; 7. c; 8. a; 9. b; 10. d.

Exercise 11

Q.1 What is the major toxic mechanism for hydrogen cyanide?
   a. Interfere with or block the active sites of the enzyme
   b. Inactivate or remove the cofactor
   c. Compete with the cofactor for a site on the enzyme
   d. Altering enzyme structure directly thereby changing the specific
      three-dimensional nature of the active site
   e. None of the above
Q.2 What is the major mechanism for toxicity of dithiocarbamate during
   alcohol consumption?
   a. Interfere with or block the active sites of the enzyme
   b. Inactivate or remove the cofactor
   c. Compete with the cofactor for a site on the enzyme
   d. Altering enzyme structure directly thereby changing the specific
      three-dimensional nature of the active site
   e. None of the above
Q.3 Which of the following substances can cause a syndrome in infants referred
   to as "blue baby"?
   a. Carbon monoxide
   b. Chlorine gas
   c. Ozone
   d. Sulfuric oxides
   e. Nitrogen compounds

Q.4 Which of the following refers to a substance that is attached to an antigen and promotes an antigenic response.
  a. Light chain
  b. Heavy chain
  c. Leukocyte
  d. Helper cell
  e. Hapten

Q.5 Which kind of cells are the primary targets of the AIDS virus?
  a. Cytoxic (killer) cell
  b. Helper T-cells (e.g., CD4)
  c. Memory cells
  d. Suppressor T-cells
  e. Delayed hypersensitivity T-cells

Q.6 The largest percent of antibodies belong to the _____ class.
  a. IgG
  b. IgE
  c. IgM
  d. IgA
  e. IgD

Q.7 Which of the following hypersensitivity reactions is most often seen in transfusion reactions?
  a. Cytotoxic
  b. Cell-mediated
  c. Immune complex
  d. Anaphylactic
  e. None of the above

Q.8 What kind of hypersensitivity is associated with asthma?
  a. Cytotoxic
  b. Cell-mediated
  c. Immune complex
  d. Anaphylactic
  e. None of the above

Q.9 What kind of the following interactions is characteristic of that for caffeine and sleeping pills?
  a. Additive
  b. Synergistic
  c. Antagonistic
  d. None of the above
  e. They do not interact with each other

Q.10 Yu-cheng disease in Taiwan is due to the toxic effect of _____.
  a. lead
  b. polychlorinated biphenyls (PCBs)

c. dioxin
d. asbestos
e. mercury

Answers
1. b; 2. b; 3. e; 4. e; 5. b; 6. a; 7. a; 8. d; 9. c; 10. b.

Exercise 12

Q.1 When were both federal regulatory and legislative efforts begun to reduce lead hazards, including the limitation of lead in paint and gasoline?
  a. 1970s
  b. 1980s
  c. 1990s
  d. 1940s
  e. 1950s

Q.2 Under the CAAA of 1990, an allowance is the right to emit how much sulfur dioxide?
  a. 100 tons
  b. 10 tons
  c. 1000 tons
  d. 1 ton

Q.3 Which of the following is not an indicator pollutant for regulation under the National Ambient Air Quality Standards (NAAQS) provisions?
  a. Sulfur dioxide (SO_2)
  b. Carbon monoxide (CO)
  c. Nitrogen oxides (NO_x)
  d. Asbestos
  e. Particulate matter (PM-10)

Q.4 Reformulated gasoline ("oxygenated fuel") with a 2% minimum oxygen content is required during the winter months in nonattainment areas for carbon monoxide. Which of the substances listed below may be added to fuel to render it oxygenated?
  a. Lead
  b. Methyl tertiary butyl ether
  c. Organic magnesium
  d. Mercury
  e. Benzene

Q.5 The federal Clean Water Act (CWA) and its amendments apply primarily to_____.
  a. protection of surface waters
  b. protection of groundwater
  c. navigable waterways
  d. boat moorings
  e. bays and estuaries

Q.6 Runoff that results from rain falling on roofs, roads, parking lots, loading docks, storage areas, and other areas exposed to rain is referred to as

_____.

a. storm water
b. effluent
c. dirty water
d. fugitive effluent
e. escaped liquid

Q.7 "Source reduction" refers to the deliberate decrease in the amounts of any hazardous substance, contaminant or pollutant that enters the environment prior to recycling, treatment, or disposal. This practice is most closely associated with what federal regulation?

a. Resource Conservation and Recovery Act (RCRA)
b. Clean Water Act
c. Clean Air Act Amendments of 1990
d. Comprehensive Environmental Response, Compensation and Liability Act (CERCLA)
e. Pollution Prevention Act of 1990

Q.8 Many companies are encouraged by the USEPA and State Environmental Protection Agencies to follow certain policies in dealing with environmental pollution. This now normally involves the use of

_____.

a. really good lawyers
b. concealment
c. cleanup
d. pollution prevention
e. witness protection programs

Q.9 There are several elements to a proactive environmental management program. Which one of the following does NOT apply.

a. Hold orientation and training sessions where environmental policy can be communicated to every employee.
b. Establish clear lines of authority with written policies for compliance and corrective measures with prompt reporting.
c. Reporting requirements and schedules for self-reporting data to regulatory agencies should be monitored.
d. Avoid providing environmental information to employees and management, so they can claim they were unaware of the law.
e. Develop a computerized information management system to coordinate corporate-wide data to identify problems, evaluate compliance, and target opportunities for future compliance planning.

Q.10 Permissible Exposure Limits are

a. promulgated by the Occupational Safety and Health Administration and have the force of law.
b. identical to and interchangeable with Short-Term Exposure Limits.

   c. authorized under the Toxic Substances Control Act.
   d. promulgated by the Environmental Protection Agency.
   e. directly adopted from the American Conference of Governmental Industrial Hygienists Threshold Limit Value list.

Answers

1. a; 2. d; 3. d; 4. b; 5. a; 6. a; 7. e; 8. d; 9. d; 10. a.

Exercise 13

Q.1 What is the process by which plants use energy from the sun to turn carbon dioxide and water into simple sugars?
   a. Photosynthesis
   b. Breathing
   c. Retrogradation
   d. Retrogression
   e. Photographic

Q.2 What is the best example(s) from the list below of an organism belonging to the first trophic level?
   a. Human
   b. Wolf
   c. Plant
   d. Large cat
   e. a and c

Q.3 Give an example of a primary consumer.
   a. Caterpillar
   b. Grasshopper
   c. Cattle
   d. Elephants
   e. All of the above

Q.4 Circle three macronutrients listed below.
   a. Sulfur
   b. Copper
   c. Carbon
   d. Oxygen
   e. Iron

Q.5 Circle all the ways carbon dioxide is released into the atmosphere.
   a. Respiratory process of animals
   b. Combustion of fossil or organic fuels
   c. Decomposition of organic matter
   d. The emissions of electric cars
   e. The heavy use of phones

Q.6 What gas makes up the largest percent of the Earth's air?
   a. Iron
   b. Nitrogen

   c. Oxygen
   d. Carbon
   e. Phosphorus
Q.7 Which substance has been identified as a respiratory tract carcinogen in humans?
   a. Kaolin
   b. Hydrogen fluoride
   c. Arsenic
   d. Cotton dust
   e. Vanadium
Q.8 Chloracne is associated with
   a. prominent hyperkeratosis of the follicular canal
   b. production of excessive sebum
   c. exposure to halogenated aliphatic hydrocarbons
   d. exposure to chlorine gas
   e. increases in serum androgen levels
Q.9 Which of the following statements is NOT true?
   a. Arsenic, benzene, and vinyl chloride are known human carcinogens.
   b. Many peroxisome proliferators cause hepatic tumors in rats and are promoting agents for hepatocarcinogenesis.
   c. Benzidine, beta-naphthylamine, and derived dyes have caused urinary bladder tumors in exposed workers.
   d. Short asbestos fibers (<2 μm long) are believed to be predominately responsible for the induction of mesotheliomas.
   e. Butylated hydroxyanisole acts as a nonmutagenic carcinogen in the forestomach of rats.
Q.10 Which of the following is characteristic of a nongenotoxic carcinogen?
   a. Has no influence on the promotional stage of carcinogenesis
   b. Would be expected to produce positive responses in in vitro assays for mutagenic potential
   c. Typically exerts other forms of toxicity and/or disrupts cellular homeostasis
   d. Generally shows little structural diversity
   e. Typically has little effect on cell turnover

Answers

1. a; 2. c; 3. e; 4. a, c, d; 5. a, b, c; 6. b; 7, c; 8, a; 9. d; 10. c.

Exercise 14

Q.1 The Resource Conservation and Recovery Act (RCRA) applies to facilities and agencies that do which of the following with hazardous waste?
   a. Generate and store
   b. Dispose of
   c. Treat

   d. Transport

   e. Any of the above

Q.2 Under RCRA definition, a waste that explodes or reacts with water or acid and is unstable is considered to be _____.

   a. ignitable

   b. corrosive

   c. reactive

   d. toxic

   e. none of the above

Q.3 Offsite shipments of hazardous waste must be labeled and marked according to requirements of what agency?

   a. Environmental Protection Agency (EPA)

   b. Department of Consumer Affairs

   c. Department of Defense (DOD)

   d. Department of Transportation (DOT)

   e. Department of Energy (DOE)

Q.4 A step in the Superfund process is to identify "PRPs" that can be required to finance cleanup activities. PRPs refer to:

   a. Potentially Remaining Parties

   b. Possible Responsible Polluters

   c. Potentially Responsible Parties

   d. Potentially Remaining Polluters

   e. none of the above

Q.5 If you are responsible for, or aware of, a substance that has been discharged or released into the environment in an amount that exceeds its listed "RQ" under SARA Title III, what must you do according to these regulations?

   a. Immediately report the release to local emergency response agencies, and state and national emergency response agencies

   b. Seek out an attorney

   c. Deny knowledge of the incident

   d. Take cover

   e. Rinse it down with a garden hose

Q.6 UN-based packaging regulations divide hazardous materials into Groups I, II, or III. The most hazardous materials fall into which group?

   a. Group I

   b. Group II

   c. Group III

   d. Nonconforming group

   e. None of the above

Q.7 According to a federal Underground Storage Tank (UST) law found under RCRA, tanks storing petroleum or hazardous chemicals are required to have leak detection systems installed by what date?

   a. 1995

   b. 2000

    c. Whenever convenient

    d. 1993

    e. Does not apply to USPS

Q.8 If only 10% of the volume of petroleum is contained in pipes underground attached to the tank, does the system still qualify as a UST under federal regulations?

    a. Yes

    b. No

Q.9 These actions may be covered by a portion of tort law that deals with acts not intended to inflict injury but where persons may be harmed by the careless and improper actions of another, such as the improper disposal of hazardous wastes.

    a. Knowing endangerment

    b. Negligent actions

    c. Knowing actions

    d. Willful avoidance

Q.10 Environmental law is a system of laws that encompass all of the environmental protections that originate from all the sources listed below except _____.

    a. United States constitution and state constitutions

    b. regulations published by federal, state, and local agencies

    c. justice of the peace rulings

    d. presidential executive orders

    e. the common law

Answers

1. e; 2. c; 3. d; 4. c; 5. a; 6. a; 7. d; 8. a; 9. b; 10. c.

14.3.3 FILL IN THE BLANKS

Exercise 15

Q.1 The process of contamination of environment (air, water, and soil) through discharge of harmful substances is known as _____.

Q.2 The size of the particles, which can reach alveoli of lungs is less than _____.

Q.3 The pollutants released directly into atmosphere either through natural or anthropogenic sources are called _____ pollutants.

Q.4 Pollutants formed due to the interaction of pollutants already present in the atmosphere are called as _____ pollutants.

Q.5 Man-made sources or anthropogenic sources constitute _____ of pollution.

Q.6 The major air pollutant is _____.

Q.7 The pollutant that is produced due to incomplete combustion is _____.

Q.8 The lethal concentration of CO in air is _____.
Q.9 The major source of CO in urban setting is _____.
Q.10 CO binds with hemoglobin forming _____.

Answers

1. POLLUTION; 2. 1 μm (particles of 5 μm or more are deposited in upper respiratory tract and between 1 and 5 μm in the terminal airways); 3. PRIMARY (e.g., carbon monoxide, carbon dioxide, etc.); 4. SECONDARY (e.g., ozone, PAN); 5. 98%; 6. CARBON MONOXIDE (CO) (CO—52%, sulfur oxide—18%, hydrocarbons—12% are the top three air pollutants); 7. CO; 8. 400 ppm; 9. AUTOMOBILES; 10. CARBOXY HEMOGLOBIN (because CO has 200 times more affinity for HB than oxygen, the oxygen-carrying capacity of blood is severely hampered).

Exercise 16

Q.1 The color of blood in CO poisoning is _____.
Q.2 The main symptom in CO poisoning is _____.
Q.3 The specific therapy for CO poisoning is _____.
Q.4 The normal concentration of carbon dioxide in atmosphere is _____.
Q.5 Symptoms of CO2 poisoning are evident at a concentration of _____ in air.
Q.6 The process of elevation of earth's temperature due to increase in greenhouse gases in the atmosphere is called _____.
Q.7 Greenhouse gas of animal origin, which is implicated in global warming is _____.
Q.8 The primary pollutants responsible for acid rains are _____.
Q.9 The level of SO2 in air, which is considered dangerous, is _____.
Q.10 _____ gas is used as preservatives in canned meat products

Answers

1. CHERRY RED (carboxy hemoglobin gives characteristic cherry red color to blood. Hence, despite of asphyxia, there is no development of cyanosis. The skin and mucosa are red); 2. HYPOXIA (brain and heart are very sensitive for hypoxia as they have high oxygen requirement); 3. OXYGEN; 4. 0.5% (5000 ppm); 5. 5%; 6. GLOBAL WARMING (important greenhouse gases are CO2, methane, water vapor, etc.); 7. methane gas (which is produced in ruminants due to bacterial fermentation); 8. SULFUR OXIDES (SO2, SO3) (sulfur oxides combine with water vapor in either air or body to form sulfurous or sulfuric acid. The other component is nitrogen oxides, which similarly form nitric acid upon contact with moisture); 9. 100 ppm; 10. SO2 (SO2 acts as a preservative; further, it masks the odor of the meat and improves its color.

Exercise 17

Q.1 "Silo-fillers disease" or "Silage gas" poisoning is caused by _____.

Q.2 The level of nitrogen oxides (NO2 and N2O4) in air, which can cause harmful effects, is _____.

Q.3 The major system affected by NO2 and SO2 poisoning is _____ system.

Q.4 Painter's syndrome is caused due to continuous exposure to _____ vapors.

Q.5 The main symptoms in chronic exposure to solvents are _____.

Q.6 The pollutant that can form ozone in the atmosphere by absorbing UV light is _____.

Q.7 The pollutant that can cause permanent damage to lungs even with short-term exposure in low concentrations is _____.

Q.8 The combination of smoke and fog results in the formation of _____ that considerably reduces visibility.

Q.9 The important contributor for development of photochemical smog is _____.

Q.10 The level of total dissolved solids in drinking water, which cause no hazard to animals, is _____.

Q.11 The species of animal that is highly sensitive for PCBs' toxicity is _____.

Q.12 PCB inhibits the synthesis of the central neurotransmitter in _____ brain.

Q.13 Feminization of male fetus is caused by _____ pollutants.

Q.14 "Cola-colored babies" are born when mothers are exposed to _____ pollutants during pregnancy.

Q.15 "Chick edema" is a characteristic clinical condition produced by _____ pollutants.

Q.16 Water-treatment processes such as chlorination lead to the production of _____ due to reaction of chlorine with organic matter.

Answers

1. NITROGEN DIOXIDE (NO2); 2. 100 ppm; 3. RESPIRATORY; 4. SOLVENT; 5. ENCEPHALOPATHY (endocrine disruption is also reported for organic solvents. Organic solvents include benzene, toluene, gasoline, petrol, and kerosene. Bad news for those who like the smell of petrol, kerosene, etc.); 6. NO2; 7. OZONE (O3); 8. SMOG; 9. PEROXY ACETYL NITRATE (PAN) (PAN is mutagenic and can cause skin cancer); 10. <1000 ppm; 11. MINK; 12. DOPAMINE; 13. PCB (PCBs are endocrine disruptors possessing estrogenic activity that causes feminization of male fetus); 14. PCB; 15. PCB; 16. TRIHALOMETHANES.

14.3.4 TRUE OR FALSE STATEMENTS (WRITE T FOR TRUE AND F FOR FALSE STATEMENT)

Exercise 18

Q.1 An inversion is a stable, slow-moving air mass that results from the formation of a cool layer of air above warmer air near the earth. _____

Q.2 Global warming can be attributed to greenhouse gases. _____

Q.3 Ozone depletion has been linked to CFCs. _____

Q.4 There are traces of helium found in the atmosphere. _____

Q.5 The combined reflective ability of cloud cover and ground surfaces are known as inversions. _____

Q.6 The troposphere is the layer of air in the 20–40 km altitude range.
_____

Q.7 Ozone is a primary pollutant. _____

Q.8 The amount of nitrogen dioxide in the atmosphere has decreased in the last 20 years. _____

Q.9 Lead has been reduced by 98% in ambient concentrations from 1970.
_____

Q.10 An oxidant is a substance that removes hydrogen from a compound.
_____

Answers

1. False; 2. True; 3. True; 4. True; 5. False; 6. False; 7. False; 8. False; 9. True; 10. True.

Exercise 19

Q.1 Carbon monoxide is a gray-colored gas with an odor like rotten eggs.
_____.

Q.2 Nasal hairs play a part in cleaning air before it reaches the lungs.
_____.

Q.3 The beginning signs of an asthma attack include sweating and rapid pulse.
_____

Q.4 During an airway spasm, the muscles of the alveoli contract and the membranes swell. _____

Q.5 There is a phenomenon called sick-building syndrome. _____

Q.6 Cat saliva is considered to be a biological contaminant. _____

Q.7 The number of asthma cases since 1982 have decreased. _____

Q.8 The New England area is considered to be an acid-sensitive region.
_____

Q.9 The Kyoto conference in 1997 suggested that the United States decrease greenhouse gas emissions 7% below 1990 levels. _____

Q.10 Acid deposition is a threat to aquatic ecosystems because it leads to reductions in fish populations. _____

Answers

1. False; 2. True; 3. False; 4. False; 5. True; 6. True; 7. False; 8. True; 9. True; 10. True.

Exercise 19

Q.1 Carcinogens refers to chemicals that primarily cause reproductive disorders. _____

Q.2 Most cancer risks are modifiable through changes in human behavior. _____

Q.3 The best estimate for the contribution of pollution to cancer risk is around 2% of the total risk. _____

Q.4 Chemical pollutants contribute substantially to cancer risk. _____

Q.5 Reservoirs are those living organisms or inanimate objects that provide the conditions where the organisms may survive, multiply, and also provide the conditions necessary for transmission. _____

Q.6 The leading cause of injury-related death in the United States involve motor vehicles accounting for nearly 4000 deaths per year with more than 40% of those deaths in the 16−19 years age group. _____

Q.7 Falls are the leading causes of accidental deaths in the home. _____

Q.8 Teratologic defects usually arise during embryonic period of development and the causative factors are usually not genetic but from exposure to chemicals or radiation. _____

Q.9 Kwashiorkor develops from a lack of vitamin C. _____

Q.10 Environmental disease refers to any pathologic process having a characteristic set of signs and symptoms that are detrimental to the well-being of the individual and are the consequence of many factors, including exposure to physical or chemical agents, poor nutrition, and social or cultural behaviors. _____

Answers

1. False; 2. True; 3. True; 4. False; 5. True; 6. False; 7. True; 8. True; 9. False; 10. True.

Exercise 20

Q.1 Protein is the basic informational macromolecule that is the basis of heredity whose chemical structure has been known for more than 45 years. _____

Q.2 Because every individual within each species is very much a representation of the information contained in the genome together with the expression of those genes in the development of that individual, all the genotypic changes are harmful or damaging. _____

Q.3 One of the most well-known cytogenetic defects is trisomy 21 or Down's disease which is characterized by the addition of an extra chromosome to chromosome number 21. _____

Q.4 Most teratogens exert their effect during certain critical time windows in the late stages of tissue and organ formation known as organogenesis. _____

Q.5 Lead has been recognized as a hazard since early civilization when it was used to store wine, to pipe water, and even as vessels in which to cook food. _____

Q.6 Once a potential toxic substance goes into our society, it automatically produces an adverse effect. _____

Q.7 External respiration refers to the exchange of gases between blood and individual cells. _____

Q.8 Sulfur oxides tend to reach deep into lung tissue, while nitrogen dioxides tend to act in the upper moist airways of the respiratory tree. _____

Q.9 The skin is the body's largest organ and consists of many interconnected tissues. _____

Q.10 Epidermis is the outer, thinner layer of the skin, and dermis is the inner and much thicker layer of the skin. _____

Answers

1. False; 2. False; 3. True; 4. False; 5. True; 6. False; 7. False; 8. False; 9. True; 10. True.

Exercise 21

Q.1 Zinc, iron, and copper are examples of macronutrients. _____

Q.2 Humans are nitrogen-based life forms. _____

Q.3 The sedimentary cycle refers to calcium, iron, and phosphorus getting leached from sedentary rocks by water erosion. _____

Q.4 The gastrointestinal tract is a major route of absorption for many toxic agents including mercury, lead, and cadmium. _____

Q.5 A toxin can produce a harmful effect upon an organ only by stimulating the normal metabolic actions of that particular organ. _____

Q.6 Many enzymes require a nonprotein component called apoenzyme and a protein component called cofactor to become active. _____.

Q.7 Cadmium and beryllium are believed to inactivate enzymes by blocking the sites on the enzyme where such cofactors as iron normally attach. _____

Q.8 When lead covalently bonds to an enzyme, its inhibition of enzymes is considered to be irreversible. _____

Q.9 The exposure of allergens can trigger a diminished immune response in some people. _____

Q.10 Chemical pollutants such as ozone can depress the immune response by inactivating alveolar macrophages. _____

Answers

1. False; 2. False; 3. False; 4. True; 5. False; 6. False; 7. False; 8. True; 9. False; 10. True.

Exercise 22

Q.1 B cells are the principle agents in cell-mediated immunity. _____
Q.2 Humoral immune responses are characterized by subcutaneous bleeding. _____

Q.3 The environmental pollutants such as ozone and fine particulates contribute to the significant rise in the numbers and severity of asthma cases. _____

Q.4 If absorbed, lead tends to be stored mostly in fatty tissue. _____
Q.5 Dioxin is considered to be one of the most toxic natural chemicals. _____

Q.6 The EPA has listed 20 µg/dL as the maximum acceptable blood lead level for fetuses and young children. _____
Q.7 Lead may impair fertility in both men and women when blood lead levels approach 50 µg/dL. _____
Q.8 The process by which plants turn carbon dioxide and water into nutrients is known as photosynthesis. _____
Q.9 Allergic contact dermatitis is a nonimmune response caused by a direct action of an agent on the skin. _____
Q.10 The primary site of kidney damage resulting from acute exposure to inorganic mercury salts is the glomerulus. _____

Answers

1. False; 2. True; 3. True; 4. False; 5. False; 6. False; 7. True. 8. True; 9. False; 10. False.

Exercise 23

Q.1 If only 20% of the volume of petroleum is contained in pipes underground attached to the tank, the system will qualify as a UST under federal regulations. _____
Q.2 A company or agency remains responsible for the proper disposal of hazardous waste even after it leaves their property. _____
Q.3 In order for an employee to be prosecuted for negligent violation (giving rise to criminal liability), the law must demonstrate the actions were intentional. _____
Q.4 A large quantity generator is defined as the one that produces 1000 kg or more of hazardous wastes in a year. _____

Q.5 In some states, used oil (such as motor oil) that is not recycled is designated a hazardous waste. _____

Q.6 A waste is considered hazardous if it has a pH greater than 10. _____

Q.7 The first step in implementing CERCLA is to locate or find the hazardous waste site(s) . _____

Q.8 The purpose of SARA Title III is to assure the public and emergency response agencies that information regarding hazardous chemicals is available to them. _____

Q.9 The DOT regulates the disposal of hazardous wastes shipped by truck. _____

Q.10 Source reduction must be reported by facilities generating over a certain amount of toxic emissions during the previous calendar year. _____

Q.11 Septic tanks, heating oil tanks, and residential fuel tanks are regulated under the federal UST law. _____

Answers

1. False; 2. True; 3. False; 4. False; 5. True; 6. False; 7. True; 8. True; 9. False; 10. True; 11. False.

FURTHER READING

Caravati, E.M., 2004. Hydrogen Sulfide. In: Dart, R.C., Caravati, E.M., McGuigan, M.A., Whyte, I.M., Dawson, A.H., Seifert, S.A., Schonwald, S., Yip, L., Keyes, D.C., Hurlbut, K.M., Erdman, A.R. (Eds.), Medical Toxicology. Lippincott Williams & Wilkins, Philadelphia, pp. 1169–1173.

Chou, S., Fay, M., Keith, S., Ingerman, L., Chappell, L., 2006. ATSDR Toxicological Profile for Hydrogen Sulfide. ATSDR, Atlanta.

Costa, D.L., Gordon, T., 2013. Air pollution. In: Klaassen, C.D. (Ed.), Casarett and Doull's Toxicology: The Basic Science of Poisons, eighth ed. McGraw-Hill, New York, pp. 1231–1272.

Dixon, R.L., 2010. Environmental toxicology. In: second reprint Gupta, P.K. (Ed.), Modern Toxicology: The Adverse Effects of Xenobiotics, Vol. 2. PharmaMed Press, Hyderabad, India, pp. 398–446.

Di Glutio, R.T., Newman, M.C., 2013. Ecotoxicology. In: Klaassen, C.D. (Ed.), Casarett and Doull's Toxicology: The Basic Science of Poisons, eighth ed. McGraw-Hill, New York, pp. 1275–1304.

Laws, E.A., 2013. Environmental Toxicology. Springer, New York, pp. 1–737. ISBN: 978-1-4614-5763-3 (Print) 978-1-4614-5764-0 (Online).

Zakrzewski, S.F., 2002. Environmental Toxicology., third ed. Oxford University Press, New York, pp. 1–448.

Veterinary toxicology

15

CHAPTER OUTLINE

Illustrated Toxicology. DOI: http://dx.doi.org/10.1016/B978-0-12-813213-5.00015-8
© 2018 Elsevier Inc. All rights reserved.

15.1 INTRODUCTION

Information with regard to general toxicology, principles of toxicology, mechanism of toxicity, biotransformation and toxicokinetics, toxicity of various xenobiotics including pesticides, metals nonmetals, solvents, vapors and gases, poisonous plants, animal and plant toxins, poisonous foods and food poisonings, target organ toxicity, environmental toxicology, and health effects of radiation has already been dealt in various chapters in this book. This chapter deals with toxicity of xenobiotics that have more relevance to veterinarians having interest in domestic and other animals.

15.2 DEFINITIONS

Q. Define veterinary toxicology.

    Veterinary toxicology deals with the cause, diagnosis, and management of established poisonings in domestic and wild animals.

Q. What are sources of animal poisoning?

    1. Accidental/malicious poisoning

    2. Certain soil imbalances can lead to pasture grasses with too much of one mineral, which can be toxic to livestock.

    3. From algae and salt to lead and household products

Q. What is malicious poisoning?

    Malicious poisoning is the unlawful or criminal killing of human beings or animals by administering certain toxic/poisonous agents. Incidence of such poisonings is quite prevalent in animals (Fig. 15.1).

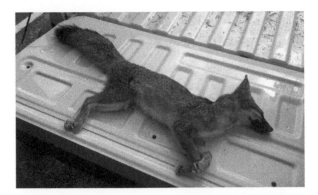

FIGURE 15.1

Malicious and cruel: to poison a dog.

Reproduced from National Park Service. (https://www.nps.gov/samo/images/gray-fox-death_1.jpg)

Q. Define accidental poisoning.

Accidental poisoning may occur when human beings or animals take toxicant accidentally or is added unintentionally in food or through in its feed, fodder, or drinking water. Such toxicants come from either natural or man-made sources. The natural sources include ingestion of toxic plants, biting or stinging by poisonous reptiles, ingestion of food contaminated with toxins, and contaminated water with minerals. Man-made sources include therapeutic agents, household products, and agrochemicals.

Q. Define tetrodotoxin.

Tetrodotoxin, also known as puffer poison, is found in many species of puffer fish, ocean sunfish, and porcupine fish. It is an amino perhydroquinazoline compound.

Q. Define saxitoxin.

Some mollusks contain neurotoxins known as saxitoxin, which are produced when certain species of algae undergo rapid growth and are ingested by mollusks.

Q. Define hemotoxicity.

Hemotoxicity is related to blood toxicity. It includes coagulopathies, cardiotoxicity, and hemolysis.

Q. Define antibiotic growth promoters.

The term "antibiotic growth promoter" is used to describe any medicine that destroys or inhibits bacteria and is administered at a low, subtherapeutic dose. The use of antibiotics for growth promotion has started with the intensification of livestock farming.

Q. What is phytobiotics?

Phytobiotics can be defined as plant-derived products added to feed to improve performance. They originate from leaves, roots, tubers or fruits of herbs, spices, and other.

Q. Define growth promotants.

Growth promotants are used to help increase the efficiency of animal production by increasing weight gain. Growth promotant is typically a small pellet that is implanted under the skin on the back of an animal's ear. The pellet releases tiny amounts of hormone and safely dissolves as the treatment is completed.

Q. Define withdrawal time.

Withdrawal time is defined as the time required after administration of a drug to a dairy cow needed to assure that drug residues in the marketable milk is below a determined maximum residue limit (MRL).

15.3 POISONOUS PLANTS

Q. How poisonous plants are responsible for toxicity in animals?

Many plants commonly used as food possess toxic parts, are toxic unless processed, or are toxic at certain stages of their lives. Some only pose a serious threat to certain animals (such as cats, dogs, or livestock) or certain types of people (such as infants, the elderly, or individuals with pathological vulnerabilities). Most of these food plants are safe for the average adult to eat in modest quantities.

15.3.1 PLANTS CONTAINING CYANIDE/CYANOGENIC PLANTS

Toxic effects of cyanides are also discussed in Chapter 7, Nonmetals and micro-nutrients, dealing with nonmetals.

Q. What is prussic acid poisoning?

Prussic acid is also known as hydrocyanic acid (HCN). Prussic acid is not normally present in plants, but under certain conditions, several common plants can accumulate large quantities of cyanogenic glycosides that can convert to prussic acid. The risk of prussic acid poisoning in livestock is increased during periods of drought, and even more so after drought breaks, when stressed, stunted plants begin to grow. Prussic acid is a potent, rapidly acting poison, which enters the bloodstream of affected animals and is transported through the body. It then inhibits oxygen utilization by the cells so that, in effect, the animal dies from asphyxia.

Q. What are sources of prussic acid poisoning?

Approximately 200 plants are known to accumulate sufficient quantities of cyanogenic glycosides to cause poisoning (Figs. 15.2 and 15.3). The plant species that commonly cause prussic acid poisoning in livestock are:

Sorghum spp. (Johnson grass, Sudan grass, and *S. bicolor*, the common cereal grain crop referred to as "*Sorghum*" or the synonyms—durra, jowari, and milo),

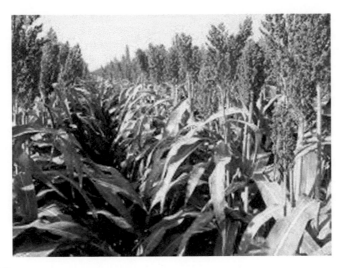

FIGURE 15.2

Sorghum plant.

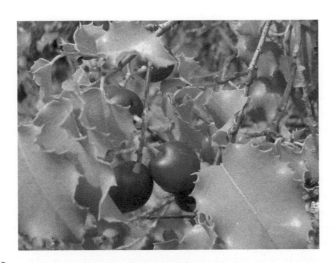

FIGURE 15.3

Prunus spp. Common name: Wild cherries, black cherry, bitter cherry, choke cherry, and pin cherry.

Acacia greggii (guajillo),
Amelanchier alnifolia (western service berry),
Linum spp. (linseeds and flaxes),
Sambucus nigra (elderberry),
Suckleya suckleyana (poison suckleya),
Triglochin maritima and *T. palustris* (marsh arrow grasses),
Mannihot esculentum (cassava),
Prunus genus until proved otherwise (apricot, peach, chokecherry, pincherry, wild black cherry, ornamental cherry, peaches, nectarines, apricots, almonds, bird cherries, black thorn, cherry laurels [commercial orchard species are often specifically bred for low cyanide content; however, ornamental members of this genus are often highly poisonous]),
Nandina domestica (heavenly or sacred bamboo),
Phaseolus lunatus (Lima beans),
Trifolium sp. (clovers; often, pasture species have been bred for low cyanide content),
Zea mays (corn),
Eucalyptus spp. (gum trees),
Hydrangea spp. (hydrangeas),
Pteridium aquilinum (bracken fern),
Bahia oppositifolia (bahia), and
Chaenomeles spp. (flowering quince).

Q. Which plant conditions are dangerous for prussic acid poisoning in animals?

Certain conditions lead to dangerous levels of cyanogenic glycosides in plants. These conditions include:

1. periods of rapid regrowth following stunting, for example, after a drought breaks, if a crop is eaten back and then allowed to regrow or if a crop is harvested for hay and then allowed to regrow (levels are highest in young plants with green, growing shoots);
2. frosted or wilted plants that have a transient increase in glycoside levels;
3. herbicide-treated plants that have a transient increase in glycoside levels;
4. high nitrogen and low phosphorus levels in the soil;
5. plant species, such as sorghum, which can contain more prussic acid than Sudan grass—varieties vary in their prussic acid potential; and
6. plants that are wet with dew or light rain.

Q. Which animal species are more susceptible to prussic acid poisoning?

Ruminant animals (cattle and sheep) are more susceptible to prussic acid poisoning than monogastric animals (horses and pigs).

Q. Why are monogastric animals less susceptible to prussic acid poisoning?

The lower pH in the stomach of the monogastric animals helps to destroy the enzymes that convert cyanogenic glycosides to prussic acid. Hence, they are less susceptible.

Q. Why some animals are more susceptible to prussic acid poisoning than others?

1. For prussic acid poisoning, high levels of cyanogenic glycosides and enzymes are necessary to metabolize them. The action of rumen microbes will metabolize cyanogenic glycosides. Therefore, poisoning is more likely in ruminant animals. Sheep are more resistant to poisoning than cattle due to the different enzyme systems in their forestomachs.

2. Hungry animals are more at greater risk as they will normally consume a larger amount of toxic material in a short time. This "overload" of prussic acid can overwhelm an animal's ability to metabolize prussic acid to the nontoxic thiocyanate. Large amounts of prussic acid can, therefore, be absorbed and lead to poisoning.

3. Travelling stock and recently introduced stock are at greater risk as they are unaccustomed to local plants. There is also evidence that localized animals become accustomed to the poison and get accustomed to tolerate increasing amounts.

Q. What is the mode of action of cyanide ions in animal toxicity?

In acute cyanide poisoning, cyanide ions (CN^-) bind to, and inhibit, the ferric (Fe^{3+}) heme moiety form of mitochondrial cytochrome c oxidase. This blocks the fourth step in the mitochondrial electron transport chain (reduction of O_2 to H_2O), resulting in the arrest of aerobic metabolism and death from histotoxic anoxia. Tissues that heavily depend on aerobic metabolism such as the heart and brain are particularly susceptible to these effects. Cyanide also binds to other heme-containing enzymes, such as members of the cytochrome p450 family, and to myoglobin. However, these tissue cyanide "sinks" do not provide sufficient protection from histotoxic anoxia.

Q. What is the lethal dose of cyanide in animals?

The acute lethal dosage of hydrogen cyanide (HCN) in most animal species is ~2 mg/kg. Plant materials containing ≥ 200 ppm of cyanogenic glycosides are dangerous.

The CN^- radicals combine with the ferric iron of cytochrome oxidase in mitochondria and inhibit the electron transport system.

Q. Describe in brief symptoms of acute cyanide poisoning in domestic animals?

Acute cyanide poisoning: Signs generally appear within 15−20 minutes to a few hours after animals consume toxic forage, and survival after onset of clinical signs is rarely >2 hours. Excitement can be displayed initially, accompanied by rapid respiration rate. Dyspnea follows shortly with tachycardia. The classic "bitter almond" breath smell may be present. Salivation, excess lacrimation, and voiding of urine and feces may occur. Vomiting may occur, especially in pigs. Muscle fasciculation is common and progresses to generalized spasms and coma before death. Animals may stagger and struggle before collapse. In other cases, sudden unexpected death may ensue. Mucous membranes are bright red but may become cyanotic terminally. Venous blood is classically described as "cherry red" because of the presence of high venous blood, pO_2; however, this color rapidly changes after death. Serum ammonia and neutral and aromatic amino acids are typically increased. Cardiac arrhythmias are common due to myocardial histotoxic hypoxia. Death occurs during severe asphyxial convulsions. The heart may continue to beat for several minutes after struggling and breathing stops.

Poachers use cyanide to kill the animals such as zebra, birds, and cheetah, and even elephants are poisoned by cyanide (Figs. 15.4 and 15.5).

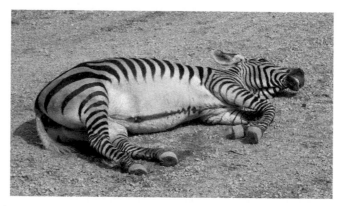

FIGURE 15.4

Poachers used cyanide to kill the animals, the picture of Zebra.

Reproduced from https://commons.wikimedia.org/wiki/File:Hartmanns_Mountain_Zebra_Resting.jpg.

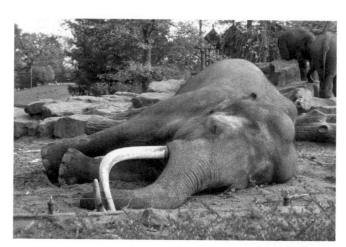

FIGURE 15.5

Elephants that was killed by cyanide poisoning.

Reproduced from https://commons.wikimedia.org/wiki/File:Sleeping_asian_elephant.jpg.

Q. Describe in brief symptoms of chronic cyanide poisoning in domestic animals.

Chronic cyanide poisoning syndrome: Chronic cyanogenic glycoside hypothyroidism will present as hypothyroidism with or without goiter. Cystitis ataxia toxidromes are typically associated with posterior ataxia or incoordination that may progress to irreversible flaccid paralysis, cystitis secondary to urinary incontinence, and hind limb urine scalding and alopecia. Death, although uncommon, is often associated with pyelonephritis. Late-term abortion and musculoskeletal teratogenesis may also occur.

15.3.2 PLANTS PRODUCING LATHYRISM

Q. What is lathyrism?

Lathyrism or neurolathyrism is a neurological disease of humans and domestic animals, caused by eating certain legumes of the genus *Lathyrus*.

Q. Give suitable examples of plants producing lathyrism.

Plants producing lathyrism (Figs. 15.6−15.8) include:

1. *Lathyrus sativus* (also known as Grass pea, Kesari Dal, Khesari Dal, or Almorta),
2. *Lathyrus cicera, L. ochrus,*
3. *Lathyrus clymenum,* and
4. *Lathyrus odoratus.*

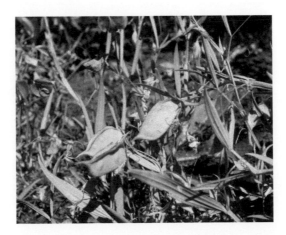

FIGURE 15.6

Lathyrus sativus plant with pods.

Reproduced from http://cropgenebank.sgrp.cgiar.org/images/other_crops/lathyrus_sp_7679_pod.jpg.

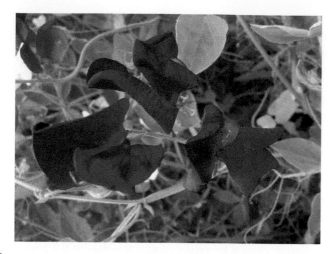

FIGURE 15.7

Lathyrus odoratus plant and seeds.

Reproduced from https://commons.wikimedia.org/wiki/File:Sweet_Pea-5.jpg.

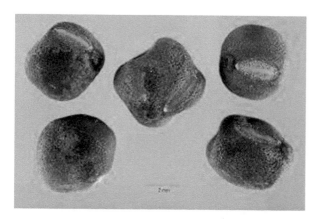

FIGURE 15.8

Lathyrus odoratus plant seeds.

http://plants.usda.gov/gallery/standard/laod_001_shp.jpg.

Q. What is odoratism or osteolathyrism?

The lathyrism resulting from the ingestion of *L. odoratus* seeds (sweet peas) is often referred to as odoratism or osteolathyrism, which is caused by a different toxin (beta-aminopropionitrile) that affects the linking of collagen, a protein of connective tissues.

Q. What is neurolathyrism?

Neurolathyrism is a neurological disease of humans and domestic animals, caused by long-term feeding/eating of seeds of certain legumes of the genus *Lathyrus*. There is gradual weakness of muscles followed by paralysis leading to death due to respiratory failure.

Q. What is the toxic principle of lathyrism?

Lathyrus grain contains high concentrations of the glutamate analog neurotoxin β-oxalyl-L-α,β-diaminopropionic acid (ODAP, also known as β-N-oxalyl-amino-L-alanine, or BOAA).

Q. What are the characteristic symptoms of lathyrism poisoning?

It is characterized by a lack of strength or inability to move the lower limbs, and may involve pyramidal tracts producing signs of upper motor neuron damage. The toxin may also cause aortic aneurysm. A unique symptom of lathyrism is the atrophy of gluteal muscles (buttocks). ODAP is a poison of mitochondria, the powerhouse of the cell, leading to excess cell death, especially in motor neurons. Children can develop bone deformity and reduced brain development.

15.3.3 PLANTS PRODUCING THIAMINE DEFICIENCY/BRACKEN FERN POISONING

Q. What is bracken fern poisoning?

Pteridium sp. of plants (Bracken fern) contain thiaminase enzyme that catalyzes thiamine and produces vitamin B deficiencies in animals. The plant is known to cause bone marrow suppression and anemia in cattle and sheep.

Q. What are the toxic principles of bracken fern?

The toxic principle is Ptaquiloside (PTA). Bracken fern is known carcinogen to produce and release allelopathic chemicals, which is an important factor in its ability to dominate other vegetation, particularly in regrowth after fire.

Q. Name some plants producing bracken fern poisoning.

Important species of bracken plant (Figs. 15.9 and 15.10) are given below:

1. *Pteridium aquilinum*—nearly cosmopolitan
2. *Pteridium arachnoideum*—Mexico, Central + South America, Galápagos
3. *Pteridium caudatum*—Mexico, Central + South America, Florida, West Indies
4. *Pteridium centraliafricanum*—Zaire, Zambia, Tanzania, Burundi
5. *Pteridium esculentum*—China, SE Asia, Australia
6. *Pteridium falcatum*—Guangxi
7. *Pteridium feei*—Mexico, Central America
8. *Pteridium lineare*—Yunnan
9. *Pteridium revolutum*—China
10. *Pteridium tauricum*—Caucasus
11. *Pteridium yunnanense*—Yunnan

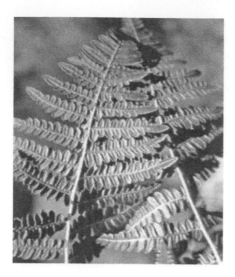

FIGURE 15.9

Pteridium aquilinum (Bracken fern).

Reproduced from https://www.ars.usda.gov/arsuserfiles/images/docs/9859_10053/Bracken%20Fern%20Photo.bmp.

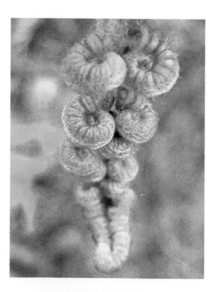

FIGURE 15.10

Young Bracken fronds curled.

https://upload.wikimedia.org/wikipedia/en/thumb/e/e2/Curled_bracken_fronds.JPG/220px-Curled_bracken_fronds.JPG.

Q. What is the mode of action of bracken fern poisoning?

The chemicals in the fern can damage blood cells and can destroy Vitamin B1. This in turn causes beriberi, a disease normally linked to nutritional deficiency. Hydrogen cyanide is released by the young fronds of bracken when eaten by mammals or insects. Two major insect-moulting hormones, alpha ecdysone and 20-hydroxyecdysone, are found in bracken. These cause uncontrollable, repeated moulting in insects ingesting the fronds, leading to rapid death.

Q. What are the symptoms of bracken fern poisoning in animals?

All parts of bracken fern are toxic, as it results in thiamine deficiency; symptoms include progressive loss of coordination, decreased appetite, weight loss, muscle tremors, constipation, weakness, depression, and blindness followed by death (within 2−10 days) (Figs. 15.11 and 15.12).

The carcinogenic compound in bracken or PTA can leach from the plant into the water supply, which may cause an increase in the incidence of gastric and esophageal cancers in bracken-rich areas. In cattle, bracken poisoning can occur in both an acute and chronic form—acute poisoning being the most common. In pigs and horses bracken poisoning induces vitamin B deficiency. Poisoning usually occurs when there is a shortage of available grasses such as in drought or snowfalls. Generally, most poisonings in horses occur in late summer, when toxicity levels are at their highest.

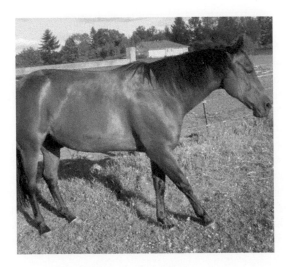

FIGURE 15.11

Bracken fern (*Pteridium aquilinum*) toxicity in horses.

Reproduced from Flickr https://www.flickr.com/photos/holyoutlaw/5834412670.

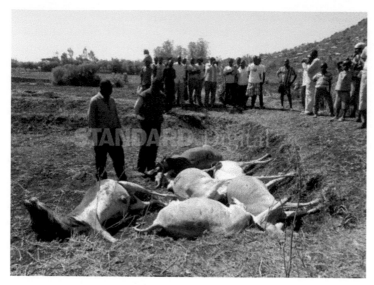

FIGURE 15.12

Carcasses of cattle that died after eating a poisonous weed known as bracken fern.

http://www.standardmedia.co.ke/article/2000154602/cattle-die-in-homa-bay-after-eating-toxic-plant-as-drought-persists.

15.3.4 PLANTS PRODUCING PHOTOSENSITIZATION

Q. What is photosensitization?

Abnormal sensitivity of unpigmented or less pigmented parts of skin to sunlight due to the presence of photodynamic substances in peripheral circulation is known as photosensitization.

Q. What is photodynamic substance?

A substance that absorbs UV light and emits energy while coming to ground state is called photodynamic substance.

Q. How photosensitization differs from sunburn and photodermatitis?

Photosensitization occurs when skin (especially areas exposed to light and lacking significant protective hair, wool, or pigmentation) becomes more susceptible to ultraviolet light because of the presence of photodynamic agents. Photosensitization differs from sunburn and photodermatitis, because both of these conditions result in pathologic skin changes without the presence of a photodynamic agent. Sometimes photosensitization in cattle and horse that resembles sunburns has been observed (Fig. 15.13).

Q. Why lesions in photosensitization are seen only in few areas of the body?

Melanin pigment protects skin from UV light. Hence, in light pigmented areas or in areas devoid of fur/wool, more UV light is absorbed leading to sunburn

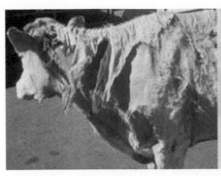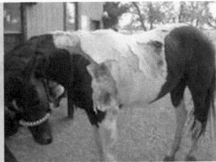

FIGURE 15.13

Photosensitization in cattle and horse that resembles sunburns.

lesions. Light pigmented areas and areas devoid of hair/wool such as face, eyelids, muzzle, coronary band, and udder are more prone for photosensitization.

Q. What is primary photosensitization?

The type of photosensitivity produced due to direct ingestion of photodynamic substances or metabolically activated agents is called primary photosensitization For example, plants belonging to species such as *Hypericum* (Fig. 15.14), *Fagopyrum* (Fig. 15.15), and *Parthenium* produce primary type of photosensitivity. Likewise, drugs such as phenothiazines, tetracyclines, sulfonamides, and acridine dyes also produce primary type of photosensitivity.

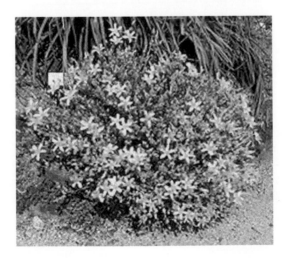

FIGURE 15.14

Hypericum sp. (St. John Wort).

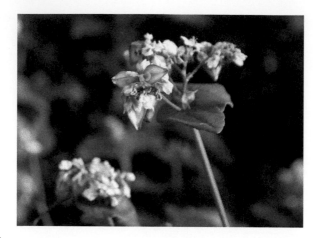

FIGURE 15.15

Fagopyrum sp.

Reproduced from https://commons.wikimedia.org/wiki/File:Japanese_Buckwheat_Flower.JPG.

Q. What is secondary/hepatogenous photosensitization?

The type of photosensitivity, which is produced due to hepatic damage consequent to ingestion of hepatotoxic substances, is called secondary/hepatogenous photosensitization (e.g., Pyrrolizidine alkaloid-containing plants—*Senecio* sp. (Fig. 15.16), *Heliotropium* sp., *Lantana camara*; Mycotoxins—Sporodesmins; Blue green algae—*Microcystis* sp. The prognosis

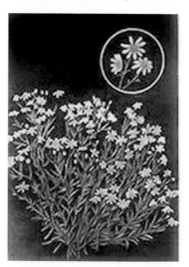

FIGURE 15.16

Senicio sp.

http://poisonousplants.ansci.cornell.edu/images/senecio2.jpg.

is poor in secondary type photosensitization because the hepatic damage is generally irreversible leading to death.

15.3.5 OTHER TOXIC PLANTS

15.3.5.1 *Lantana plant*

Q. How does Lantana plant poisoning occur in animals?

Animals in pastures with sufficient forage will often avoid Lantana plant (Fig. 15.17), perhaps because of its pungent aroma and taste, but animals unfamiliar to the plant may ingest enough to affect them. Fifty to ninety percent of animals newly exposed may be affected. Foliage and ripe berries contain the toxic substances with the toxins being in higher concentrations in the green berries. Species affected include cattle, sheep, horses, dogs, guinea pigs, and rabbits.

Q. What are common toxic principles in Lantana plant?

Lantana plant contains lantadene A and B (the major toxins involved in poisoning) as well as other structurally and toxicologically related pentacyclic triterpene acids, including reduced lantadene A, dihydrolantadene A, and icterogenin.

Q. What are clinical signs of Lantana plant poisoning?

Lantana is also called Red sage, Wild sage, Yellow Sage, and Shrub Verbena. Triterpenoids (liver toxins) are found in all parts of the plant. Symptoms include depression, vomiting, diarrhea, weakness, and

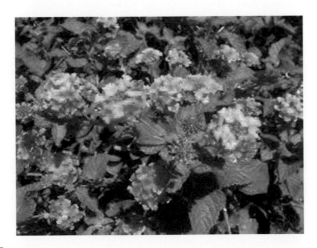

FIGURE 15.17

Lantana camara.

https://encrypted-tbn3.gstatic.com/images?q = tbn:ANd9GcRpqqJ2Ulc1omPTNIRRrLC_PX1HuJ-M-2bTD9zGpmXPuNBiqLpGkg.

possible liver failure (which occur more commonly with farm animals). The plant is also toxic to dogs and cats. Liver failure is more common in livestock.

The major clinical effect of Lantana toxicosis is photosensitization, the onset of which often takes place in 1−2 days after consumption of a toxic dose (1% or more of animal's body weight). Jaundice is usually prominent, animals usually become inappetent, and they often exhibit decreased digestive tract motility and constipation. Other signs may include sluggishness, weakness, and transient, sometimes bloody diarrhea. In acute cases, death occurs in 2−4 days. Subacute poisoning is more common and may result in death after 1−3 weeks of illness and weight loss. Raw photosensitized surface areas are susceptible to invasions by blow fly maggots and bacteria. In severely affected cattle, lesions may appear at the muzzle, mouth, and nostrils. Ulceration may be present in the cheeks, tongue, and gums, whereas swelling, hardening, peeling of mucous membranes, and deeper tissues occur in the nostrils.

Dogs usually do not ingest a fatal dose (Fig. 15.18), but unless the dog is treated immediately, he can deteriorate and die within 1−3 weeks. A fatal dose causes death in 2−4 days.

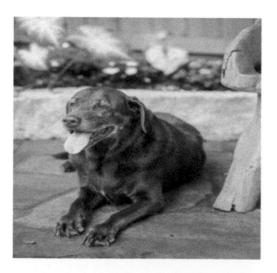

FIGURE 15.18

Poisonous Lantana plant that affect dog.

http://hgtvhome.sndimg.com/content/dam/images/grdn/fullset/2013/3/13/0/Original_lgummere-dog.jpg.rend.
hgtvcom.1280.1707.suffix/1452646785201.jpeg.

15.3.5.2 *Tansy mustard (*Descurainia pinnata*)*

Q. Describe in brief characteristics of tansy mustard plant.

The plant belongs to mustard family (Brassicaceae) and grows up to 2 ft tall, usually single-stemmed, leafy throughout, and covered with fine gray hairs; leaves are alternate and pinnately divided into numerous small segments; flowers are small, yellow, and occur in long clusters at the ends of the stem; fruits are long, round, slender, two-celled capsules filled with numerous small, waxy seeds (Fig. 15.19).

Q. What is the toxic principle of tansy mustard?

The toxin is unknown. Some symptoms suggest that sulfur may play a role.

Q. What are signs of poisoning of tansy mustard in animals?

Despite similarity of the symptoms with those produced in one type of selenium poisoning, tansy mustard does not contain enough selenium to produce the disease. In cattle, the first symptom is a partial or complete blindness. This is followed by an inability to use the tongue or to swallow. The disease is popularly termed "paralyzed tongue" or "wooden tongue." Because of blindness, animals may wander aimlessly until exhausted or stand pushing against a solid object in their path for hours. Because of the inability to swallow, animals may be observed standing at water unable to drink or unsuccessfully grazing forage. Animals become thinner and weaker and will die if not treated.

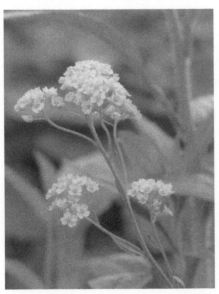

FIGURE 15.19

Tansy mustard *(Descurainia pinnata)*.

Reproduced from Pxhere https://pxhere.com/en/photo/1351550.

15.3.5.3 Cotton seed toxicity

Q. What is cotton seed toxicity?

Excess pigment found in cottonseed products cause cumulative toxicity. Immature ruminants and pigs are most susceptible. Prolonged exposure causes weight loss, weakness, and loss of appetite. Gossypol is a phenolic compound present in cotton seed (*Gossypium* spp.). Cotton seed meal is a byproduct of cotton that is used for animal feeding because it is rich in oil and proteins. However, gossypol toxicity limits the use of cotton seed in animal feed. It is of most concern in domestic livestock, especially preruminants or immature ruminants and pigs; mature ruminants are more resistant to gossypol's toxic effects. However, gossypol toxicosis can affect high-producing dairy cows with high feed intake, dairy goats, and other mature ruminants fed excess gossypol for long periods.

15.3.5.4 Castor bean toxicity

Q. What is castor bean toxicity?

Castor seed is the source of castor oil. Castor oil and its derivatives are used in the manufacturing of soaps, lubricants, hydraulic and brake fluids, paints, dyes, coatings, inks, cold-resistant plastics, waxes and polishes, nylon, pharmaceuticals, and perfumes The seeds contain between 40% and 60% oil that is rich in triglycerides. Approximately 90% of fatty acid chains are ricinoleates. Oleate and linoleates are the other significant components. The seed also contains ricin, a water-soluble toxin, which is also present in lower concentrations.

15.3.5.5 Ragwort poisoning

Q. What is Ragwort plant?

It is a yellow-flowered ragged-leaved European plant of the daisy family, which is a common weed of grazing land and is toxic to livestock (Fig. 15.20).

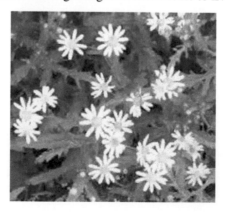

FIGURE 15.20

Senecio squalidus L. (Ragwort plant).

Q. Describe in brief toxicity of Ragwort.

Ingestion of Ragwort (*Senecio jacobaea*) for a long period leads to weight loss and diarrhea. Affected cattle are often dull and depressed and may show persistent straining leading to prolapse of the rectum.

15.3.5.6 Tetrapterys plant poisoning

Q. How does plant tetrapterys cause poisoning?

The ingestion of plants of the genus *Tetrapterys*, family *Malpighiaceae*, causes primarily degenerative and fibrotic changes in the myocardium and related signs of cardiac failure. The natural disease occurs only in cattle over 1 year of age in southeastern Brazil and only in pastures where *Tetrapterys* spp. occur and after the cattle have stayed for 1−2 months on the pasture.

Q. What is the toxic principle of tetrapterys?

The main principle toxin in tetrapterys plant is *T. multiglandulosa* that leads to pendulous and multinodular enlargement of the brisket area in cattle.

15.4 NITRATE AND NITRITE POISONING

Q. What are the sources of nitrate intoxication in animals?

1. Nitrate-accumulating weeds include pigweed (*Amaranthus* spp.), dock (*Rumex* spp.), nightshades (*Solanum* spp.; Fig. 15.21) and lambsquarter (*Chenopodium* spp.; Fig. 15.22). Potentially troublesome crop plants include corn, sorghum, oats, barley, beet tops, and wheat.

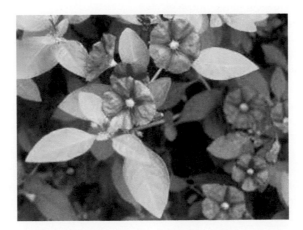

FIGURE 15.21

Solanum species—Nightshades.

https://upload.wikimedia.org/wikipedia/commons/3/3a/Lycianthes_rantonnei.jpg.

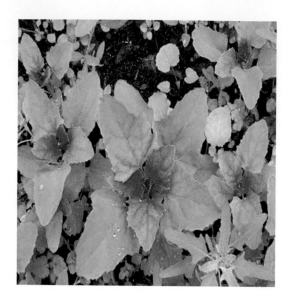

FIGURE 15.22

Chenopodium species.

http://upload.wikimedia.org/wikipedia/commons/b/b2/Chenopodium_album_a1.jpg.

2. Nitrate is also found in fertilizers and is a common contaminant of water. Thus, exposure to these sources can cause intoxication if exposure is of sufficient magnitude.

Q. How do plants accumulate nitrate?

Under certain adverse environmental conditions (drought), many weed and crop plants accumulate nitrate to potentially toxic concentrations.

Q. What is difference between sodium nitrate and nitrite?

Sodium nitrate and sodium nitrite, two common preservatives used in foods, are often used interchangeably. Sodium nitrite has two oxygen atoms and one nitrogen atom (NO_2^-). Sodium nitrate has one more oxygen atom (NO_3^-).

Q. What is nitrate poisoning?

Nitrate poisoning is a condition that may affect ruminants consuming certain forages or water that contain an excessive amount of nitrate. This disease is often called brown blood disease as it turns the gills of fish from a bright red to a dark brown-like color, and is caused by having a too high level of nitrite intake.

Q. What are the circumstances that cause nitrate and nitrate toxicosis?

1. Most commonly from ingestion of plants that contain excess nitrate, especially by hungry animals engorging themselves and taking in an enormous body burden of nitrate.

2. Confounding interactions with nonprotein nitrogen, monensin, and other feed components may exacerbate effects of excessive nitrate content in livestock diets, especially when coupled with management errors.
3. Accidental ingestion of fertilizer or other chemicals.
4. Ponds that receive extensive feedlot or fertilizer runoff.
5. Crops that readily concentrate nitrate include cereal grasses (especially oats, millet, and rye), corn (maize), sunflower, and sorghums. Weeds that commonly have high nitrate concentrations are pigweed, lamb's quarter, thistle, Jimson weed, fireweed (*Kochia*), smartweed, dock, and Johnson grass.
6. Anhydrous ammonia and nitrate fertilizers and soils naturally high in nitrogen tend to increase nitrate content in forage.

Q. Which animal species are susceptible to nitrate poisoning?

Many species are susceptible to nitrate and nitrite poisoning, but cattle are affected most frequently. Ruminants are especially vulnerable because the ruminal flora reduces nitrate to ammonia, with nitrite (~10 times more toxic than nitrate) as an intermediate product. Nitrate reduction (and nitrite production) occurs in the cecum of equids but not to the same extent as in ruminants. Young pigs also have gastrointestinal (GI) microflora capable of reducing nitrate to nitrite, but mature monogastric animals (except equids) are more resistant to nitrate toxicosis because this pathway is age-limited.

Q. What are the signs of toxicity of nitrate poisoning?

Toxic signs of nitrite poisoning usually appear suddenly because of tissue hypoxia and low blood pressure as a consequence of vasodilation. Vasodilation and hypotension observed in nitrate poisoning are due to smooth muscle relaxation. Rapid, weak heartbeat with subnormal body temperature, muscular tremors, weakness, and ataxia are early signs of toxicosis when methemoglobinemia reaches 30%–40%. Brown, cyanotic mucous membranes develop rapidly as methemoglobinemia exceeds 50%. Dyspnea, tachypnea, anxiety, and frequent urination are common. Some monogastric animals, usually because of excess nitrate exposure from nonplant sources, exhibit salivation, vomiting, diarrhea, abdominal pain, and gastric hemorrhage. Affected animals may die suddenly without appearing ill, in terminal anoxic convulsions within 1 hour or after a clinical course of 12–24 hour or longer. Acute lethal toxicoses almost always are due to development of ≥ 80% methemoglobinemia.

Q. Describe the mechanism of action of nitrate and nitrite poisoning.

In biological system two major pathways contribute to systemic NO formation (Fig. 15.23). The most well-known pathway is the production of NO from L-arginine in the presence of oxygen by isoforms of the enzyme NO synthase (L-arginine-NO pathway).

Q. What is the treatment for methemoglobinemia?

Methylene blue is used to treat severe methemoglobinemia. The pathway of methemoglobinemia treatment is shown in Fig. 15.24. Methylene blue may

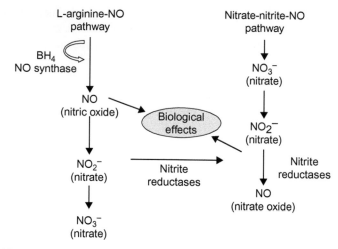

FIGURE 15.23

Two primary pathways for nitric oxide (NO) production, the L-arginine–NO and nitrate–nitrite–NO pathways.

http://jap.physiology.org/content/jap/116/5/463/F1.large.jpg.

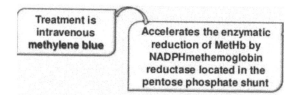

FIGURE 15.24

Treatment of poisoning of methemoglobinemia.

be dangerous in patients who have or may be at risk for a blood disease called G6PD deficiency and should not be used.

15.5 AMMONIA POISONING

Q. How does ammonia poisoning occur in animals?

It is caused by abrupt addition of feed-grade urea or ammonium salts to the ruminant diet.

Mature ruminants are most susceptible, as they convert nonprotein nitrogen to ammonia, which is toxic. Toxic symptoms include muscle tremors, weakness, difficulty breathing, and death.

15.6 OXALATE POISONING (SEE CHAPTER 7: NONMETALS AND MICRONUTRIENTS)

Q. What are oxalates?

Oxalates belong to a group of substances known as antinutrients. Antinutrients are, as their name would suggest, compounds that prevent the nutritive value of foods from being effective, by preventing the absorption of nutrients, by being toxic themselves, or by one or more methods of action.

Q. What is oxalate poisoning?

High levels of toxins, commonly known as oxalic acid, cause oxalate poisoning. Oxalic acid is produced naturally in the body when ascorbic acid and glycine are metabolized. These low levels formed are excreted in the urine in measurable amounts.

Q. Which plants are known as oxalate accumulators?

Many of the species are known as wood sorrels as they have an acidic taste reminiscent of the unrelated sorrel proper (*R. acetosa*). Some species are called yellow sorrels or pink sorrels after the color of their flowers instead (Figs. 15.25 and 15.26). Other species are colloquially known as false shamrocks, and some are called sour grasses. For the genus as a whole, the term "oxalises" is also used. These plant species are also known as oxalate accumulators.

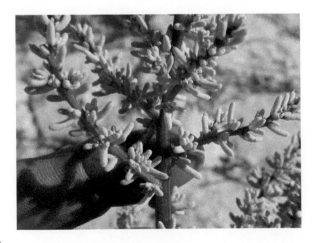

FIGURE 15.25

Oxalate accumulator plant *H. glomeratus*.

Reproduced from https://commons.wikimedia.org/wiki/File:Halogeton_glomeratus_(3939414465).jpg.

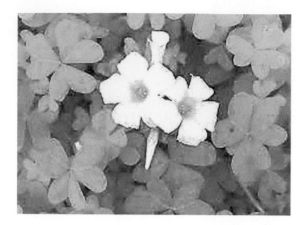

FIGURE 15.26

O. pescaprae (oxalate accumulator)

Q. How oxalates do the damage?

Oxalates present in plants (Fig. 15.27), and some animal foods bind with minerals in the body, such as magnesium, potassium, calcium, and sodium, creating oxalate salts. Most of these salts are soluble and pass quickly out of the body. However, oxalates that bind with calcium are practically insoluble and these crystals solidify in the kidneys (kidney stones) or the urinary tract, causing pain and irritation. These crystals can then easily settle out as sediments from the urine, causing kidney stones.

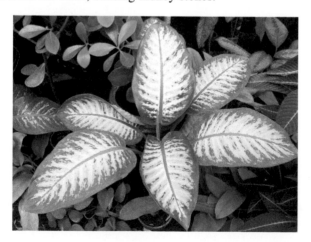

FIGURE 15.27

Dieffenbachia (oxalate accumulator).

15.7 METALS AND NONMETALS
15.7.1 LEAD POISONING

Toxic effects of lead are also discussed in Chapter 6, Metals and Micronutrients.

Q. What is lead poisoning

Lead poisoning is a type of metal poisoning caused by increased levels of the heavy metal lead in the body.

Q. How does lead poisoning take place in animals?

Lead poisoning of cattle on pasture is fairly common when old batteries and other lead-containing trash is left available to them. Like most toxic heavy metals, lead interferes with a variety of body processes and is toxic to many organs and tissues, including the heart, bones, intestines, kidneys, and reproductive and nervous systems. The brain is the organ most sensitive to lead exposure. Lead interferes with the development of the nervous system and is therefore particularly toxic to children, causing potentially permanent learning and behavior disorders including violence. Symptoms include abdominal pain, confusion, headache, anemia, irritability, and in severe cases seizures, coma, and death.

Q. What is the mechanism of lead toxicity?

The mechanism of lead-induced toxicity is not fully understood. The prime targets to lead toxicity are the heme synthesis enzymes and thiol-containing antioxidants and enzymes (superoxide dismutase, catalase, glutathione peroxidase, glucose 6-phosphate dehydrogenase, and antioxidant molecules like GSH). The low blood lead levels are sufficient to inhibit the activity of these enzymes and induce generation of reactive oxygen species and intensification of oxidative stress. Oxidative stress plays an important role in pathogenesis of lead-induced toxicity and pathogenesis of coupled disease. The primary target of lead toxicity is the central nervous system. There are different cellular, intracellular, and molecular mechanisms of lead neurotoxicity such as induction of oxidative stress, intensification of apoptosis of neurocytes, and interfering with Ca $(2+)$-dependent enzyme like nitric oxide synthase.

15.7.2 COPPER (CU) POISONING

Toxic effects of copper are also discussed in Chapter 6, Metals and Micronutrients.

Q. What is the source of copper poisoning in animals?

Acute Cu toxicity results from ingestion of high Cu feeds, Cu salts, pesticides, poultry litter, and other high Cu intakes of 20−100 mg/kg in sheep and young calves, and 200−800 mg/kg in adult cattle. Chronic Cu toxicity occurs when high levels of Cu are ingested over a period of time, but at doses below the acutely toxic level.

Q. Which animals are susceptible to copper poisoning and why?

Usually poisoning occurs due to improperly formulated mineral mixes or certain plants causing mineral imbalances. Signs in affected animals include depression, lethargy, weakness, recumbence, rumen stasis, anorexia, thirst, dyspnea, pale mucous membranes, hemoglobinuria, and jaundice. Several days or weeks before the hemolytic crisis, liver enzymes, including alanine transferase (ALT) and aspartate transaminase (AST), are usually increased. Sheep are the most susceptible species and result from accidental feeding of feedstuffs intended for other livestock. Sheep's liver cells have a high affinity for Cu, and they excrete Cu into the bile at a very low rate, leading to a buildup of liver Cu concentration over time.

Q. Which breed is more susceptible to copper toxicosis?

Some animals show genetic variations. For example, Bedlington Terrier (a breed of dog) is highly susceptible to copper toxicosis due to genetic predisposition (Fig. 15.28). This breed has autosomal recessive gene that cause retention of copper due to failure of excretion.

Q. What are signs and symptoms of copper deficiency?

Signs are related to liver damage and include diarrhea, pain, dehydration, jaundice, and blood in the urine. Copper deficiency is likely to occur in winter on free-draining or peaty soils, especially when there has been lots of rain. Young stock suffers poor growth (Fig. 15.29) and loss of coordination of the hind limbs, and adult cattle gets diarrhea (scours).

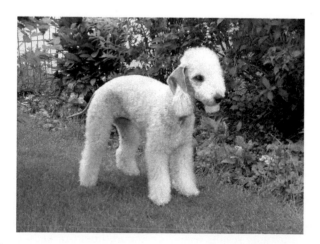

FIGURE 15.28

Bedlington Terrier—genetic predisposition for copper accumulation.

Reproduced from https://commons.wikimedia.org/wiki/File:Boutchie_apres_championnat_004.JPG.

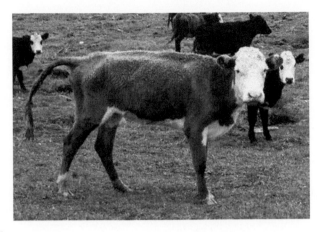

FIGURE 15.29

Copper deficiency in cattle.

http://www.teara.govt.nz/files/p17537pc.jpg.

15.7.3 SELENIUM POISONING

Toxic effects of selenium are also discussed in Chapter 7, Non-Metals and micronutrients.

Q. What are the sources of selenium poisoning in animals?

Following are the sources of selenium poisoning in animals.

1. Plants
   a. Obligate accumulator or indicator plants
   b. Facultative accumulator plants
   c. Nonaccumulator plants
2. Feed supplements
3. Injectable selenium supplements
4. Industrial and commercial practices
5. Selenium containing shampoos
6. Sea foods

Q. Which selenium plants are called obligate (primary) accumulators or indicator plants?

The types of plants that physiologically require selenium and accumulate high levels of selenium are called obligate (primary) accumulators or indicator plants. For example, *Astragalus* spp. (Fig. 15.30), *Stanleya* spp. (Fig. 15.31), and *Oonopsis* spp. Animals avoid these plants as they are not palatable, but in scarcity they are consumed leading to toxicity. The level of selenium found in obligate accumulators is 100−1500 ppm.

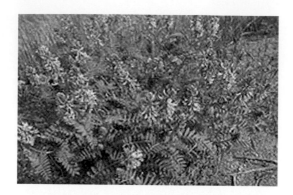

FIGURE 15.30

Astragalus sp. (Milk vetches) obligate (primary) accumulator.

https://upload.wikimedia.org/wikipedia/commons/thumb/9/92/Astragalus_bisculatus.jpg/330px-
Astragalus_bisculatus.jpg.

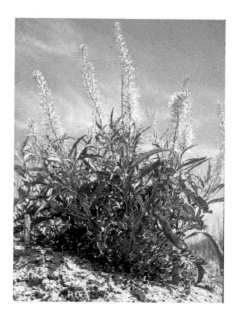

FIGURE 15.31

Stanleya sp. (Princes plumes) obligate (primary) accumulator.

https://csuvth.colostate.edu/poisonous_plants/images/web159-1.jpg

Q. Which selenium plants are called facultative accumulators? Give examples

The types of plants that do not require selenium but accumulate high levels of selenium if present in soil are called facultative accumulators. For example, *Acacia* spp., *Atriplex* spp., *Artemisia* spp. (Fig. 15.32), and *Aster* spp. (Fig. 15.33). As these plants are more palatable, toxicity is often seen in

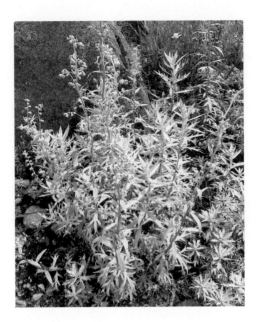

FIGURE 15.32

Artimesia sp. selenium facultative accumulator plant.

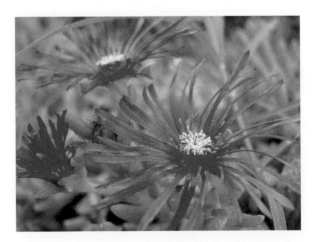

FIGURE 15.33

Aster sp. (Asters) selenium facultative accumulator plant.

animals. The level of selenium found in facultative accumulators is 25−100 ppm.

Q. What is selenium toxicity?

Selenium is a nonmetal that functions as both toxicant and an essential element. Selenium poisoning occurs when animals ingest excessive amounts of selenium. In its most severe form, it causes blindness and staggering. In can also cause cracked hooves and lameness.

Subacute toxicity is called blind staggers and caused by the accumulation of 2−5 ppm of selenium in dry matter content.

Q. What is "alkali disease" in animals?

Chronic toxicity caused by selenium is called alkali disease or bobtail disease. The minimum lethal dose of selenium for the horse is 3.3 mg/kg of body weight. This disease is common in cattle and horses and exhibit weight loss, hair loss (especially obvious in the mane and tail), and lameness in all four limbs. The coronary bands are painful to palpation, and the band may separate with excretion of necrotic tissue from the defect (Fig. 15.34). In severe cases the hoof wall may slough off.

Q. What is "blind staggers" disease in animals?

In "blind staggers" (common in cattle and sheep), animals develop a staggering gait, wander aimlessly, and "head press." The disease occurs when animals graze on plants that accumulate a toxic amount of the selenium. Some plants require selenium, and these selenium-accumulating plants are considered "indicator species." These indicator species include locoweeds and

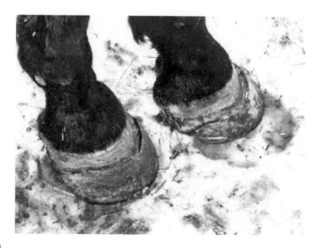

FIGURE 15.34

Chronic selenium toxicosis leads to separation of the hoof wall.

http://www.rockymountainrider.com/articles/2013/images/1013%20Selenium%20photo%205.jpg.

milk vetches, woody aster, prince's plume, and golden weed. They can all be highly toxic due to their selenium content.

15.7.4 FLUORIDE POISONING

Toxic effects of fluoride are also discussed in Chapter 7, Non-Metals and micronutrients.

Q. What is fluorosis?

   Fluorosis is a chronic condition caused by excessive intake of fluorine compounds, marked by mottling and staining of the teeth, and, if severe, calcification of the ligaments and abnormalities of the skeleton are observed.

Q. How are animals exposed to excess fluoride?

   Animals are exposed to excess fluorides through the ingestion of high-fluoride rock phosphates used as nutritional supplements by the ingestion of forages contaminated with excess fluorides from industrial pollutants or volcanic emissions or through water containing excess fluorides from industrial pollution or dissolved from natural sources.

Q. How does fluorosis ingestion affect animals?

   Fluoride ingestion is detrimental to the animals. Acute fluoride poisoning of cattle can result in clinical signs of depression, weakness, and ataxia with postmortem findings of gastroenteritis and degenerative changes in the renal tubular epithelium. Effects vary from animal to animal. Normally fluoride is required for enamel formation but excess fluoride before complete formation of enamel can damage tooth due to oxidation. Brown or black discoloration of teeth seen in fluorosis is due to oxidation of enamel (Fig. 15.35).

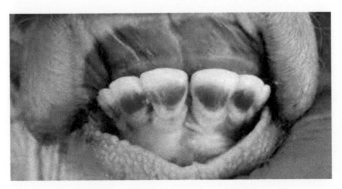

FIGURE 15.35

Severe form of dental fluorosis (deep yellowish coloration) in a calf.

https://encrypted-tbn3.gstatic.com/images?q = tbn:
ANd9GcRotDD6D2TwWd4V09fLD5CO84_EP5a4t6qsZUQW1XfDL4niLc3C.

Clinical signs develop slowly and can be confused with other chronic problems. Some animals often show nonspecific intermittent stiffness and lameness which appear to be associated with periosteal overgrowth leading to spurring and bridging near joints as well as ossification of ligaments, tendon sheaths, and tendons (Fig. 15.36). The clinical presentation may easily be confused with other conditions, such as degenerative arthritis, but the lesions associated with fluorosis are not primarily associated with articular surfaces.

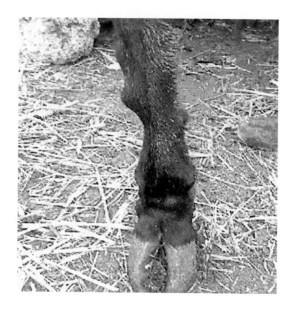

FIGURE 15.36

Fluorosis in animals—skeletal form.

https://upload.wikimedia.org/wikipedia/commons/thumb/c/cf/Fluwor%C3%B4ze_egzostozes1-800h.jpg/
220px-Fluwor%C3%B4ze_egzostozes1-800h.jpg.

15.7.5 SULFUR POISONING

Toxic effects of sulfur are also discussed in Chapter 7, Nonmetals and micronutrients, non-metalics.

Q. Describe sulfur poisoning in animals.

In animals acute oral poisoning with elemental sulfur results in formation of hydrogen sulfide, as well as many other potential metabolites. The gastric and respiratory effects are postulated to be due to the coagulative effects of rumen-produced sulfurous acids and the irritating effects of hydrogen sulfide, respectively. Sulfate-induced selenium deficiency can cause poor growth, weakness, poor immune function, poor reproductive function, damage to the cardiac or skeletal muscles, and death.

15.7.6 MOLYBDENUM POISONING

Toxic effects of molybdenum are also discussed in Chapter 6, Metals and Micronutrients.

Q. What is molybdenum poisoning?

It is caused by imbalance in copper/molybdenum ratios in soil. Ruminants, especially young cattle, are most susceptible.

Q. What are the signs and symptoms of molybdenum toxicity in animals?

In animals due to Cu deficiency, melanin production is reduced due to decrease in the activity of Cu containing enzyme tyrosinase. This enzyme converts tyrosine into melanin. In buffaloes, spectacle eye (Fig. 15.37) is prominently visible due to light colored hair and depigmentation around eyes in molybdenum poisoning.

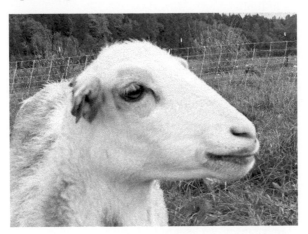

FIGURE 15.37

Spectacle-eye appearance—Molybdenum poisoning.

http://www.toxinfo.co.in/files/spectacled%20appearance.jpg.

15.7.7 COBALT DEFICIENCY (VITAMIN B12 DEFICIENCY)

Toxic effects of cobalt are also discussed in Chapter 6, Metals and Micronutrients.

Q. Why animals need cobalt?

All ruminants (including sheep, cattle, and goats) require cobalt in their diet for the synthesis of vitamin B12. Vitamin B12 is essential for energy metabolism and the production of red blood cells. Normally microorganisms in the rumen are able to synthesize vitamin B12 needs of ruminants if the diet is adequate in cobalt. Cobalt deficiency in soils can cause vitamin B12 deficiency in livestock.

Q. What are the symptoms of cobalt deficiency?

Cobalt deficiency causes lack of appetite, lack of thrift, severe emaciation, weakness, anemia, decreased fertility, and decreased milk and wool production, weeping eyes, leading to a matting of wool on the face. Sheep are more susceptible to cobalt deficiency than cattle. Cobalt deficiency also impairs the immune function of sheep, which may increase their vulnerability to infection with worms.

15.7.8 MANGANESE DEFICIENCY

Q. What are common manganese deficiency symptoms in animals?

The prominent symptoms in animals include:
1. stiffening of limbs,
2. defective ovulation,
3. reduced fertility, and
4. high infant mortality.

Q. What is the role of manganese in the body?

Manganese is an activator of enzyme reactions concerned with carbohydrate, protein, and lipid metabolism.

15.7.9 SALT POISONING/DEFICIENCY

Q. How does salt poisoning occur in animals?

Salt poisoning occurs when animal ingests high concentrations of salt or is deprived of water, especially in hot weather or in cold weather when water freezes. Soil imbalances can lead to toxicity.

Q. What are signs and symptoms of salt poisoning?

Salt poisoning in dogs and cats results in clinical signs of vomiting, diarrhea, inappetence, lethargy, walking drunk, abnormal fluid accumulation within the body, excessive thirst or urination, potential injury to the kidneys, tremors, seizures, coma, and even death when untreated. Poultry, feeder pigs, and ruminants are more susceptible. Blindness, deafness, or paralysis may result.

Q. What is salt deficiency?

Salt deficiency can lead to pica in animals (Fig. 15.38). Pica can be a serious problem because items such as rubber bands, socks, rocks, and string can severely damage or block your dog's intestines.

Q. What type of pathognomonic histological appearance is seen in brain after salt poisoning in pigs?

Perivascular cuffing of eosinophils is observed in cerebral cortex and meninges, which is known as eosinophilic meningoencephalitis (Fig. 15.39).

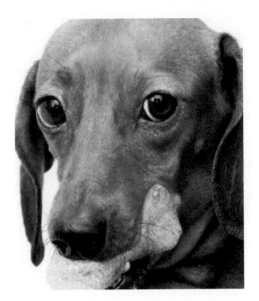

FIGURE 15.38

Pica can be a serious problem because items such as rubber bands, socks, rocks, and string can severely damage or block your dog's intestines.

https://animalwellnessmagazine.com/wp-content/uploads/345.jpg.

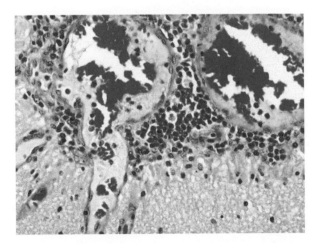

FIGURE 15.39

Perivascular cuffing of eosinophils (Eosinophilic Meningoencephalitis) in cerebral cortex and meninges after salt poisoning.

https://www.askjpc.org/wsco/wsc/images/2008/082201-1.jpg.

15.8 PESTICIDE POISONING

Toxic effects of pesticide poisoning are also discussed in Chapter 5, Pesticides (Agrochemicals).

Q. Which pesticides are commonly used for malicious poisoning in animals?
1. Organophosphorus insecticides
2. Carbamates
3. Rodenticides
4. Fumigants such as aluminum phosphide and zinc phosphide
5. Pyrethroid insecticides

Q. How animals are exposed to pesticides?

The most common exposure scenarios for pesticide-poisoning cases are:
1. accidental,
2. suicidal poisonings,
3. occupational exposure,
4. by exposure to off-target drift, and
5. through environmental contamination, e.g., aerial spray. (Fig. 15.40).

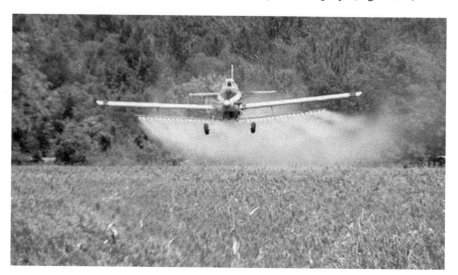

FIGURE 15.40

Spray of herbicides for the control of weeds.

http://sustainablepulse.com/wp-content/uploads/2014/01/crop-duster-560x322.jpg.

15.9 POISONOUS FUNGI

Toxic effects of fungi are also discussed in Chapter 10 Poisonous Food and Food Poisonings.

15.9.1 DEFINITIONS

Q. Define mycotoxins.

Mycotoxins are toxic byproducts (secondary metabolites) produced by fungi. There are 400 mycotoxins produced by 350 species of fungi.

Q. Which animals are susceptible to mycotoxins?

It is a worldwide problem caused by ingestion of moldy feed, corn, or certain varieties of mold-infected pasture grass and forage (e.g., fescue grass, rye, and sweet clover). All species of livestock, horses, and poultry are susceptible. Ingestion of these toxins can lead lameness, paralysis, listlessness, jaundice, and internal bleeding.

Q. Which mycotoxins are considered more serious threat to animals?

Mycotoxins such as aflatoxins, ochratoxin A, fumonisins, certain trichothecenes, zearalenone, and fusarium are considered the most serious threat to human health, animals, and birds due to their potential of carcinogenic, hepatogenic, teratogenic, mutagenic, and other serious effects leading to economic losses.

15.9.2 AFLATOXICOSES

Q. Which species of *Aspergillus* are important that produce aflatoxins?

Aflatoxins are produced primarily by some strains of *A. Flavus* and by most, if not all, strains of *A. parasiticus*, plus related species, *A. nomius* and *A. niger* (Figs. 10.8−10.10).

Q. What are aflatoxins?

Aflatoxins are toxic metabolites produced by certain fungi in/on foods and feeds. They are probably the best known and most intensively researched mycotoxins in the world.

Q. What are major aflatoxins responsible for toxicity in animals?

There are four major aflatoxins: B1, B2, G1, G2 plus two additional metabolic products, M1 and M2, which are of significance as direct contaminants of foods and feeds.

Q. What are signs and symptoms of aflatoxin poisoning in animals?

Aflatoxicosis is primarily a hepatic disease. Aflatoxins cause liver damage, decreased milk and egg production, recurrent infection as a result of immunity suppression (e.g., salmonellosis). These toxins result in embryo toxicity in animals that consume low dietary concentrations. The young ones are most susceptible; all ages are affected but in different degrees for different species. Other signs of aflatoxicosis in animals include gastrointestinal dysfunction, reduced reproductivity, reduced feed utilization and efficiency, anemia, and jaundice. Nursing animals may be affected as a result of the conversion of aflatoxin B1 to the metabolite aflatoxin M1 excreted in milk of dairy cattle.

Aflatoxin B1, aflatoxin M1, and aflatoxin G1 have been shown to cause various types of cancer in different animal species. However, only aflatoxin B1 has been identified as a carcinogen.

15.9.3 FACIAL ECZEMA

Q. What is facial eczema?

Facial eczema is a type of sunburn (photosensitization) affecting exposed areas of pale skin of sheep (Fig. 15.41) and cattle due to liver damage. It is caused by a poisonous substance called "sporidesmin," which is produced on pasture plants by the fungus *Pithomyces chartarum*, which lives in dead vegetative material in pastures, especially perennial ryegrass. Facial eczema is an example of "secondary photosensitization," in which the skin lesions are really the secondary result of liver damage, rather than the direct result of a plant toxin.

Q. What are the clinical symptoms of facial eczema in animals?

The clinical symptoms of facial eczema are distressing: restlessness, frequent urination, shaking, persistent rubbing of the head against objects (e.g., fences, and trees), drooping and reddened ears, swollen eyes, and avoidance of sunlight by seeking shade. Exposed areas of skin develop weeping dermatitis and scabs that can become infected and attractive to blow fly causing myiasis.

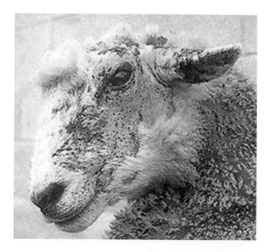

FIGURE 15.41

A sheep showing clinical symptoms of facial eczema.

https://upload.wikimedia.org/wikipedia/commons/8/8b/A_sheep_with_facial_eczema.jpg.

15.9.4 FESCUE TOXICOSIS

Q. What is fescue toxicosis?

Most tall fescue (*Festuca arundinacea*) is infected with a fungal endophyte. The endophyte produces toxins that cause a number of problems for grazing animals, although sheep appear to be less affected than cattle and horses (Fig. 15.42). However, sheep are prone to "fescue foot," hyperthermia, poor wool production, and reproductive problems, as well as lowered feed intake and the resulting poor weight gains. Stockpiled fescue is less toxic.

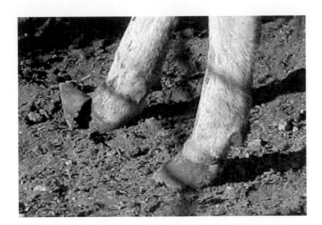

FIGURE 15.42

Fescue toxicosis in horse.

https://encrypted-tbn1.gstatic.com/images?q = tbn:ANd9GcQyK0-
Q6f41E2NhvO7JmwWR4Ru_daPxnapvOjdTIG4ey7KMNOD6.

15.9.5 ZEARALENONE

Q. Which toxin(s) is produced by Zearalenone?

Zearalenone (ZEN), also known as RAL and F-2 mycotoxin, is a potent estrogenic metabolite produced by some *Fusarium* and *Gibberella* species, *F. verticillioides*, and *F. incarnatum*. These species produce toxic substances of considerable concern to livestock and poultry producers, namely deoxynivalenol, T-2 toxin, HT-2 toxin, diacetoxyscirpenol, and zearalenone.

Q. Why pigs and cattle differ in their susceptibility to zearalenone?

Zearalenone toxins are produced by *Fusarium* spp. (Fig. 15.43). In pigs, the major metabolite of Zearalenone is α-zearalenol, which has greater affinity for estrogen receptors than β-zearalenol, which is formed in cattle. Hence, pigs are more susceptible than cattle.

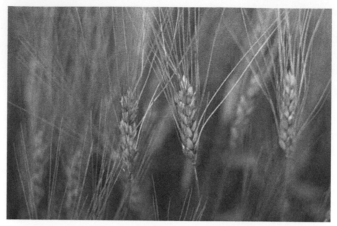

FIGURE 15.43

Fusarium roseum—source of zearalenone toxins.

http://www7.inra.fr/hyp3/images/6032317.jpg.

Q. What is the toxic potential of Zearalenone?

Zearalenone produces an estrogenic effect in that it will stop ovulation in ewes and can cause reduced lambing percentages from 5% to 50% and is considered as the main cause of a long drawn out tupping season.

15.9.6 TRICHOTHECENES

Q. Which fungi species are responsible for trichothecene toxins?

Trichothecenes are a very large family of chemically related mycotoxins produced by various species of *Fusarium*, *Myrothecium*, *Trichoderma*, *Trichothecium*, *Cephalosporium*, *Verticimonosporium*, and *Stachybotrys*. After direct dermal application or oral ingestion, the trichothecene mycotoxins can cause rapid irritation to the skin or intestinal mucosa. These mycotoxins are known to cause a rapid inhibition of protein synthesis and polyribosomal disaggregation. The most important trichothecene mycotoxin in the United States is deoxynivalenol (DON), a common contaminant of wheat, barley, and maize. DON is sometimes called vomitoxin because of its deleterious effects on the digestive system of monogastric animals. Thus, these toxins cause inflammation of the gut lining and produce scouring, poor growth and are the main cause of ill thrift in lambs.

Q. What is alimentary toxic aleukia (ATA)?

Trichothecene mycotoxin known as T-2 toxin may contaminate small grains. T-2 toxin causes a fatal disease of humans known as ATA, a disease that was particularly problematic in Russia in the 1940s. Symptoms of ATA in humans include skin pain, vomiting, diarrhea, complete degeneration of bone marrow, and eventually death. Broiler chickens fed low doses of T-2 toxin may demonstrate symptoms of weight loss, feather malformation, and yellowing of the beak and legs.

15.9.7 RYEGRASS STAGGERS

Q. What is ryegrass staggers disease?

Endophytes (fungi that live inside the plant) that produce the mycotoxin Lolitrem B is responsible for ryegrass staggers. This disease can be a serious problem in livestock grazing perennial ryegrass pasture during the summer and autumn months. It is most commonly seen in sheep and cattle, but horses, deer, and alpaca are also susceptible. While ryegrass staggers have not been recorded in goats, they may also be susceptible but may not develop symptoms due to their different grazing/browsing habits. Affected animals develop muscle tremors and incoordination, which worsens with stress and external stimuli (Fig. 15.44). They may have a stiff gait, which can progress eventually to paralysis. This is not the same disease as grass tetany (which is sometimes referred to as grass staggers). Ryegrass staggers is caused by a group of toxins that accumulates in the leaf sheaths of perennial ryegrass, whereas grass tetany is caused by low blood magnesium.

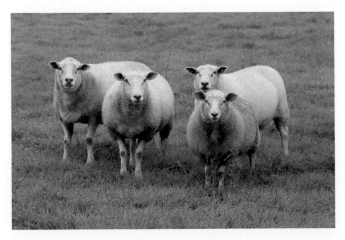

FIGURE 15.44

Mycotoxins produced by the endophytes living within ryegrass cells could affect livestock, causing them to tremble and lose coordination.

Reproduced from https://pixabay.com/en/sheep-flock-of-sheep-flock-pasture-1763376/.

15.9.8 ERGOTISM

Q. What is ergotism?

Poisoning produced by eating food affected by ergot is known ergotism. It causes headache, vomiting, diarrhea, and gangrene of the fingers and toes traditionally due to the ingestion of the alkaloids produced by the *Claviceps purpurea* fungus (Fig. 10.4) that infects rye and other cereals, and more recently by the action of a number of ergoline-based drugs. It is also known as ergotoxicosis, ergot poisoning, and Saint Anthony's Fire. Ergot poisoning is a proposed explanation of bewitchment.

Q. Which animal species are affected by ergot?

Historically rye was commonly affected by the ergot fungus; however, wheat, barley, oats, brome, fescue, blue, Timothy, and other grasses can also be infected. All animals are susceptible to ergot but cattle are often most affected. The fungus produces toxic compounds called ergot alkaloids.

Q. What are signs and symptoms of ergot poisoning?

The fungus produces toxic compounds called ergot alkaloids that are vasoactive causing severe vasoconstriction of small arteries.

- The extremities of cattle are most often affected, causing loss of the tips of ears and tail.
- Depending on the level of ingestion, feet and legs can be affected as well, causing signs of lameness with potential swelling observed in the fetlocks and hock joints, and, in severe cases, loss of hooves.
- Changes in blood flow can also affect thermoregulation and result in heat intolerance.
- Cattle will commonly develop a rough hair coat, lose weight, and have extended periods of time standing in water or shade if available (Fig. 15.45).

15.9.9 DEGNALA DISEASE

Q. How Degnala disease is produced?

Degnala disease (which is believed to be a mycotoxicosis) has clinical syndrome similar to chronic ergotism and is characterized by the development of edema, necrosis, and gangrene of the legs, tail, ears, etc. (Fig. 15.46).

As a result, in the dependent parts of ear, tail, foot blood supply is obstructed and ultimately tissues die of anoxia.

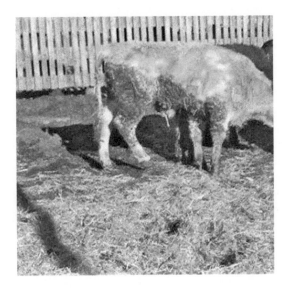

FIGURE 15.45

Severe cases of ergot poisoning may no longer be able to walk and must be euthanized on site.

http://static.agcanada.com/wp-content/uploads/sites/5/2014/07/ergot-poisoning_Univer_RGB-300x300.jpg.

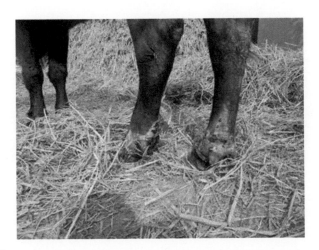

FIGURE 15.46

Degnala disease in Buffaloes.

http://images.engormix.com/e_articles/2185_78,201.jpg.

15.10 ALGAL POISONING

Toxic effects of algal poisoning are also discussed in Chapter 10, Poisonous Food and Food Poisonings.

Q. What is algal poisoning?

Algal poisoning is an acute, often fatal condition caused by high concentration of toxic blue algae (more commonly known as cyanobacteria—literally blue—green bacteria) in drinking water as well as basin water used in agriculture, recreation, and agriculture (Fig. 15.46).

Q. How do animals get poisoned by algae?

Severe illness and fatalities of livestock, pets, wildlife, birds, and fish (Fig. 10.12) occur in almost all countries of the world. Most poisonings occur due to consumption of water contaminated with cyanobacteria that contains harmful toxins (Fig. 15.47).

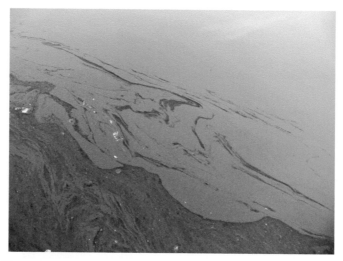

FIGURE 15.47

Toxic blue—green algae.

Reproduced from https://commons.wikimedia.org/wiki/File:CyanobacteriaLamiot2009_07_26_290.jpg.

15.11 POISONOUS AND VENOMOUS ORGANISMS

Toxic effects of poisonous and venomous organisms are also discussed in Chapter 9, Poisonous and Venomous Organisms.

Q. What are animal toxins?

A toxin is a poisonous substance produced within living cells or organisms; synthetic toxicants created by artificial processes are thus excluded.

Q. What is the nature of animal toxins?

Toxins can be small molecules, peptides, or proteins that are capable of causing disease on contact with or absorption by body tissues interacting with biological macromolecules such as enzymes or cellular receptors. Toxins vary greatly in their toxicity, ranging from usually minor (such as a bee sting) to almost immediately deadly (such as botulinum toxin).

15.11.1 BLISTER BEETLE POISONING

Q. What is cantharidin toxicosis?

It is caused by blister beetles (Fig. 15.48). It is also known as Blister Beetle Poisoning or Cantharidin toxicosis in Equines. There are more than 200 species of blister beetles, each varying in size, shape, and color, but the most common is genus *Epicauta* that commonly contaminates alfalfa hay causing toxicosis in horses, sheep, or cattle. Signs include salivation due to oral ulcers, abdominal pain, shock, and blood in the urine.

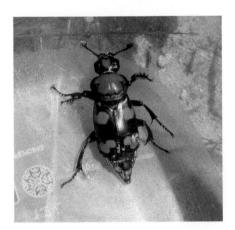

FIGURE 15.48

Blister beetle—*Lytta magister*.

Reproduced from https://commons.wikimedia.org/wiki/File:American_Burying_Beetle_(7489198288).jpg.

15.11.2 TICKS

The adult ticks are found on a variety of domesticated species such camels, cattle, goats, sheep, and even dogs. The ticks also are found on various species of wildlife throughout the distribution range, but the adults are generally found on the larger mammals (Fig. 15.49).

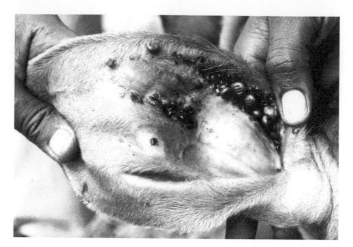

FIGURE 15.49

Tropical bont ticks, *Amblyomma variegatum* Fabricius, feeding on the calf ear. Note the large "nutmeg" size of the females.

Reproduced from https://commons.wikimedia.org/wiki/File:Rhipicephalus-appendiculatus-calf-ear.jpg.

15.12 MICROBIAL TOXINS

Toxic effects of microbial toxins are also discussed in Chapter 10, Poisonous Food and Food Poisonings.

Q. What are microbial toxins?

Microbial toxins are toxins produced by microorganisms, including bacteria and fungi. Microbial toxins promote infection and disease by directly damaging host tissues and by disabling the immune system. Some bacterial toxins, such as Botulinum neurotoxins, are the most potent natural toxins known.

Q. What are Botulinum neurotoxins?

Botulism, also known as botulinus intoxication, is a serious illness that causes paralysis, caused by the *botulinum* toxin. The toxin is caused by *Clostridium botulinum*, a type of bacterium.

Q. What are Tetanus toxins?

Clostridium tetani produces tetanus toxin (TeNT protein), which leads to a fatal condition known as tetanus in many vertebrates (including humans) and invertebrates.

Q. What are Staphylococcal toxins?

Immune evasion proteins from *Staphylococcus aureus* have a significant conservation of protein structures and a range of activities that are all directed at the two key elements of host immunity, complement, and neutrophils.

These secreted virulence factors assist the bacterium in surviving immune response mechanisms.

15.13 RESIDUE TOXICOLOGY

The use of veterinary drugs in food-producing animals has the potential to generate residues in animal-derived products (meat, milk, eggs, and honey) and poses a health hazard to the consumer.

Q. What do you mean by tissue residue?

Tissue residue is the concentration of a chemical or compound in an organism's tissue or a portion of an organism's tissue. Tissue residue is used in aquatic toxicology to help determine the fate of chemicals in aquatic systems, bioaccumulation of a substance, bioavailability of a substance, account for multiple routes of exposure (ingestion, absorption, and inhalation), and address an organism's exposure to chemical mixtures.

Explanation: A tissue residue approach to toxicity testing is considered a more direct and less variable measure of chemical exposure and is less dependent on external environmental factors than measuring the concentration of a chemical in the exposure media. Tissue residue approaches are used for chemicals that bioaccumulate or for bioaccumulative chemicals.

Q. Which substances or chemicals are known to have persistence in the body? Give suitable examples.

The majority of these substances are organic compounds that are not easily metabolized by organisms and have long environmental persistence. Examples of these chemicals include polychlorinated dibenzodioxins, furans, biphenyls, DDT and its metabolites, and dieldrin.

Q. What do you mean by veterinary drug residues?

Veterinary drug residues are the very small amounts of veterinary medicines that can remain in animal products and therefore make their way into the food chain. These include any degradation products, which are the result of the medicine breaking down into its component parts.

Q. Define maximum residue limits

Maximum Residue Limit or Maximum Residue Level (MRL) is the maximum amount of a pesticide or drug (mainly veterinary pharmaceuticals) residue that is legally permitted or recognized as acceptable in or on food commodities and animal feeds. Although both the terms have the same meaning, in practice, the term maximum residue limit is used for the pesticide residue, whereas the term maximum residue level is applicable for the drug residue.

Q. What does withdrawal symptom mean?

The unpleasant physical reaction that accompanies the process of ceasing to take an addictive drug is known as withdrawal symptom.

Or

Abnormal physical or psychological features that follow the abrupt *discontinuation* of a drug that has the capability of producing physical dependence is called withdrawal symptom. For example, common opiates *withdrawal symptoms* include sweating, goose bumps, vomiting, anxiety, insomnia, and muscle pain.

Q. What is tolerance/maximum residue levels (MRLs)?

MRLs for pesticide residues and residues of veterinary drugs are the maximum concentrations of residues to be legally permitted in or on a food. MRLs for pesticides may also be applicable to animal feeds.

Q. Who sets maximum residue levels (MRLs)?

The scientific advice developed by JMPR and JECFA aims to provide maximum residue levels for individual crops, plant, and animal products, based on the results of scientific studies, so that these levels can be used by the relevant Codex committee to develop the draft MRLs, which may be adopted by the CAC.

Q. What are the factors that influence the occurrence of residues in animal products?

There are many factors influencing the occurrence of residues in animal products such as drug's properties and their pharmacokinetic characteristics, physicochemical or biological processes of animals and their products. The most likely reason for drug residues might be due to improper drug usage and failure to keep the withdrawal period.

Q. What is the public health significance of drug residues?

The major public health significances of drug residue are development of antimicrobial drug resistance, hypersensitivity reaction, carcinogenicity, mutagenicity, teratogenicity, and disruption of intestinal normal flora. The residual amount ingested is in small amounts and not necessarily toxic. However, there is limited information on the magnitude of veterinary drug residue worldwide.

Q. Who sets the withdrawal times and levels for drug residues in animal's products?

Center for Veterinary Medicine (CVM) of Food and Drug Administration (FDA) sets the withdrawal times and limits for approved food animal drugs.

Q. Who sets the withdrawal times and limits for pesticide residues in animal's products?

Environment Protection Agency (EPA) sets the withdrawal times and limits for pesticide residues in plant and animal products.

Q. How withdrawal time can be extrapolated from pharmacokinetic parameters?

Withdrawal time $= 10 \times T_{1/2}$ ($T_{1/2}$ = half-life of the drug).

Q. What is the difference between "Maximum residue level" and "Maximum residue limit"?

"Maximum residue level" is used for drugs, whereas "maximum residue limit" is used for pesticides.

Q. What are the techniques used for the detection of residues in foods?

Techniques such as ELISA, HPLC, LC, GC, and Paper chromatography are being used.

Q. What are the general classes of veterinary drugs that are found in animal products as residues?

The general classes of veterinary drugs found in animal products are antimicrobials, antiinflammatory, growth promoters, antiparasitic and insecticides, and tranquilizers.

Q. Which is the most common type of drug residue in animal products?

Antibiotics are the most frequently found drug residues followed by antiinflammatory drugs.

Q. What are the hazards of drug residues in animal products?

The hazards of drug residues in animal products are as follows:

1. Aesthetic issues: The presence of drugs in animal is not appealing for consumer.
2. Allergic reactions: Certain drug residues like Penicillin can cause allergic reaction in sensitive individuals at a level of 10 IU (0.6 µg).
3. Development of antibiotic resistance in microorganisms.
4. Direct toxic effects—cancer, reproductive, and developmental effects. For example:
   a. Clenbuterol residues were reported to have caused tachycardia, muscle tremor, headache, nausea, and fever and chills in humans.
   b. Furazolidone and its metabolites are banned by FDA as they were reported to cause cancer in humans.
5. Deleterious effects of hormone residues in humans. For example:
   a. Diethyl stilbesterol: Vaginal clear cell adenocarcinoma in female off springs exposed in utero; structural abnormalities of uterus.
   b. International export barriers: Export of animal products need to comply with international standards for drug residues.

15.14 QUESTION AND ANSWER EXERCISES

15.14.1 SHORT QUESTIONS AND ANSWERS

Exercise 1

Q.1 In arsenic poisoning, why milk is considered unfit, whereas meat is passed for human consumption?

Arsenic gets methylated and rapidly excreted through urine, milk, sweat, etc. Hence, milk is considered unfit for consumption. As arsenic tends to accumulate only in visceral organs and not in muscles, flesh of surviving animal is considered fit for human consumption.

Q.2 Give reasons as to why mercury poisoning is not common in animals?

Hg compounds are completely replaced by better alternatives in medicinal, agricultural, and industrial use. Hence, Hg poisoning is not common in animals (predatory animals at the end of food chain are more likely to accumulate Hg, which causes poisoning).

Q.3 Why young animals are more susceptible for mercury poisoning?

Developing nervous system is more susceptible to mercury. Hence, young ones are more susceptible.

Q.4 Why milk from lead-affected animals is dangerous for young ones?

Considerable amount of lead is excreted in milk (about 5% of blood concentration). Because young animals have greater capacity to absorb lead than adults, milk from lead-affected animals is dangerous to young ones.

Q.5 Why lead poisoning is more common in veterinary cases?

Lead is ubiquitous in nature. Most of the animals live at a closer level to soil and hence get more exposure. Furthermore, habits like frequent digging of soil seen in dogs and cats increase exposure. Ultimately, increasing vehicular and industrial pollution is the major reason for lead toxicosis.

Q.6 Animals with depraved appetite (pica) are more commonly affected with lead poisoning. Why?

In pica, animals tends to lick walls, chew on dry peelings of paint, eat wall posters, etc. Because paints are lead-based, the animals are affected with lead poisoning. Even children chewing on toys painted with cheap lead paints are also reported to be affected with lead toxicosis.

Q.7 Why acute lead toxicosis is not common?

More than 90% of ingested lead is eliminated from gastrointestinal tract without absorption. Furthermore, even after absorption, only <1% of lead is in free form. Hence, acute lead toxicosis is not common.

Q.8 Is it true that lead directly enters bone and gets deposited?

NO. Initially, lead is distributed to various soft tissues and later gets redistributed to bone from these soft tissues.

Q.9 Why milk from lead-affected animals is dangerous for young ones?

Considerable amount of lead is excreted in milk (about 5% of blood concentration). Because young animals have greater capacity to absorb lead than adults, milk from lead-affected animals is dangerous to young ones.

Q.10 Why only whole blood is recommended for estimation of lead?

Majority of lead (90%) is bound to hemoglobin in RBC. Hence, plasma or serum samples are not appropriate.

Exercise 2

Q.1 Is arsenic cumulative in animals?

No. Arsenic is rapidly detoxified and is completely eliminated in a few days.

Q.2 In which species of animals, organic arsenicals cause nervous symptoms?

In swines. Nervous symptoms include ataxia and incoordination.

Q.3 In arsenic poisoning, why milk is considered unfit, whereas meat is passed for human consumption?

Arsenic gets methylated and is rapidly excreted through urine, milk, sweat, etc. Hence, milk is considered unfit. As arsenic tends to accumulate only in visceral organs and not in muscles, flesh of surviving animal is considered fit for human consumption.

Q.4 Give reasons as to why mercury poisoning is not common in animals?

Hg compounds are completely replaced by better alternatives in medicinal, agricultural and industrial use. Hence, Hg poisoning is not common in animals.

Q.5 Why young animals are more susceptible for mercury poisoning?

Developing nervous system is more susceptible to mercury. Hence young ones are more susceptible.

Q.6 Why acute lead toxicosis is not common?

Because more than 90% of ingested lead is eliminated from GIT without absorption. Furthermore, even after absorption, only <1% of lead is in free form. Hence, acute lead toxicosis is not common.

Q.7 Why lead poisoning is more common in veterinary cases?

Lead is ubiquitous in nature. Most of the animals live at a closer level to soil and hence get more exposure. Furthermore, habits like frequent digging of soil seen in dogs and cats increase exposure. Ultimately, increasing vehicular and industrial pollution is the major reason for lead toxicosis.

Q.8 Animals with depraved appetite (pica) are more commonly affected with lead poisoning. Why?

In pica, animals tend to lick walls, chew on dry peelings of paint, eat wall posters, etc. Because paints are lead-based, the animals are affected with lead poisoning. Even children chewing on toys painted with cheap lead paints are also reported to be affected with lead toxicosis.

Q.9 Why molybdate salts are given as supportive therapy in copper poisoning?

Molybdenum has inverse relationship with copper, increasing its elimination. Hence, molybdate salts are used in copper poisoning.

Q.10 How zinc administration decreases development of copper toxicity?

Zinc induces the synthesis of mucosal metallothioneins in GIT, which bind to copper and prevent Cu absorption. Hence, zinc supplementation decreases the development of copper toxicity.

Exercise 3

Q.1 Among ruminants, why cattle are more susceptible than sheep for nitrate poisoning?

The rumen of sheep is effective in converting nitrites to ammonia, which is used for protein synthesis. However, in cattle, the rumen is not as effective as sheep. Hence, in cattle, high nitrites accumulate resulting in poisoning.

Q.2 Why nonruminants are not affected by nitrates from plant sources?

The conversion of nitrates to nitrites does not occur in nonruminants (lack of rumen microflora). Hence, nonruminants are not affected. However, pigs are most sensitive to ingestion of preformed nitrites.

Q.3 Why plant accumulate nitrates in toxic proportions?

Plants absorbs nitrates from soil due to physiological requirement. However, any change in environmental conditions that affect the utilization of nitrates leads to nitrate accumulation. For example, lack of rainfall—no leaching of nitrates from soil; low temperature—inhibits nitrate reductase activity; and high temperature—excessive absorption from soil.

Q.4 Why chopping, cutting, or chewing plants increases cyanide toxicity?

Cyanogenic glycosides are present in epidermal cells, whereas the enzyme β-glycosidase is present in mesenchymal cells. Hence, chopping, cutting, or chewing ruptures the cells releasing the enzyme that releases HCN.

Q.5 Why ruminants are more susceptible to cyanogenic glycoside poisoning?

The pH, water content, and microflora of rumen facilitate the release of cyanide from cyanogenic glycosides. Hence, ruminants are more susceptible to cyanogenic glycoside poisoning.

Q.6 Why nonruminants are not affected by cyanogenic glycosides?

Acidic pH destroys β-glycosidase enzyme, which is responsible for the release of HCN. Hence, nonruminants are not affected by cyanogenic glycosides.

Q.7 Why ruminants are less susceptible for oxalate poisoning?

Rumen has the ability to convert soluble oxalates into insoluble form. Hence, ruminants are less susceptible for oxalate poisoning. But if the rumens ability for conversion is exceeded, oxalate poisoning occurs.

Q.8 What is mode of action of botulinum?

Neurotoxin produces functional paralysis. It inhibits release of Ach and some other neurotransmitters from vesicles. The toxin binds to surface proteins and inhibit exocytosis of vesicles in response to $Ca++$, which in turn inhibits release of neurotransmitters at the junction.

Q.9 Why urinary bladder tumors are common in cattle in bracken fern poisoning?

Ptaquiloside is converted into an active carcinogen dienone in alkaline medium. As the urine in cattle is alkaline, the conversion of ptaquiloside to dienone occurs, leading to development of urinary bladder tumors.

Q.10 Despite the presence of lectins, why barley is nontoxic to animals?

The structure of lectins contains A and B chains lined by disulfide bond. The presence of both chains is necessary for producing toxicity. But barley is not toxic due to the presence of only A chain.

Exercise 4

Q.1 Why strychnine is least toxic to chicken and pigeons?

In birds and pigeon, strychnine is absorbed very slowly. Hence, strychnine is least toxic to chicken and pigeons. However, other avian species are easily affected.

Q.2 Why organochloride (OC) insecticides are being discouraged/banned?

OC insecticides are not degradable and are persistent in the environment. And due to high lipid solubility, they accumulate in the food chain and enter human and animal bodies. Hence, OC compounds are being discouraged.

Q.3 Despite the presence of lectins, why barley is non-toxic to animals?

The structure of lectins contains A and B chains lined by disulfide bond. The presence of both chains is necessary for producing toxicity. But barley is not toxic due to the presence of only A chain.

Q.4 Why selenium toxicity is more commonly seen in arid and semiarid climatic zones?

In arid and semiarid climatic zones, due to less rainfall, selenium is not leached from the top layers of the soil. Hence, chances of selenium accumulation are more common.

Q.5 Why cracked and overgrown hooves are seen in selenium poisoning?

Selenium replaces sulfur in sulfur-containing amino acids, such as cysteine and methionine, which leads to structural abnormalities in proteins. Hence, overgrown and cracked hooves are seen.

Q.6 Why the pH of the blood is acidic in urea poisoning?

Liver detoxification of ammonia to urea requires bicarbonate (HCO_3-), which depletes blood HCO_3- buffer leading to acidosis. Blood pH changes from 7.4 to 7.0.

Q.7 What is aflatoxicosis?

Aflatoxicosis is a disease associated with Aflatoxins. The disease is common in livestock, domestic animals, and humans throughout the world. The occurrence of aflatoxins is influenced by certain environmental factors.

Q.8 How can you reverse the adverse effects of excess molybdenum?

Treatment with supplemental copper can often reverse the adverse effects of excess molybdenum. Conversely, treatment of Wilson disease with molybdenum compounds is used to reduce copper burden. Molybdenum treatment may also be beneficial for angiogenesis, inflammation, and other disorders associated with excess copper.

Q.9 Why selenium toxicity is more commonly seen in arid and semiarid climatic zones?

In arid and semiarid climatic zones, due to less rainfall, selenium is not leached from the top layers of the soil. Hence, chances of selenium accumulation are more common.

Q.10 Why cracked and overgrown hooves are seen in selenium poisoning?
Selenium replaces sulfur in sulfur-containing amino acids such as cysteine and methionine, which leads to structural abnormalities in proteins. Hence, overgrown and cracked hooves are seen.

15.14.2 MULTIPLE CHOICE QUESTIONS (CHOOSE THE BEST STATEMENT, IT CAN BE ONE, TWO OR ALL OR NONE)

Exercise 5

Q.1 A concentration of 0.01 % is equivalent to how many parts per million (ppm)?
a. 1 ppm
b. 10 ppm
c. 100 ppm
d. 1000 ppm
e. 10,000 ppm

Q.2 A blood lead concentration reported as 80 g/dL is the same as:
a. 0.08 ppm
b. 0.8 ppm
c. 8 ppm
d. 80 ppm
e. 800 ppm

Q.3 If the toxic level of a drug in feed is 100 ppm for a 20-kg pig, what is the estimated toxicity of the drug on a milligram per kilogram of body weight basis? Assume the feed is air dried and the pig eats feed at the rate of 6% of its body weight daily.
a. 2 mg/kg
b. 4 mg/kg
c. 6 mg/kg
d. 8 mg/kg
e. 10 mg/kg

Q.4 Induction of emesis is recommended as a detoxification procedure in dogs ingesting any of the following except:
a. antifreeze (ethylene glycol)
b. acetaminophen
c. kerosene
d. liquid aspirin
e. chocolate

Q.5 The antidotal agent N-acetylcysteine is indicated for treatment of poisoning with:
a. cholecalciferol rodenticides
b. acetaminophen
c. brodifacoum

d. chlorpyrifos

e. copper

Q.6 Inorganic arsenic toxicosis is manifested clinically as

    a. icterus, anemia, and hemoglobinuria

    b. anurosis, incoordination, and constipation

    c. cardiomyopathy, hydrothorax, and ascites

    d. photosensitization, dermatitis, and hair loss

    e. vomiting, gastroenteritis, diarrhea, and dehydration

Q.7 Which combination of a/mineral additives is most useful in preventing chronic copper toxicosis in sheep?

    a. Selenium and molybdenum

    b. Selenium and sulfate

    c. Zinc and molybdenum

    d. Sulfate and molybdenum

    e. Arsenic and sulfate

Q.8 Deficiency of which element in the sow predisposes baby pigs to toxicosis by injectable iron preparations?

    a. Copper

    b. Chromium

    c. Magnesium

    d. Selenium

    e. Zinc

Q.9 Selenium absorption by crop plants is favored by soil that is:

    a. acidic, wet, and poorly drained

    b. acidic, semi-arid, and well drained

    c. alkaline, well aerated, and well drained

    d. alkaline, wet, and poorly aerated

    e. acidic or alkaline, wet, and poorly aerated

Q.10 In ruminants. urea toxicosis is characterized by:

    a. ruminal alkalosis, systemic acidosis and elevated blood ammonia levels

    b. ruminal acidosis, systemic alkalosis and elevated blood ammonia levels

    c. ruminal alkalosis, systemic alkalosis and elevated blood ammonia levels

    d. ruminal acidosis, systemic alkalosis and decreased blood ammonia levels

    e. ruminal alkalosis, systemic alkalosis and elevated blood urea nitrogen levels

Answers

1. c ($1 \times 10^2 \times 100/1 \times 10^6$); 2. b; 3. c; 4. c; 5. b; 6. e; 7. d.; 8. d; 9. c; 10. a.

Exercise 6

Q.1 In cattle chronic fluoride toxicosis causes:

    a. diarrhea, pale hair coat, lameness, and hoof overgrowth

    b. icterus, hemoglobinuria, and photosensitization

    c. emaciation, hair loss, and lameness

    d. rumen stasis, nephrosis, and constipation

    e. lameness, exostosis, and excessive dental wear

Q.2 Which organic synthetic herbicide is often considered dangerous because it induces accumulation of nitrites in some weed species?

    a. Paraquat

    b. Glyphosate

    c. Lindane

    d. 2,4-dichlorophenoxy acetic acid

    e. Pentachlorophenol

Q.3 Which category of insecticidal compounds presents a problem of persistent residues in fatty tissues of animals?

    a. Carbamates

    b. Organochlorines

    c. Organophosphates

    d. Pyrethrins

    e. Juvenile hormones

Q.4 If acute organophosphate insecticide poisoning is suspected, what is the best initial sample to obtain from a live animal for initial diagnostic testing?

    a. Serum

    b. Whole blood

    c. Urine

    d. Stomach contents

    e. Fat biopsy

Q.5 Cholinesterase inhibitor pesticides typically cause all of the following except:

    a. salivation

    b. miosis

    c. dyspnea

    d. blindness

    e. bradycardia

Q.6 When applied to organophosphate insecticide poisoning, the term aging refers to:

    a. loss of insecticidal activity with time

    b. isomerization of the organophosphate to a more toxic chemical form

    c. hydrolysis of the cholinesterase organophosphate bond induced by oxime drugs

    d. a chemical change that increases the stability of the organophosphate cholinesterase bond

    e. altered toxicity of organophosphates from spontaneous hydrolysis of ester groups

Q.7 Newer anticoagulant rodenticides, also known as second-generation anticoagulants, are important in veterinary medicine because they:
a. have been developed to be toxic in rats but not in other classes of mammals
b. have effects that are readily treated by synthetic vitamin K injection
c. are more potent or longer acting than first generation anticoagulants, requiring prolonged therapy
d. are more readily detected by chemical analysis than first-generation rodenticides
e. do not interact with other drugs or chemicals

Q.8 A group of swine shows paralysis, hoof (corollary band) and hair lesions, and lesions of focal symmetric poliomyelomalacia. The most likely cause of these signs is toxicosis involving:
a. arsenic
b. copper
c. lead
d. selenium
e. zinc

Q.9 Overheated Teflon-coated frying pans release vapors that are especially toxic to
a. cats
b. dogs
c. gerbils
d. parakeets
e. reptiles

Q.10 Which clinicopathologic value is least likely to be abnormal 2−24 hours after a dog is bitten by a rattlesnake?
a. Serum amylase activity
b. Serum creatine phosphokinase activity
c. Serum-γ-glutamyltransferase activity
d. Platelet count
e. Prothrombin time

Answers
1. e; 2. d; 3. b; 4. b; 5. d; 6. d; 7. c; 8. d; 9. d; 10. a.

Exercise 7

Q.1 The parts of the plant that does not accumulates fluoride is
a. seed
b. stem
c. leaf
d. flower

Q.2 Fluoride interferes with the following element(s) in the body:
a. Calcium
b. Magnesium
c. Manganese
d. Phosphorus

Q.3 Which form of fluorosis is seen if the animal is exposed to fluorine during early stages of life?
   a. Skeletal
   b. Dental
   c. Both
   d. Not affected

Q.4 Which of the following form of phosphorus is toxic?
   a. White
   b. Red
   c. Yellow
   d. Black

Q.5 The following form of selenium is/are soluble:
   a. Elemental (0)
   b. Selenide (+2)
   c. Selenite (+2)
   d. Selenate (+6)
   e. Organo selenium

Q.6 The following plant(s) is/are nitrate accumulators:
   a. Cereal grasses
   b. Maize
   c. Sunflower
   d. Sorghum

Q.7 The following method of storing forage reduces nitrate content:
   a. Hay making
   b. Silage making
   c. Composting
   d. Straw making

Q.8 Maximum accumulation of nitrates is seen in the following part of the plant:
   a. Tip
   b. Leaves
   c. Upper 1/3 of stem
   d. Lower 1/3 of stem

Q.9 The most resistant species to DNOL poisoning is
   a. cattle
   b. dog
   c. cat
   d. horse

Q.10 Methoxychlor is less toxic than
   a. DDT
   b. perthane
   c. heptachlor
   d. endrin

Answers

1. a; 2. a, b, and c (Interaction with calcium leads to hypocalcemia and interference with magnesium causes hypomagnesaemia causing seizure); 3. c (If the animal is exposed in late stages of life, only skeletal form is observed, but if exposure takes place in early stages of life, both forms are seen); 4. a and c (white and yellow phosphorus are soluble and readily absorbed, hence cause toxicity, whereas red phosphorus is insoluble, hence is nontoxic); 5. c, d, and e (Selenite ($+2$) and Selenate ($+6$) are soluble and hence cause toxicity in animals); 6. a, b, c, and d; 7. b (the process of fermentation reduces nitrate content in forages); 8. d. (parts closer to soil accumulate more nitrates); 9. a; 10. c.

Exercise 8

Q.1 Exposure to fumes of which of the following metals is most likely to cause acute chemical pneumonitis and pulmonary edema?
- **a.** Lead
- **b.** Zinc
- **c.** Cadmium
- **d.** Copper
- **e.** Magnesium

Q.2 Which of the following is NOT true about arsine?
- **a.** It is a gas at room temperature
- **b.** It produces acute intravascular hemolysis
- **c.** It has a garlic-like odor
- **d.** Acute renal failure is a common man infestation of arsine poisoning
- **e.** Significant hepatotoxicity often occurs as part of arsine poisoning

Q.3 Which of the following is NOT commonly associated with mercury vapor poisoning?
- **a.** Acute, corrosive bronchitis
- **b.** Interstitial pneumonitis
- **c.** Tremor
- **d.** Increased excitability
- **e.** Vomiting and bloody diarrhea

Q.4 Which form of mercury was the predominant cause of Minamata Bay disease?
- **a.** Metallic mercury
- **b.** Mercuric salts
- **c.** Mercurous salts
- **d.** Organic mercury compounds
- **e.** Mercury was not the causative agent

Q.5 Which is the only arsenic that can cause blindness?
- **a.** Arsenic trioxide
- **b.** Arsenic pentoxide
- **c.** Arsine
- **d.** Arsinilic acid

Q.6 Copper has inverse interrelationship with the following element(s)
   a. Iron
   b. Molybdenum
   c. Sulfur
   d. Both b and c

Q.7 In lead poisoning, basophilic stipplings (BS) are commonly seen in this species:
   a. Cattle
   b. Sheep
   c. Dog
   d. Horse

Q.8 Which of the following forms of Hg is more toxic?
   a. Elemental
   b. Monovalent
   c. Divalent
   d. Organic

Q.9 Mercury can cross the following barriers in the body
   a. Blood—brain barrier (BBB)
   b. Placental barrier (PB)
   c. Both
   d. No barrier

Q.10 The following properties can be attributed to methylmercury (Organic Hg)
   a. Mutagenic
   b. Carcinogenic
   c. Embryotoxic
   d. Teratogenic

Answers

1. c; 2. e; 3. e; 4. d; 5. d; 6. d; 7. c (BS are remnants of RNA seen in RBC, which take up basophilic stain. However, BS are not pathognomonic for lead); 8. d (Organic form of Hg is more toxic than inorganic form due to higher lipid solubility); 9. c (As Hg can cross BBB causing neurological symptoms and crossing PB leads to accumulation in fetus and abortions); 10. a, b, c, and d.

Exercise 9

Q.1 During extraction of oil from castor seeds, the toxic principle ricin is only present in
   a. oil
   b. seed cake
   c. Both
   d. None

Q.2 Which of the following part of bracken fern is more toxic?
   a. Rhizome
   b. Stem

    c. Leaves

    d. Tips

Q.3 Abrin is a _____

    a. toxalbumin

    b. toxglobulin

    c. polypeptide

    d. carbohydrate

Q.4 The imbalance of following electrolyte is observed in oleander poisoning:

    a. Sodium

    b. Potassium

    c. Magnesium

    d. Calcium

Q.5 The contraindications in strychnine poisoning are

    a. ketamine

    b. morphine

    c. emesis

    d. All

Q.6 The toxicity produced by excessive ingestion of urea in cattle is due to

    a. urea itself

    b. ammonia

    c. urea as well as ammonia

Q.7 Fluoroacetate inhibits synthesis of

    a. norepinephrine

    b. acetylcholine

    c. citric acid

    d. pyruvic acid

Q.8 Organochlorine insecticides protect against the acute toxicity of several organophosphorus insecticides by

    a. stimulating enzymatic detoxification of organophosphates

    b. increasing noncatalytic binding sites of organophosphates

    c. stimulating enzymatic detoxification as well as increasing noncatalytic binding sites of organophosphates

Q.9 Ethylene dibromide in high concentrations produces

    a. lung edema

    b. nephritis

    c. hepatitis

Q.10 Carbamate insecticides interact with

    a. esteratic site of acetylcholine enzyme (AChE)

    b. anionic site of AChE

    c. esteratic as well as anionic site of AChE

Answers

    1. a (Ricin is not extracted in oil but is retained in seed cake); 2. a (All parts of bracken fern are toxic; however, rhizome is more toxic); 3. a; 4. b (Hyperkalemia produced in cardiac glycoside toxicity is fatal); 5. d (Ketamine

causes motor stimulation; morphine—respiratory depression and emesis leads to seizure development); 6. b; 7. c; 8. c; 9. a; 10. a.

Exercise 10

Q.1 Organochlorine insecticides protect against the acute toxicity of several organophosphorus insecticides by
  a. stimulating enzymatic detoxification of organophosphates
  b. increasing noncatalytic binding sites of organophosphates
  c. stimulating enzymatic detoxification as well as increasing noncatalytic binding sites of organophosphates

Q.2 Ethylene dibromide in high concentrations produces
  a. lung edema
  b. nephritis
  c. hepatitis

Q.3 Carbamate insecticides interact with
  a. esteratic site of acetylcholine enzyme (AChE)
  b. anionic site of AChE
  c. esteratic as well as anionic site of AChE

Q.4 Red squill is obtained from the plant
  a. *Urginea maritima*
  b. *Strophanthus* sp.
  c. *Croton tiglium*
  d. *Cassia fistula*

Q.5 Cypermethrin-induced toxicity is laboratory animals is also known as
  a. Turner's syndrome
  b. T-syndrome
  c. X-disease
  d. CS syndrome

Q.6 The diagnostic symptom of chronic pyrethroid toxicity is
  a. muscular twitching
  b. grinding of teeth
  c. hypothermia
  d. irritation

Q.7 The avian toxicant 4-aminopyridine is toxic to dogs and causes clinical effects similar to those of
  a. arsenic
  b. ethylene glycol
  c. lead
  d. organophosphates
  e. strychnine

Answers

1. c; 2. a; 3. a; 4. a; 5. d; 6. a; 7. e.

Exercise 11

Q.1 Convulsion in acute poisoning can be treated by:
  a. morphine
  b. barbiturates
  c. d-tubocurarine
  d. chloral hydrate

Q.2 Vitamin K is recommended in the treatment of poisoning due to
  a. sweet clover
  b. Zineb
  c. *Prunus* sp.
  d. *Lotus* sp.

Q.3 Band formation in the hooves is seen in poisoning due to
  a. fluorides
  b. ergotism
  c. lead
  d. selenium

Q.4 BAL is the specific antidote against poisoning by
  a. selenium
  b. copper
  c. lead
  d. lewisite

Q.5 Alopecia and diarrhea are the prominent symptoms in poisoning with
  a. copper
  b. molybdenum
  c. *Leucaena leucocephala*
  d. Two of the above
  e. None of the above

Q.6 Liver damage occurs in poisoning with
  a. *Lantana*
  b. Pyrrolizidine alkaloids
  c. copper
  d. All of the above
  e. None of the above

Q.7 Garlic-like odor of rumen content is indicative of
  a. phenol poisoning
  b. phosphorus poisoning
  c. hemlock poisoning
  d. cyanide poisoning

Q.8 Cyanotic mucous membranes are seen in poisoning with
  a. nitrate/nitrite
  b. chlorates
  c. carbon monoxide
  d. Only one of the above

    e. None of the above
    f. All of the above

Q.9 The concentration of arsenic in liver/ kidney associated with toxicity is
    a. 3–5 ppm
    b. 10–20 ppm
    c. 20–50 ppm
    d. None of the above

Q.10 The most appropriate sample to be collected in case of nitrate/ nitrite poisoning is
    a. blood
    b. rumen contents
    c. fodder
    d. CSF
    e. aqueous humor
    f. All of the above

Q.11 Which of the following reason(s) contribute to the susceptibility of ruminants for urea poisoning
    a. Urease present in plants
    b. Alkaline pH of rumen
    c. Acidic pH of stomach
    d. Urease activity of rumen

Q.12 Which of the following age group is more resistant to urea toxicity?
    a. Calf
    b. Heifer
    c. Bull
    d. Cow

Answers

1. b; 2. a; 3. d; 4. d; 5. b and c; 6. d; 7. b; 8. f; 9. a; 10. d; 11. a and b (The primary diet of ruminants is plants, which also contain urease enzyme, increasing the conversion of urea into ammonia. Furthermore, alkaline pH of rumen facilitates this conversion. In nonruminants, the pH of stomach is acidic and the diet is not primarily from plants, hence they are least susceptible); 12. a (In young ruminants the rumen microbial is not well developed hence less urease activity is seen).

15.14.3 FILL IN THE BLANKS

Exercise 12

Q.1 The metallic poison, which is considered as "king of poisons and poison of kings" is _____.

Q.2 The treatment of molybdenum poisoning involves administration of _____.

Q.3 The most toxic gaseous form of arsenic which is released during charging of storage batteries is _____.

Q.4 Among the arsenicals, the least toxic form is _____.

Q.5 Drinking water containing more than _____ of arsenic is considered potentially toxic to large animals.

Q.6 The specific antidote for arsenic poisoning is _____.

Q.7 The water-soluble derivative, which is considered superior to BAL is _____.

Q.8 The treatment of molybdenum poisoning involves administration of _____.

Q.9 Acute zinc deficiency causes _____ in children.

Q.10 The common source of mercury poisoning in animals is through _____.

Answers

1. ARSENIC (Arsenic (and Thallium) causes severe GIT irritation. Hence, arsenic is considered "King of poisons." Because arsenic was extensively used by kings to eliminate competitors, it is also known as "Poison of kings"); 2. COPPER SALTS (e.g., Copper sulfate); 3. ARSINE; 4. ORGANIC ARSENICALS; 5. 0.25%; 6. BRITISH ANTI-LEWISITE (BAL) or DIMERCAPROL; 7. MESODIMERCAPROSUCCINIC ACID (MDSA) and DI-MERCAPTO-SUCCINIC ACID (DMSA); 8. Copper salts (e.g., Copper sulfate); 9. erosive dermatitis; 10. Food (Predatory animals at the end of food chain are more likely to accumulate Hg, which causes poisoning).

Exercise 13

Q.1 Sheep may be affected with arsenic toxicity due to the managemental practice of _____ for controlling ectoparasites.

Q.2 The species of animal that is more sensitive to arsenic poisoning is _____.

Q.3 Arsenic undergoes _____ biotransformation reaction in the body.

Q.4 The mechanism of toxicity of arsenic involves binding to _____.

Q.5 During acute arsenic toxicity, the primary symptom is _____.

Q.6 The nature of diarrhea in acute arsenic poisoning is described as _____.

Q.7 In chronic arsenic poisoning, _____ colored mucosa is characteristic.

Q.8 Samples that should be collected in suspected cases of arsenic toxicity are _____ and _____.

Q.9 The level of arsenic in visceral organs, indicative of arsenic poisoning is _____.

Q.10 The diagnosis of oxalate crystals in _____ and _____ is indicative of oxalate poisoning.

Answers

1. DIPPING (Generally, arsenic containing compounds [e.g., sodium arsenite; lead arsenate] are used for dipping); 2. CAT; 3. METHYLATION; 4. SULFYDRYL GROUPS (−SH) (e.g., Lipoic (thioctic) acid); 5. GASTROENTERITIS; 6. RICE WATERY; 7. BRICK RED; 8. HAIR and NAILS; 9. >3 ppm; 10. KIDNEY and RUMEN EPITHELIUM.

Exercise 14

Q.1 The primary source for molybdenum in animals is through _____.

Q.2 The species of animal which is more susceptible to molybdenum poisoning is _____.

Q.3 Molybdenum toxicosis occurs primarily in the deficiency of _____ mineral intake.

Q.4 The ideal ratio of copper to molybdenum should be _____.

Q.5 The level of molybdenum, which causes toxicity, irrespective of copper content is _____.

Q.6 Molybdenum is primarily excreted through _____.

Q.7 In molybdenum poisoning, deficiency of _____ mineral is observed.

Q.8 Peat scours or treat or shooting diarrhea is a characteristic symptom of _____.

Q.9 Light colored hair and depigmentation around eyes in molybdenum poisoning causes _____ appearance.

Q.10 Molybdenosis in sheep is manifested as _____ or _____.

Answers

1. GRAZING (Molybdenum poisoning is referred to as Molybdenosis or Treat. The term "treat" refers to watery foul smelling diarrhea, which is characteristic in molybdenosis); 2. CATTLE; 3. COPPER; 4. 6:1 (ratio of <2:1 Cu to Mo can cause molybdenum toxicosis); 5. >10 ppm; 6. URINE (Biliary excretion accounts for about 20% of the excretion); 7. COPPER (Hence, most of the symptoms in Mo poisoning resemble copper deficiency); 8. MOLYBDENOSIS (Peat scour or treat refers to foul smelling watery feces with gas bubbles. Molybdenum complexes with catechols and inactivates them. Hence, the natural bacteriostatic activity of GIT is lost, which lead to infection and diarrhea); 9. SPECTACLE-EYE (Due to Cu deficiency, melanin production is reduced due to decrease in the activity of Cu containing enzyme tyrosinase. This enzyme converts tyrosine into melanin. Spectacle eye is prominently visible in buffaloes); 10. ENZOOTIC ATAXIA or SWAY BACK (Mo causes Cu deficiency. Cu-dependent enzymes like cytochrome oxidase, necessary for synthesis of phospholipids in myelin. Hence, in Cu deficiency, defective nerves are formed, which cause sway back).

Exercise 15

Q.1 The anemia caused by copper toxicosis is _____ type.

Q.2 Gunmetal kidneys are characteristic in _____ poisoning.

Q.3 The major symptoms of copper toxicosis are _____ and
_____.

Q.4 In copper poisoning, elevation of liver marker enzymes
_____ is seen prior to _____ (about
3−6 weeks before).

Q.5 If hemolytic crisis develops in copper poisoning, the prognosis
is _____.

Q.6 Lead inhibits "heme" synthesis through the inhibition of the enzyme
_____.

Q.7 In dogs, the predominant symptoms of lead poisoning are
_____.

Q.8 The characteristic histological picture in tubular cells of kidney in lead
poisoning is the presence of _____.

Q.9 Neurological symptoms accompanied by GIT symptoms possibly indicate
_____ poisoning.

Q.10 The predominant manifestation of lead poisoning in cattle is
_____.

Answers

1. HEMOLYTIC (Hemolysis of RBC releases hemoglobin causing hemoglobin-uria); 2. COPPER (Hemoglobin released during hemolysis clogs the renal tubules and leads to darkening and necrosis of kidneys. Hence, gunmetal-like kidneys are seen); 3. HEPATOTOXICITY and HEMOLYTIC ANAEMIA; (Hepatotoxicity precedes the development of hemolytic anemia. Once liver is damaged; Cu is released into blood causing rapid hemolysis); 4. AST, SDH, and LDH and HEMOLYTIC CRISIS (Although marker enzymes are elevated, the level of Cu in blood is not increased until a day to two before development of hemoly-sis); 5. GRAVE; 6. δ-AMINO LEVULINIC ACID SYNTHETASE (ALA-D synthase); 7. GASTROINTESTINAL; 8. INTRANUCLEAR INCLUSION BODIES. (Eosinophilic); 9. LEAD; 10. NEUROLOGICAL SYMPTOMS.

Exercise 16

Fill in blanks

Q.1 Oxalate poisoning in animals occurs commonly through _____
consumption.

Q.2 The most important oxalate containing plants, which cause oxalate
poisoning are _____ and _____.

Q.3 *Halogeton* species contains _____ % of oxalates on dry matter basis.

Q.4 The species of fungus, which is rich in oxalates and can cause oxalate
poisoning, is _____.

Q.5 The most commonly affected species for oxalate poisoning is _____.

Q.6 Pastures containing _____ % oxalates is toxic for sheep.

Q.7 The important element with which oxalates interact in the body is _____.

Q.8 The primary clinical sign in oxalate poisoning is _____.

Q.9 The deposition of insoluble calcium oxalate crystals in renal tubules causes _____.

Q.10 The common site of urinary obstruction due to oxalate crystals in bulls and rams is _____.

Answers

1. PLANTS; 2. *Halogeton glomeratus* and *Oxalis pescaprae*; 3. 34; 4. ASPERGILLUS; 5. SHEEP; 6. 2; 7. CALCIUM; 8. HYPOCALCEMIA; 9. OXALATE NEPHROSIS; 10. SIGMOID FLEXURE (In rams, the oxalate crystals also deposit in urethral process).

Exercise 17

Fill in blanks

Q.1 Death in fluoride toxicity is due to _____ and _____.

Q.2 The chronic disease which occurs due to continuous ingestion of small doses of fluoride is _____.

Q.3 In case of fluorosis, treatment with _____ salts is usually followed.

Q.4 Supplementation with _____ mineral supplements can cause fluorosis.

Q.5 The fatal toxicosis which can occur from gases and dust from volcanic eruptions is_____.

Q.6 Acute fluoride poisoning is common in _____, whereas chronic poisoning is common in _____ species of animals.

Q.7 The maximum tolerable level of fluoride in forage for herbivorous animals is _____.

Q.8 The level of fluoride in drinking water, which can cause fluorosis in animals is _____.

Q.9 In the body, fluoride accumulates in and _____.

Q.10 Fluoride is gradually excreted from the body through _____.

Answers

1. HYPERKALEMIA and HYPOCALCEMIA; 2. FLUOROSIS (Fluorosis is endemic in at least 22 countries worldwide and in many areas of Andhra Pradesh and Telangana states); 3. CALCIUM (Ca salts are mainly used as supportive therapy. However, no specific antidote for fluoride toxicity); 4. ROCK PHOSPHATE (The optimum ratio of fluoride to phosphorus in rock phosphates should be 1:100); 5. FLUORINE INTOXICATION; 6. DOGS; HERBIVORES (Dogs are poisoned from fluoride containing pesticides, whereas herbivores from eating

contaminated pastures); 7. 40–50 ppm (A level of 50 ppm should not be exceeded in the ration of animals); 8. >2 ppm (Dental defects are seen at 5 ppm, wear and tear at 10 ppm, and systematic effects at 30 ppm); 9. BONE, TEETH. (Bone acts as sink for fluoride similar to lead. However, accumulation in teeth only occurs during formative stages i.e., young age only); 10. URINE.

Exercise 18

Q.1 In oxalate poisoning, administration of _____ salts is carried out as a part of treatment.

Q.2 Fluoride causes the formation of _____ in the acidic medium of stomach, which is responsible for the corrosive action.

Q.3 Hyperkalemia occurring in fluoride poisoning is due to the inhibition of _____ enzyme.

Q.4 Brown or black discoloration of teeth seen in fluorosis is due to oxidation of _____, which is defective in tooth.

Q.5 In fluorosis, defects in bones are due to replacement of _____ groups with fluoride in hydroxyapatite structure.

Q.6 Chronic fluorosis is manifested in _____ and _____ forms.

Q.7 The prognosis in case of phosphorus poisoning is _____.

Q.8 The samples of choice to be collected in suspected cases of fluoride poisoning are _____ and _____.

Q.9 In fluorosis, the density of bones is _____.

Q.10 The soft tissue that accumulates highest amount of fluorine in the body is _____.

Answers

1. CALCIUM (Calcium salts are used to correct hypocalcaemia observed in oxalate poisoning); 2. HYDROFLUORIC ACID; 3. Na+ -K+ ATPase; 4. ENAMEL (Fluoride is required for enamel formation but excess before complete formation of enamel can damage tooth due to oxidation); 5. HYDROXYL; 6. SKELETAL and DENTAL; 7. GUARDED to GRAVE; 8. BONE and URINE (Affected cattle have 3000 ppm and sheep have 5000 ppm of fluoride in bone against a normal value of 200–600 ppm. In urine >15 ppm is suggestive of fluorosis); 9. INCREASED (Fluoride binds with Ca by replacing hydroxyl groups in bones causing an increased mineralization and bone density); 10. PINEAL GLAND.

Exercise 19

Fill in the Blanks

Q.1 Nitrate is first converted to _____ in rumen by micro flora.

Q.2 The use of _____ fertilizers increases the concentration of nitrates in plants.

Q.3 The herbicide which increases nitrate content in plants is _____.

Q.4 High nitrate content is present in drinking water from _____ source.

Q.5 The species of animals that are more susceptible to nitrate poisoning are _____.

Q.6 The concentration of nitrates in plants, which is toxic to animals is _____% or _____ ppm.

Q.7 Drinking water containing more than _____ ppm of nitrates can cause poisoning.

Q.8 The nitrate content in young plants is _____ than mature plants.

Q.9 The presence of _____ bacteria in water increases nitrate toxicity.

Answers

1. NITRITE (Nitrites [NO_2^-] are 10 times more toxic than nitrates [NO_3-]); 2. NITRATE; 3. 2,4-D; 4. DEEP WELL (Deep well water contains around 1700−3000 ppm of nitrates due to seepage from surface soil); 5. RUMINANTS; 6. 1 or 10,000 (on dry matter basis, a concentration of 0.5% nitrates is toxic in plant material); 7. 1500; 8. MORE; 9. COLIFORM.

Exercise 20

Q.1 The growth of plants/algal blooms in ponds causes _____ in nitrate content of water.

Q.2 The deficiency of molybdenum/sulfur/phosphorus in soil causes _____ in nitrate accumulation in plants.

Q.3 The deficiency of copper/cobalt/ manganese in soil causes _____ in nitrate accumulation in plants.

Q.4 The addition of _____ to feeds improves tolerance to nitrate toxicity.

Q.5 The antibiotic used as feed additive, which enhances conversion of nitrates to nitrites causing poisoning is _____.

Q.6 Watering of animals immediately after consuming on nitrate rich plants _____ the chances of nitrate poisoning.

Q.7 Nitrite ion enters erythrocytes in exchange for _____ ion.

Q.8 Nitrite combines with hemoglobin (in 1:2 ratio) to form _____.

Q.9 The color of blood in nitrate poisoning is _____.

Q.10 Physiologically formed methemoglobin (1%−2%) is converted back to hemoglobin in the body by the enzymes _____.

Answers

1. DECREASE; 2. INCREASE; 3. DECREASE; 4. SOLUBLE CARBOHYDRATES (TDN) (Carbohydrates are necessary for rumen microflora for the conversion of nitrites into ammonia, which is utilized for protein synthesis); 5. MONENSIN; 6. DECREASES (As nitrates and nitrites are eliminated through urine. On the contrary, watering after consumption of cyanogenic plants increases cyanide toxicity); 7. CHLORIDE; 8. METHEMOGLOBIN (Ferrous (Fe^{2+}) is oxidized to ferric (Fe^{3+}) in methemoglobin, which decreases oxygen carrying capacity of blood);

9. CHOCOLATE BROWN (Due to methemoglobin formation); 10. DIAPHORASE—I and II (Diaphorase-I is NAD dependent, whereas DIAPHORASE-II is NADP dependent).

Exercise 21

Q.1 Formation of _____ of methemoglobin produces symptoms of nitrate poisoning.

Q.2 Vasodilation and hypotension observed in nitrate poisoning is due to smooth muscle relaxation caused by _____.

Q.3 The respiration in nitrate poisoning is _____.

Q.4 Chronic nitrate poisoning leads to the development of _____ in sheep.

Q.5 The preferred antemortem sample to be collected in nitrate poisoning is _____.

Q.6 The specific treatment for nitrate poisoning is _____.

Q.7 Methylene blue is oxidized to _____ during the conversion of methemoglobin to hemoglobin.

Q.8 The conversion of methemoglobin to hemoglobin by methylene blue depends on the availability of _____.

Q.9 The use of _____ is contraindicated in nitrate toxicity to improve blood pressure and heart function.

Q.10 The use of _____ metal chelator is contraindicated in selenium toxicity.

Answers

1. 20%–40%; 2. NITRIC OXIDE (NO); 3. RAPID (Rapid respiration is a prominent clinical sign in nitrate poisoning); 4. GOITER (Nitrate interferes with iodine metabolism); 5. PLASMA (Serum cannot be used as nitrate are retained in blood clot); 6. METHYLENE BLUE (Reducing agents such as ascorbic acid are also used); 7. LEUCOMETHYLENE BLUE; 8. NADPH2; 9. ADRENERGIC AGONISTS (Adrenergic agonists increase oxygen demand but in nitrate poisoning, the oxygen carrying capacity of blood in severely hampered); 10. DIMERCAPROL (BAL).

Exercise 22

Q.1 The type of climates in which selenium toxicity is more common is _____ climates.

Q.2 The pH of the soil, which favors selenium accumulation is _____.

Q.3 The metabolite of selenium excreted through urine is _____.

Q.4 Cytotoxicity of selenium is due to the generation of _____ at cellular level.

Q.5 The nonenzymatic antioxidant depleted by selenium is _____.

Q.6 In selenium poisoning, the characteristic odor observed is _____.

Q.7 The vitamin that can aggravate selenium poisoning is _____.

Q.8 Subacute toxicity of selenium is also known as _____.

Q.9 Chronic selenium toxicity is also called as _____.

Q.10 In cattle, cracked and overgrown hooves are the main symptoms of _____ poisoning.

Answers

1. ARID AND SEMIARID; 2. ALKALINE (>7.0); 3. TRIMETHYL SELENONIUM; 4. FREE RADICALS; 5 GLUTATHIONE (GSH); 6. GARLIC-LIKE (Recollect, phosphorus also produces garlic-like odor); 7. VITAMIN E; 8. BLIND STAGGERS; 9. ALKALI DISEASE; 10. SELENIUM.

Exercise 23

Q.1 In horses, loss of hair from the mane is the main symptom of _____ poisoning.

Q.2 The most toxic from of selenium is _____.

Q.3 Organo selenium is formed due to the replacement of _____ by selenium in amino acids.

Q.4 The level of selenium in plants, which is toxic to animals is _____.

Q.5 The type of plants that physiologically require selenium and accumulate high levels of selenium are called _____.

Q.6 The level of selenium found in obligate accumulators is _____.

Q.7 The type of plants that do not require selenium but accumulate high levels of selenium if present in soil are called _____.

Q.8 The level of selenium found in facultative accumulators is _____.

Q.9 The type of plants that do not require selenium but accumulate low levels of selenium if present in soil are called _____.

Q.10 The level of selenium found in nonaccumulators is _____.

Answers

1. SELENIUM; 2. ORGANO SELENIUM (The magnitude of toxicity of selenium is Organo selenium > Selenite = Selenate > Selenide > Elemental Selenium); 3. SULFUR (Sulfur containing amino acids being cysteine and methionine); 4. 5 ppm AND ABOVE; 5. OBLIGATE (PRIMARY) ACCUMULATORS or INDICATOR PLANTS; (e.g., *Astragalus* sp., *Stanleya* sp., and Oonopsis sp. Animals avoid these plants as they are not palatable, but in scarcity they are consumed leading to toxicity); 6. 100−1500 ppm; 7. FACULTATIVE ACCUMULATORS (e.g., *Acacia* spp., *Aster* spp., *Astriplex* spp., and *Artemisia* spp. As these plants are more palatable, toxicity is often seen in animals); 8. 25−100 ppm; 9. NON-ACCUMULATORS. (e.g., Maize,

Wheat, and Barley. These plants are more palatable than other accumulators and hence chances of toxicity are more); 10. 1−25 ppm.

Exercise 24

Q.1 Cyanide from plant sources is present in the form of _____.
Q.2 The accumulation of _____ in plants predisposes to cyanide formation.
Q.3 The enzyme present in plants, which releases hydrocyanic acid from cyanogenic glycosides is _____.
Q.4 The species of animals, which are more susceptible to cyanogenic glycoside poisoning are _____.
Q.5 Among ruminants, the more susceptible species for cyanogenic glycosides is _____.
Q.6 The cyanogenic glycosides present in bitter almond and wild cherry is _____.
Q.7 The cyanogenic glycosides present in sorghum and Sudan grass is _____.
Q.8 The cyanogenic glycosides present in linseed and wild clover is _____.
Q.9 The part of the plant, which contains more cyanogenic glycosides is _____.
Q.10 The level of HCN in plants, which can cause cyanide poisoning in animals is _____.

Answers

1. CYANOGENIC GLYCOSIDES (Cyanogenic glycosides are present in epidermal cells); 2. NITRATES (Cyanide is formed by the reaction of nitrates with amino acids); 3. β-GLYCOSIDASE (β-glycosidase is present in mesochymal cells); 4. RUMINANTS; 5. CATTLE (Due to large rumen, which has more microflora releasing more HCN); 6. AMYGDALINE; 7. DHURRIN; 8. LINAMARINE; 9. LEAF; 10. 200 ppm AND ABOVE.

Exercise 25

Q.1 Young plants contain _____ cyanogenic glycosides than mature plants.
Q.2 The use of _____ fertilizers increases cyanide toxicity.
Q.3 Spraying of the weedicide _____ can increase cyanide content in plants.
Q.4 The soils that favor cyanide accumulation in plants are high in _____ and low in _____ content.
Q.5 Watering animals after feeding on cyanogenic plants _____ toxicity.
Q.6 The metabolite of cyanide, which is excreted through urine is _____.
Q.7 Cyanide is converted to nontoxic thiocyanate by the enzyme _____.

Q.8 Good reserves of _____ in the body reduce the toxic effects of cyanide toxicity.

Q.9 Cyanide inhibits cellular respiration by binding with _____.

Q.10 The color of blood in cyanide poisoning is _____.

Answers

1. MORE; 2. NITRATE (Nitrate fertilizers increases nitrate content in plants, which is subsequently converted to cyanide by combining with amino acids); 3. 2,4-D (2,4-D increases nitrate content and consequently the cyanide content); 4. NITROGEN, PHOSPHORUS; 5. INCREASES (Water causes hydrolysis of cyanogenic glycosides releasing HCN); 6. THIOCYANATE; 7. RHODANESE; 8. SULFUR; 9. CYTOCHROME OXIDASE (cyta3) (Cyanide has more affinity towards metalloporphyrin (Fe)-containing enzymes); 10. BRIGHT RED (As oxygen stays in blood due to nonutilization by tissues, blood is bright in color).

Exercise 26

Q.1 The characteristic smell of ruminal contents, which can suggest cyanide poisoning is _____ smell.

Q.2 Chronic form of cyanide toxicity observed in humans due to consumption of cassava root is called as _____.

Q.3 The level of cyanide in rumen contents, which is indicative of cyanide poisoning is _____.

Q.4 The specific treatment for cyanide toxicity is _____ followed by _____.

Q.5 In selenium toxicity, depleted glutathione levels can be restored by administering _____ during treatment.

Q.6 In selenium poisoning, the level of selenium detected in blood is _____ and in hooves is _____.

Q.7 In cattle, cracked and overgrown hooves are the main symptoms _____ poisoning.

Q.8 In horses, loss of hair from the mane is the main symptom of _____ poisoning.

Q.9 The important natural source of selenium apart from plants is _____.

Q.10 The maximum permissible amount of cotton seed cake that can be added to ration of cattle is _____ (total dose).

Answers

1. BITTER ALMOND (The smell of cyanide is similar to bitter almonds, which also contains cyanide. Eighteen bitter almonds can kill a human being but the variety used in household purpose is the domesticated sweet version); 2. KONZO; 3. 10 ppm; 4. SODIUM THIOSULPHATE ($NaNO_3$ converts hemoglobin into methemoglobin, which removes cyanide from cytochrome oxidase into blood; Na_2SO_3 helps in the conversion of cyanide to nontoxic thiocyanate, which is easily excreted

through urine); 5. ACETYL CYSTEINE; 6. 1−4 ppm, 5−20 ppm; 7. SELENIUM; 8. SELENIUM; 9. VOLCANIC GASES; 10. 1 kg (Furthermore, the feeding of cotton seed cake should be interrupted after 2−3 months for 3−4 weeks).

Exercise 27

Q.1 The death in zinc phosphide poisoning is due to the release of _____.

Q.2 Cherry red color of mucous membrane is indicative of _____ poisoning.

Q.3 Deep yellow color of urine is seen in _____ poisoning, whereas brown black color is indicative of _____ poisoning.

Q.4 The toxic principle of *Cannabis sativa* is _____.

Q.5 The cyanogenetic glycoside in *Sorghum* sp. is _____ and that in *Prunus* sp. is _____.

Q.6 _____ and _____ are used in the treatment of cyanide poisoning.

Q.7 Fagopyrin from *Fygopyrum esculentum* is responsible for causing _____ in cattle.

Q.8 Chronic copper poisoning in sheep occurs when the grazing pasture contains _____ of copper on dry matter basis.

Q.9 Ammonia exerts its toxic effect by inhibition of _____.

Q.10 Cyanide in smaller quantity is detoxified by an enzyme _____.

Answer

1. Phosphine gas; 2. Cyanide; 3. Picrate, Acorn; 4. Tetrahydro cannabinol; 5. Dhurrin, Prunasin; 6. Sodium nitrite and sodium thiosulphate; 7. Primary photosensitization; 8. 15−20 ppm; 9. Citric acid cycle; 10. Rodonase.

Exercise 28

Q.1 _____ and _____ are mostly sent to the chemical examiner for confirming chronic arsenic poisoning.

Q.2 _____ is a OP compound used as anthelmintic.

Q.3 In cyanide poisoning _____ and _____ are the organs to be dispatched for chemical analysis.

Q.4 Deltamethrin is classified as _____ on the basis of the chemical nature.

Q.5 Libermann's test is employed for confirming _____ poisoning

Q.6 Major route of excretion of DDT in cattle is through _____ which causes health hazard in human beings.

Q.7 _____ and _____ cause anoxia by combining hemoglobin.

Q.8 _____ is a Dinitroaniline compound, which is used as herbicide.

Q.9 DDT was discovered and studied by _____, while organophosphorus insecticides by _____.

Q.10 _____ is used to treat rodenticide poisoning because of its anticoagulant action.

Answers

1. Horn and Hair; 2. Coumaphos; 3. Liver and Lung; 4. Type-II pyrethroid; 5. carbolic acid (phenol); 6. Milk; 7. Carbon monoxide and nitrite; 8. Pendimethalin; 9. Paul Muller, Gerhard Schrader; 10. Vitamin K.

Exercise 29

Q.1 The species of animal that is more susceptible to secondary photosensitization due to pyrrolizidine alkaloids is _____.

Q.2 *Lantana camara* causes _____ photosensitization.

Q.3 Abnormal sensitivity of unpigmented or less pigmented parts of skin to sunlight due to the presence of photodynamic substances in peripheral circulation is known as _____.

Q.4 The type of photosensitivity produced due to direct ingestion of photodynamic substances or metabolically activated agents is called _____ photosensitization.

Q.5 The photodynamic substance, formed due to bacterial break down of chlorophyll, which is responsible for secondary photosensitization is _____.

Q.6 Secondary photosensitization in *Lantana camara* is mainly due to _____.

Q.7 The phytoconstituents of *L. camara*, which cause bile duct occlusion and liver damage are _____.

Q.8 Hepatic lesions such as _____ and _____ are diagnostic in differentiation primary and secondary photosensitization.

Q.9 The primary visible lesion in photosensitization is _____.

Q.10 The prognosis is poor in _____ type photosensitization.

Answers

1. PIG; 2. SECONDARY; 3. PHOTOSENSITIZATION; 4. PRIMARY (e.g., Plants: Hypericin—*Hypericium* sp., Fagopyrin—*Fagopyrum* sp., *Parthenium* sp., Drugs—phenothiazines, tetracyclines, sulphonamides, and acridine dyes); 5. PHYLLOERYTHRIN; 6. BILE DUCT OCCLUSION; 7. LANTADENE A and B; 8. FIBROSIS, BILIARY HYPERPLASIA; 9. SUNBURNS; 10. SECONDARY (The hepatic damage is generally irreversible leading to death).

Exercise 30

Q.1 Gossypol-induced infertility is due to _____ effect on ovary.

Q.2 Bracken fern poisoning is caused due to the consumption of the plant _____.

Q.3 The enzyme present in bracken fern, which breaks down vitamin _____
is _____.

Q.4 Aplasia of bone marrow due to bracken fern toxicity is observed in
_____ species of animals.

Q.5 The aplastic anemia causing and carcinogenic factor present in bracken fern
is _____.

Q.6 In alkaline pH, ptaquiloside is converted in to active carcinogenic form
_____.

Q.7 The co-carcinogen present in bracken fern, which causes malignant tumors
in mouth, esophagus, and rumen along with papilloma virus, is
_____.

Q.8 The most susceptible species for bracken fern poisoning are _____ and
_____.

Q.9 Anemia is absent in bracken fern poisoning in _____ species.

Q.10 The main symptom of bracken fern poisoning in cattle is _____.

Answers

1. LUTEOLYTIC; 2. *Pteridium aquilinum*; 3. B1, THIAMINASE (Other thiaminase containing plants include Horse tail, Australian nardoo fern, rock fern);
4. RUMINANTS; 5. PTAQUILOSIDE; 6. DIENONE; 7. QUERCETIN;
8. HORSE, CATTLE; 9. HORSE (The main symptoms in horses are neurological); 10. APLASTIC ANEMIA.

Exercise 31

Q.1 Organochlorine insecticides such as DDT tend to accumulate in
_____ (organ of the body).

Q.2 Organochlorine insecticides such as DDT and BHC tend to be more toxic
in oily vehicles due to _____.

Q.3 The group of heterogeneous substances, which are used to control pests, are
known as _____ PESTICIDES.

Q.4 Chlorinated hydrocarbons are known as _____ insecticides.

Q.5 The most susceptible species for OC insecticide poisoning is _____.

Q.6 OC insecticides accumulate mainly in _____ tissue of the body.

Q.7 The only OC insecticide that does not accumulate in adipose tissue is
_____.

Q.8 The OC compound, which is degraded by microbes, is
_____.

Q.9 The only isomer of benzene hexachloride (BHC), which is biodegradable,
is _____ (gamma isomer).

Q.10 OC compounds produce CNS excitation by prolonging
_____ phase of action potential.

Answers

1. ADIPOSE TISSUE; 2. INCREASED ABSORPTION; 3. PESTICIDES; 4. ORGANOCHLORINE (OC); 5. CAT; 6. ADIPOSE; 7. ENDOSULFAN (Endosulfan is also biodegradable and not persistent in environment). 8. ENDOSULFAN (Endosulfan has a sulfur ring in its structure, which is susceptible for microbial degradation. However, endosulfan is banned in 2011 worldwide but is still used in some developing countries); 9. LINDANE (Gamma isomer); 10. DEPOLARIZATION (Depolarization is prolonged by extending opening of Na+ channels and closing of K+ channels. Aliphatic OC compounds such as DDT and methoxychlor follow this mechanism).

Exercise 32

Q.1 OPIDN (OP-induced delayed neuropathy) is caused due to inhibition of _____ enzyme.

Q.2 The main symptoms in OP poisoning are _____ symptoms.

Q.3 In OPIDN, the main symptom is _____ type of paralysis.

Q.4 Diagnosis of OP toxicity is carried out by measuring _____ activity in blood.

Q.5 The specific antidote for OP poisoning is _____.

Q.6 Oxime reactivators (2-PAM, DAM) should be used within 24- to 36-hour time before aging of _____ occurs.

Q.7 Use of atropine is contraindicated in _____ as it causes cyanosis.

Q.8 Insecticides that cause reversible inhibition of AChE are _____.

Q.9 Carbamates bind with AChE at _____ and _____ sites.

Q.10 Oxime reactivators are ineffective in reactivating AChE in _____ insecticide poisoning.

Answers

1. NEUROTOXIC ESTERASE (NTE), (also called Neuropathy Target Esterase); 2. CHOLINERGIC (Salivation, Lacrimation, Urination, and Defecation); 3. ASCENDING FLACCID (Hence, OPIDN is also known as dying back axonopathy. Mostly, large myelinated peripheral nerves are more affected); 4. AChE (Less than 25% activity of AChE is confirmative of OP poisoning. In birds, estimation of BuChE is important); 5. ATROPINE (Atropine inhibits cholinergic symptoms by blocking muscarinic receptors); 6. AChE; 7. CATS; 8. CARBAMATES; 9. ANIONIC and ESTERATIC; 10. CARBAMATE (Carbamates bind with both site of AChE; hence, there is no binding site for oxime reactivators).

Exercise 33

Q.1 The least toxic carbamate that is used in veterinary use is _____.

Q.2 The specific antidote for carbamate poisoning is _____.

Q.3 Pyrethroids are natural insecticides obtained from _____ flowers.

Q.4 The most widely used household insecticides are _____.

Q.5 Type I pyrethroids resemble _____ in their structure and activity.

Q.6 Type II pyrethroids contain group _____ in their structure and are more active and toxic.

Q.7 The first commercially available pyrethroid used till date for repelling mosquitoes is _____.

Q.8 The species that is highly susceptible to pyrethroids toxicity is _____.

Q.9 The relationship between toxicity of pyrethroids and temperature is _____.

Q.10 Pyrethroids cause CNS stimulation through inhibiting closure of _____ channels.

Answers

1. CARBARYL; 2. ATROPINE; 3. CHRYSANTHEMUM (The use of marigold flowers is a common folk practice to prevent insects in food grains. The active ingredient in marigold is pyrethrin. Hence, synthetic compounds resembling it are called "pyrethroids"); 4. SYNTHETIC PYRETHROIDS (Least toxic and rapidly biodegradable. These agents are used in mosquito repellants such as Good Night, All Out; and Ant and cockroach repellants—Baygon, Cross line, etc.); 5. NATURAL PYRETHRINS (e.g., Allethrin, Pyrethrin, and Permethrin); 6. α-CYANO (e.g., Deltamethrin, Cypermethrin, Fenvalerate); 7. ALLETHRIN; 8. FISH; 9. INVERSE (As ambient temperature decreases, the toxicity increases and vice versa); 10. VOLTAGE-GATED SODIUM (This leads to increased influx of Na + that leads to prolonged depolarization).

Exercise 34

Q.1 Bait shyness and tolerance develops very rapidly for rodenticide _____.

Q.2 The main symptom in ANTU poisoning is _____.

Q.3 The rodenticide red squill is obtained from the plant _____.

Q.4 The toxic glycosidic principle present in red squill is _____.

Q.5 Scillirosides are present in highest concentration in _____ part of the plant.

Q.6 The action of GIT microflora on scilliroside glycosides releases the aglycon portion _____.

Q.7 The action of scillirosides glycosides is similar to _____.

Q.8 _____ are used to control weeds.

Q.9 The most widely used herbicide is

_____.

Q.10 Herbicides enhance the palatability of certain toxic plants by increasing the content of _____.

Answers

1. ANTU; 2. PULMONARY EDEMA; 3. *Urginea maritima* (In south India, toxicity due to Indian squill (*Urginea indica*) is more common); 4. SCILLIROSIDE; 5. BULB; 6. SCILLIROSIDIN; 7. DIGITALIS (The symptoms are cardiac arrhythmia and cardiac arrest); 8. HERBICIDES; 9. 2, 4-D (2, 4-dichlorophenoxy-acetic acid); 10. NITRATES.

Exercise 35

Q.1 Long-term consumption of bracken fern causes _____ tumors in cattle.

Q.2 Enzootic hematuria due to bracken fern poisoning is seen in _____ species.

Q.3 Bracken fern produces permanent blindness in _____ species.

Q.4 The diagnosis of bracken fern poisoning involves estimation of _____ level in blood.

Q.5 The specific treatment for bracken fern induced thiamine deficiency is

_____.

Q.6 The species of animal which is more sensitive for 2, 4-D is

_____.

Q.7 The manufacturing contaminants that make 2, 4-D extremely toxic are

_____.

Q.8 The herbicides that are potent uncouplers of oxidative phosphorylation are _____.

Q.9 Urine is chrome-yellow in color and turns black upon exposure to air in

_____.

Q.10 The most toxic among the herbicides are _____.

Answers

1. URINARY BLADDER; 2. CATTLE; 3. SHEEP; 4. THIAMINE (Normal thiamine (B1) content in blood of cattle is 8.5 µg/dL which is reduced to 2.5 µg/dL); 5. THIAMINE (vitamin B1) (However, no specific treatment is available for bone marrow aplasia and tumors in cattle); 6. DOG; 7. DIOXINS;

8. DINITROPHENOLS; 9. DINITROPHENOL; 10. BIPYRIDYL GROUP (e.g., Paraquat, Diquat).

Exercise 36

Q.1 Chelating agent used to treat copper poisoning is _____.

Q.2 The species of animal, which is more susceptible of copper poisoning, is _____.

Q.3 The species, which is highly resistant to copper poisoning, is _____.

Q.4 The ratio of copper to _____ in feeds should ideally be 6:1.

Q.5 The breed of dog that is highly susceptible to copper toxicosis due to genetic predisposition is _____.

Q.6 The deficiency of _____ micromineral predisposes to copper toxicity.

Q.7 The specific transport proteins for copper in the body are _____ and _____.

Q.8 The primary organ for accumulation (storage) of copper in the body is _____.

Q.9 The major route of elimination for copper from body is _____.

Q.10 Molybdenum and sulfur reduce toxicity of copper by increasing _____.

Q.11 The anemia caused by copper toxicosis is _____ type.

Q.12 Gunmetal kidneys are characteristic in poisoning.

Q.13 In copper poisoning, elevation of liver marker enzymes (AST, SDH, and LDH) is seen prior to _____ (about 3−6 weeks before).

Q.14 If hemolytic crisis develops in copper poisoning, the prognosis is _____.

Answers

1. D-PENICILLAMINE; 2. SHEEP; 3. CHICKEN; 4. MOLYBDENUM (A ratio of Cu to Mo of 10:1 can cause copper toxicosis); 5. BEDLINGTON TERRIER (Autosomal recessive gene causes copper retention due to failure of excretion of copper); 6. MOLYBDENUM; 7. TRANSCUPERIN. CERULOPLASMIN (Transcuperin and albumin transports Cu from blood to liver. However, Transcuperin is specific but is less abundant. Ceruloplasmin transports from liver to peripheral tissues. About 90% of Cu in circulation is in bound form with ceruloplasmin); 8. LIVER; 9. BILIARY; 10. EXCRETION; 11. HEMOLYTIC (Hemolysis of RBC releases hemoglobin causing hemoglobinuria); 12. COPPER (Hemoglobin released during hemolysis clogs the renal tubules and leads to darkening and necrosis of kidneys. Hence, gunmetal-like kidneys are seen); 13. HEMOLYTIC CRISIS (Although marker enzymes are elevated, the level of Cu in blood is not increased until 1−2 days before development of hemolysis); 14. GRAVE.

Exercise 37

Q.1 Nonnutritive substances added to food to improve the physical, organoleptic, nutritive properties, or shelf life are called as _____.

Q.2 Standards relating to food production and safety are covered by
_____.

Q.3 Agents, which prevent oxidative damage of food, are called as
_____.

Q.4 The most toxic and suspected carcinogens among the food additives are
_____.

Q.5 The rare adverse effect of the coloring agent Tartrazine in humans
is _____.

Q.6 The flavoring agent that produces characteristic "candy-shop" aroma and
which is banned by FDA due to carcinogenic potential is _____.

Q.7 The flavor enhancing agent that produces "umami" type taste in foods is
_____.

Q.8 "Chinese restaurant syndrome" is caused by the food additive
_____.

Q.9 The oldest artificial sweetener used in foods is _____.

Q.10 The most common artificial sweetener approved by FDA for use in
pharmaceutical products and foods is _____.

Answers

1. FOOD ADDITIVES; 2. CODEX ALIMENTARIUS COMMITTEE;
3. ANTIOXIDANTS; 4. COLORING AGENTS; 5. ALLERGY OR
ANAPHYLAXIS; 6. SAFROLE; 7. MONOSODIUM GLUTAMATE (MSG);
8. MONOSODIUM GLUMATE (MSG) (Symptoms include headache, flushing, tingling, numbness around mouth, and palpitations. However, as exact association with
adverse effects have not been found, MSG is still used); 9. SACCHARIN (Saccharin
was reported to produce epithelia hyperplasia of urinary bladder in male rats.
However, as association between saccharin and cancer in humans in normal doses was
not established, saccharin is approved by WHO); 10. ASPARTAME (Breakdown of
aspartame produces phenylalanine and hence should be avoided by persons with
"Phenylketonuria." Sugar-free products such as Diet coke contain aspartame).

Exercise 38

Q.1 Vitamin C can react with benzoic acid, added as a preservative in foods, to
form _____.

Q.2 The substances that are added to animal feeds form improving quality of
feeds or improving animal performance are called as
_____.

Q.3 Feed additives that increase growth rate and feed conversion in animals are
called _____.

Q.4 The most commonly used group of antibiotics approved for use as growth
promoters in food producing animals are _____.

Q.5 The most sensitive species animal for ionophores toxicity is _____.

Q.6 The most common symptom in chronic ionophore antibiotic toxicity is
_____.

Q.7 The approved antibiotic, which should not be used simultaneously with other feed additives or growth promoters, is _____.

Q.8 The use of Zinc bacitracin is contraindicated in _____ animals.

Q.9 Apart from dietary sources, animals get exposed to urea from _____.

Q.10 Excessive use of ammonium nitrate and urea fertilizers in plants can result in _____ poisoning in animals.

Answers

1. BENZENE; 2. FEED ADDITIVES; 3. GROWTH PROMOTERS; 4. IONOPHORE ANTIBIOTICS (Monensin, lasalocid, and salinomycin are the commonly used ionophore antibiotics); 5. HORSE (Horses are 10 times more sensitive than cattle); 6. CARDIOMYOPATHY; 7. ZINC BACITRACIN; 8. LACTATING; 9. FERTILIZERS; 10. NITRATE.

Exercise 39

Q.1 Excessive ammonia inhibits _____ cycle in body decreasing energy production.

Q.2 _____ can be a serious problem because items such as rubber bands, socks, rocks, and string can severely damage or block your dog's intestines.

Q.3 The treatment in urea poisoning includes infusion of 5% _____ and _____ into rumen.

Q.4 Intravenous infusions containing _____ are contraindicated in urea poisoning due to induction of hyperglycemia.

Q.5 The toxic principle produced from the interaction of ammonia with reducing sugars in feeds is _____.

Q.6 4-Methyl imidazole (4-MI) present in ammoniated feeds produces CNS symptoms in cattle known as _____.

Q.7 Salt poisoning is commonly associated with deprivation of _____.

Q.8 The most susceptible species for salt poisoning are _____ and _____.

Q.9 Salt causes toxicity due to the development of _____ or _____ in blood and CSF.

Q.10 The major symptoms evident in salt poisoning are _____.

Answers

1. TCA/KREBS; 2. pica; 3. ACETIC ACID (VINEGAR) and COLD WATER (Acetic acid reduces ruminal pH and decreases conversion of urea to ammonia. Cold water reduces rumen temperature there by decreasing urease activity); 4. GLUCOSE/DEXTROSE; 5. 4-METHYL IMMIDAZOLE (4-MI) (NH3 is used similar to urea treatment to improve the N2 content of roughages); 6. BOVINE BONKER'S SYNDROME; 7. WATER (Hence, salt poisoning is termed aptly as water deprivation–induced salt poisoning); 8. POULTRY and PIGS

(Poultry have poor sense of taste and indiscriminate feeding behavior); 9. HYPEROSMOLALITY or HYPERTONICITY; 10. NERVOUS SYMPTOMS.

Exercise 40

Q.1 Urea is added to the diets of ruminants as a source of _____.

Q.2 The lethal dose of urea in cattle is _____.

Q.3 Urea can be used in the diets of ruminants and horses due to the presence of _____ microbial enzyme in rumen and cecum, respectively.

Q.4 The feed component that is required for efficient utilization of urea is _____.

Q.5 The recommended ratio of urea to molasses for straws and other high fiber diets is _____.

Q.6 In horses, the site of conversion of urea to ammonia is _____.

Q.7 The nervous symptoms found in salt poisoning is due to the development of _____ in brain.

Q.8 Dragging of hind limbs and knuckling of fetlock joints is characteristic feature of _____ poisoning in cattle.

Q.9 The level of sodium in plasma and CSF, which is diagnostic of salt poisoning is _____.

Q.10 The prognosis in case of salt poisoning is _____.

Answers

1. NITROGEN (Urea contains 46.7% nitrogen and 1 g of urea is equivalent to 2.92 g of protein); 2. 1−1.5 g /day/animal (4 g/day/animal in horses); 3. UREASE (Urease converts urea in to ammonia that is used for microbial amino acid synthesis); 4. CARBOHYDRATES or TOTAL DIGESTIBLE NUTRIENTS (TDN) (Carbohydrates (CHO) provide carbon skeleton for the production of amino acids. In cases of CHO deficiency, urea toxicity occurs due to unutilized ammonia); 5. 1:5; 6. CECUM (The urease activity in horses is about 25% that of cattle); 7. CEREBRAL EDEMA; 8. SALT; 9. >1 mEq/L (Furthermore, the level in CSF should be more than plasma); 10. GRAVE (Less than 50% of affected animals survive with treatment; recumbent and convulsing animals definitely die irrespective of treatment).

15.14.4 TRUE OR FALSE STATEMENTS (WRITE (T) FOR TRUE AND (F) FOR FALSE)

Exercise 41

State whether following sentences are True or False.

Q.1 Sodium arsenate is less toxic than sodium arsenite.

Q.2 Synthetic pyrethroids are more toxic than naturally occurring pyrethrins.

Q.3 Like mammalian species, pyrethroids are less toxic to aquatic organisms.

Q.4 Phosphine released from aluminium phosphide is less acutely toxic than methyl bromide.

Q.5 Specific antidote for diquat poisoning is atropine.

Q.6 Phase I reactions are detoxification reactions in the true sense.

Q.7 Mitochondrial fraction of the cell is a part of the microsomal fraction.

Q.8 Echothiophate is an organochlorine compound that interacts with both anionic and esteric site of AChE to produce stable complex.

Q.9 Mammals are less susceptible to OP poisoning because of presence of enzyme carboxylesterase.

Q.10 Warfarin is not a coumarine derivative used in rodent control.

Answers

1. T; 2. F; 3. T; 4. F; 5. F; 6. F; 7. F; 8. F; 9. T; 10. F.

Exercise 42

State whether following sentences are True or False.

Q.1 Oxygen therapy is advocated in cases of diquat poisoning.

Q.2 Fatty and emaciated animals are more sensitive to organochlorine insecticides.

Q.3 ANTU can produce fatal poisoning in dogs when stomach is full.

Q.4 Cholinesterse reactivator that cannot cross the blood−brain barrier is DAM.

Q.5 Extensive use of 2,4-D decreases the nitrate content of barley plants.

Q.6 Zineb breaks down to form ethylene thiourea in mammalian body.

Q.7 2-PAM is used as antidote to treat poisoning due to carbaryl.

Q.8 TCDD is nontoxic.

Q.9 The mechanism of toxicoses of phenoxy herbicides is well understood.

Q.10 Rotenone is obtained from plant Chrysanthemum.

Answers

1. F; 2. T; 3. T; 4. F; 5. F; 6. T; 7. F; 8. F; 9. F; 10. F.

Exercise 43

State whether following sentences are True or False.

Q.1 Dinitrophenol herbicide imparts yellowish green color to tissues and urine.

Q.2 Red squill is a very good rodenticide.

Q.3 Barbiturate is a drug of choice to control miosis in animals.

Q.4 Pyrethrins are produced from extracts of plant genus *Nicotiana*.

Q.5 Nicotine is used in the treatment of organophosphorus poisoning.

Q.6 Pentachlorophenol is a safe fungicide due to its poor absorption through intact skin.

Q.7 Fluoroacetate causes citrate accumulation in the cells.

Q.8 Sulfur is an inorganic insecticide.

Q.9 Coumaphos is an OP compound used as Anthelmintic.

Q.10 Deltamethrin is classified as Type-I pyrethroid on the basis of chemical nature.

Answers

1. T; 2. F; 3. F; 4. F; 5. F; 6. F; 7. T; 8. F; 9. T; 10. F.

Exercise 44

State whether following sentences are True or False.

Q.1 Fenthion is a directly acting OP insecticide.
Q.2 Dinitrophenol herbicide imparts yellowish green color to tissues and urine.
Q.3 Oxygen therapy is advocated in cases of diquat poisoning.
Q.4 Fatty and emaciated animals are more sensitive to organochlorine insecticides.
Q.5 Carbon tetrachloride is used for the treatment of fascioliasis.
Q.6 Cholinesterase inhibition due to carbamate poisoning is temporary.
Q.7 Sodium arsenate is less toxic than sodium arsenite.
Q.8 Synthetic pyrethroids are more toxic than naturally occurring pyrethrins.
Q.9 Organochlorine insecticides penetrate less through intact skin.
Q.10 Sodium arsenate is less toxic than sodium arsenite.

Answers

1. F; 2. T; 3. F; 4. T; 5. T; 6. T; 7. T; 8. F; 9. F; 10. T.

Exercise 45

State whether following sentences are True or False.

Q.1 Phase I reactions are detoxification reactions in the true sense.
Q.2 Mitochondrial fraction of the cell is a part of the microsomal fraction.
Q.3 Echothiophate is an organochlorine compound, which interacts with both anionic and esteric site of AChE to produce stable complex.
Q.4 Mammals are less susceptible to OP poisoning because of presence of enzyme carboxylesterase.
Q.5 Warfarin is not a coumarine derivative used in rodent control.
Q.6 Concentrated sulfuric acid does not char the organic matter.
Q.7 Fluoroacetate causes citrate accumulation in the cells.
Q.8 Warfarin is not a coumarine derivative used in rodent control.
Q.9 Concentrated sulfuric acid does not char the organic matter.
Q.10 Fluoroacetate causes citrate accumulation in the cells.

Answers

1. F; 2. F; 3. F; 4. T; 5. F; 6. F; 7. T; 8. F; 9. F; 10. T.

15.14.5 CORRECT THE STATEMENTS

Exercise 46

State whether the following statements are True or False, if false, correct the statement.

Statement	Correct answer
Q.1 Porphyria is a congenital type of photosensitization.	True
Q.2 Spraying of 2,4-D in sugar beet is a predisposing factor for cyanide poisoning.	False; Nitrite
Q.3 Kidney is the tissue of choice for detection of most metals and sulfonamides.	True
Q.4 ANTU is less toxic when stomach is full than when it is empty.	False; more toxic
Q.5 The toxicity of fluorocitrate is due to its conversion in body to highly toxic fluoroacetate.	False; fluoroacetate converted to fluorocitrate
Q.6 Biphasic reaction is a characteristic of carbamate poisoning.	False; OP
Q.7 Cyanide poisoning could be detected if fresh rumen content contains 10 ppm HCN.	False; More than 10 ppm
Q.8 Charring of the organs is an indicative of sulfuric acid poisoning.	True
Q.9 Denatured spirit at 1 mL/g of the tissue could be used to preserve the tissues for dispatching for an analysis.	False; Ethanol
Q.10 Pasture contaminated with 25–50 ppm of fluoride is not dangerous for grazing animals.	False; Dangerous

Exercise 47

State whether the following statements are True or False, if false, correct the statement.

Questions	Correct answer
Q.1 The chronic selenium poisoning is also known as blind staggers.	False; Alkali disease
Q.2 Malathion is less toxic than paraquat insecticide.	True
Q.3 Trivalant arsenic compounds are less toxic than pentavalant arsenicals.	False; more toxic
Q.4 Rice water stool is a characteristic feature of mercury poisoning.	False; Arsenic
Q.5 Ochratoxin is primarily a hepatotoxic mycotoxin.	False; Nephrotoxic
Q.6 Lantadene A and B from *Lantana camara* causes secondary photosensitization.	True
Q.7 Hyperthermia is one of the clinical symptoms exhibited in poisoning due to organophosphate compounds.	False; due to OC compounds
Q.8 Selenium toxicity occurs when the pasture contains more than 5 ppm of selenium.	True

(*Continued*)

Continued

Questions	Correct answer
Q.9 *Aster* sp. is an example of an indicator plant that contains high concentration of selenium.	False; Facultative accumulator
Q.10 The toxicity of nitrates is 6—10 times more than nitrite.	False; nitrites are 6—10 times more toxic

15.14.6 MATCH THE STATEMENTS

Exercise 48

Match the statement of column one with another column having the following pairs.

1. Basophilic stippling	a. BAL
2. Penicillamine chelates	b. Atropine
3. Drug of choice in carbamate poisoning	c. Copper
4. Rubratoxin	d. Estrogenic mycotoxin
5. Antidote in nitrate poisoning	e. Lameness
6. Arsenic	f. Lead
7. Zearalenone	g. Hepatic cirrhosis
8. *Sorghum* sp.	h. Cyanogenic glycoside
9. Pyrrolizidine alkaloid	i. Penicillium rubrum
10. Fluorosis	j. Methylene blue

Answers

1. Basophilic stippling	f. Lead
2. Penicillamine chelates	c. Copper
3. Drug of choice in carbamate poisoning	b. Atropine
4. Rubratoxin	i. Penicillium rubrum
5. Antidote in nitrate poisoning	j. Methylene blue
6. Arsenic	a. BAL
7. Zearalenone	d. Estrogenic mycotoxin
8. *Sorghum* sp.	h. Cyanogenic glycoside
9. Pyrrolizidine alkaloid	g. Hepatic cirrhosis
10. Fluorosis	e. Lameness

FURTHER READING

Chattopadhyay, Madhab K., 2014. Use of antibiotics as feed additives: a burning question. Front. Microbiol. 2014 (5), 334, Published online 2014 Jul 2. doi: 10.3389/fmicb.2014.0033. https://en.wikipedia.org/wiki/Feed_additive.

Costa, Lucio, G., 2013. Toxic effects of pesticides. In: Klaassen, C.D. (Ed.), Casarett and Doull's Toxicology: The Basic Science of Poisons, 8th ed McGraw-Hill, New York, pp. 883–930.

Gupta, P.K., 1986. Pesticides in the Indian Environment. Interprint, New Delhi.

Gupta, P.K., 1988. Veterinary Toxicology. Cosmo Publications, New Delhi, India (Chapter 6).

Gupta, P.K., 1988. Veterinary Toxicology. Cosmo Publications, New Delhi, India (Chapter 9).

Gupta, P.K., 2010a. Epidemiology of anticholinesterase pesticides: India. In: Satoh, T., Gupta, R.C. (Eds.), Anticholinesterase Pesticides: Metabolism, Neurotoxicity, and Epidemiology. John Wiley & Sons, Inc., Hoboken, New Jersey, USA, pp. 417–431.

Gupta, P.K., 2010b. Pesticides. In: Gupta, P.K. (Ed.), Modern Toxicology: The Adverse Effects of Xenobiotics, Vol. 2. PharmaMed Press, Hyderabad, India, pp. 1–60. , 2nd reprint.

Gupta, P.K., 2014. Essential Concepts in Toxicology. BSP Pvt Ltd, Hyderabad, India (Chapter 17).

Gupta, P.K., 2016a. Fundamental in Toxicology: Essential Concepts and Applications in Toxicology. Elsevier/BSP, USA (Chapter 17).

Gupta, P.K., 2016b. Herbicides and Fungicides. In: Gupta, R.C. (Ed.), Reproductive and Developmental Toxicology, 2nd edition Academic Press/Elsevier, Amsterdam, pp. 655–677.

Gupta, P.K., 2018a. Toxicity of Herbicides. In: Gupta, R.C. (Ed.), Veterinary Toxicology: Basic and Clinical Principles, 3rd edition Academic Press/Elsevier, San Diego, pp. 533–568.

Gupta, P.K., 2018b. Toxicity of fungicides. In: Gupta, R.C. (Ed.), Veterinary Toxicology: Basic and Clinical Principles, 3rd edition Academic Press/Elsevier, San Diego, pp. 569–582.

Gupta, R.C. (Ed.), 2018c. Veterinary Toxicology: Basic and Clinical Principles. 3rd edition Academic Press/Elsevier, San Diego.

Lützow M., 2004. Residues of veterinary drugs without ADI/MRL: what Codex and WTO rules apply? In: Technical workshop on residues of veterinary drugs without ADI/MRL, Bangkok (Thailand), August 24–26, 2004.

Clinical toxicology

16

CHAPTER OUTLINE

16.1 DEFINITIONS

Q. Define clinical toxicology.

Clinical toxicology is the discipline within toxicology, which is concerned with the impact of drugs and other chemicals on humans.

Q. Define forensic toxicology.

Forensic toxicology is the use of toxicology and other disciplines such as analytical chemistry, pharmacology, and clinical chemistry to aid medical or legal investigation of death, poisoning, and drug use.

Q. Define analytical toxicology.

Analytical toxicology is the detection, identification, and measurement of foreign compounds (xenobiotics) in biological and other specimens.
Analytical methods are available for a very wide range of compounds: these may be chemicals, pesticides, pharmaceuticals, drugs of abuse, and natural toxins.

Q. Define the term envenomation.

Envenomation is the infusion of venom into another creature by the means of biting or stinging it.

Illustrated Toxicology. DOI: http://dx.doi.org/10.1016/B978-0-12-813213-5.00016-X

16.2 ANALYTICAL TOXICOLOGY

Q. What are the objectives of analytical toxicology?

Analytical toxicology is aimed at providing support to clinical toxicology. In brief clinical toxicology includes DIMPLE which means:

1. Diagnosis (D)

2. Identification of poisons (I)

3. Management and treatment of poisoning (M)

4. Prognosis (P)

5. Law enforcement (L)

6. Education and research (E)

All the six indications mentioned above can be remembered by the mnemonic DIMPLE.

Q. When conducting an investigation, what type of question (s) is to be asked?

These include:

1. What was the route of administration?

2. What was administered dose?

3. Is concentration enough to have caused death or injury or altered the victim's behavior enough to cause death or injury?

Q. Describe the steps to be followed in an analytical toxicological investigation.

The steps to be followed in an analytical toxicological investigation are given below:

Phases and Steps

Step 1	Based on circumstantial evidence—biochemical and blood investigation
Step 2	Based on medical history—decide priorities for the analysis
Step 3	Analytical phase
Step 4	Interpretation of the results
Step 5	Perform additional analysis on the original samples or on further samples from the patient, if necessary

Q. What are general precautions to be followed by any investigator in toxicology laboratory?

1. Strong acids or alkalis should always be added to water and not vice versa.

2. Strong acids and alkalis should never be preserved together.

3. Organic solvents should not be heated over a naked flame but in water bath.

4. Use fume cupboards/hoods when organic solvents are heated.

16.3 CLINICAL TOXICOLOGY

Q. What are the most common poisons in children?

1. Cosmetics and personal care products

2. Cleaning substances and laundry products

   3. Pain medicines
   4. Foreign bodies such as toys, coins, and thermometers
   5. Topical preparations
   6. Vitamins
   7. Antihistamines
   8. Pesticides
   9. Plants
   10. Antimicrobials
Q. Which are the most common poisons in adults?
   1. Pain killer medicines
   2. Sedatives, hypnotics, and antipsychotics
   3. Antidepressants
   4. Cardiovascular drugs
   5. Cleaning substances (household)
   6. Alcohols
   7. Pesticides
   8. Bites and envenomations (ticks, spiders, bees, snakes)
   9. Anticonvulsants
   10. Cosmetics and personal care products
Q. Which are the most common routes of poisoning?
      Substances can enter the body in three ways:
   1. ingestion (swallowing),
   2. inhalation (breathing in), or
   3. exposure of body surfaces (e.g., skin, eye, and mucous membrane).

16.4 DIAGNOSIS

Q. What are the basics of diagnosis?
   1. Medical history
   2. Physical examination
   3. Differential diagnosis
   4. Investigation and final diagnosis
Q. What type of information is essential and helpful from poisoned patients?
      The information should include:
   1. the presence of preexisting conditions or allergies,
   2. whether the patient is currently using any medications or substances of any kind,
   3. whether the patient is pregnant, in case of female, and
   4. historical information obtained from family, friends, law enforcement and medical personnel, and any observers.
Q. Which chelating agent is preferred for mild lead poisoning and what is the dose?
      Succimer is the agent of choice for asymptomatic, mild lead poisoning ($45-70$ μg/dL in children, $70-100$ μg/dL in adults) because it is available p.o. and has a low side effect profile.

Q. Which chelating agent is recommended for acute lead poisoning with signs of encephalopathy?

Dimercaprol + Calcium EDT

Q. How does carbon monoxide cause normal appearing or pink-colored skin?

Carbon monoxide causes normal appearing or pink-colored skin due to its ability to increase hemoglobin's affinity for oxygen, resulting in hyperoxygenated red blood cells.

Q. What is the characteristic odor associated with different poisonings?

Characteristic odor associated with different poisoning is summarized in Table 16.1.

Table 16.1 Characteristic Odor and Potential Poisons

Odor	Potential Poison
Bitter	Almonds, cyanide
Rotten eggs	Hydrogen sulfide, mercaptans
Garlic	As, organophosphates DMSO, Thallium
Mothballs	Naphthalene, camphor
Vinyl	Ethchlorvynol
Winter green	Methylsalicylate
Phenolic	Phenol and phenolic disinfectants
Stale tobacco	Nicotine
Shoe polish	Nitrobenzene
Sweet	Chloroform and other halogenated hydrocarbons

Q. Give at least a few examples of some poisonous drugs showing pupillary manifestations such as miosis, mydriasis, and nystagmus.

Chemicals/drugs that are responsible for pupillary manifestations such as miosis, mydriasis, and nystagmus are summarized in Table 16.2.

Table 16.2 Chemicals/Drugs Responsible for Pupillary Manifestations

Miosis (Papillary Constriction)	Mydriasis (Papillary Dilatation)	Nystagmus
Barbiturates	Alcohol (constricted in coma)	Alcohol
Caffeine	Amphetamines	Barbiturates
Carbamate	Antihistamines	Carbamazepine
Carbolic acid (phenol)	Carbon monoxide	Phencyclidine
Clonidine	Cocaine	Phenytoin
Methyldopa	Cyanide	
Nicotine	Datura	
Opiates	Ephedrine	
Organophosphates		
Parasympathomimetics		

Q. Give examples of some common symptoms observed with drug poisonings.
Selected drugs showing common symptoms with drug poisoning are summarized in Table 16.3.

Table 16.3 Selected Drugs Showing Common Symptoms with Drug Poisoning

Respiratory depression	Diazepam, opioids
Irregular pulse	Salbutamol, quinine, antimuscarinics, tricyclin antidepressants
Hypothermia	Alcohol, barbiturates, benzodiazepines (BZD)
Hyperthermia	Antimuscarinics, antidepressants, (MAO inhibitors, cocaine, amphetamine, opioids, alcohol, BZD
Coma	Hypoglycemic agents, aminophylline
Constricted pupils	Opioids, antipsychotics (haloperidol, quetiapine, olanzapine, organophosphosphates
Dilated pupil	Anticholinergic drugs (atropine, hyoscine, scopolamine, LSD)

Q. Give some examples of urine color versus toxin substance.
Observation of the urine passed may also give some clue about the type of poison ingested by the patient. Color of urine versus toxin is summarized in Table 16.4.

Table 16.4 Color of Urine versus Toxin

Urine Color	Toxin/Substance
Green or blue	Methylene blue
Gray-black	Phenols or cresols
Opaque appearance which settles on standing	Primidone cresols
Orange or orange-red	Rifampicin, iron (especially after giving desferrioxamine

16.5 TREATMENT OF POISONING

Q. What are steps to general management of poisoning?
The following concepts are central to approaching a toxicosis patient:

- Ensure airway so that breathing and circulation are adequate
- Remove unabsorbed material
- Limit the further absorption of toxicant
- Hasten toxicant elimination

The initial survey should always be directed at the assessment of and correction of the life-threatening problems; if present, attention must be paid to the airways, breathing, circulation, and central nervous system (CNS).

Q. In cases of poisoning, what is the aim of treatment?

    The aim is to decrease the slope of ascending phase (AP) and increasing slope of descending phase (DP). When the slope of AP is decreased, it takes longer time for the toxicant to be absorbed (A). And increasing the slope of DP causes rapid elimination (B) in a short time (Fig. 16.1).

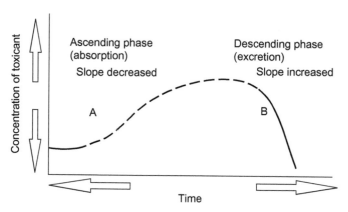

FIGURE 16.1

Time vs concentration curve of toxicant in body during treatment.

Q. What are the different methods of removal of poisons from the body?

    The different methods of removal of poisons from the body are summarized in Table 16.5.

Table 16.5 Methods of Removal of Poisons from the Body

Poisoning	Suggested Methods of Removal
Ingested	Gut decontamination
Inhaled	Provide fresh air, artificial respiration
Injected	Give first aid, followed by specific antidote, diuretics, dialysis, etc.

Q. What are principal lines of treatment?

    Principal lines of treatment include:

1. decontamination,

2. emesis, and

3. symptomatic line of treatment.

Q. What is decontamination?

    Decontamination refers to:

1. skin/eye decontamination,

2. gut evacuation, and

3. administration of activated charcoal.

Q. What are methods used to increase elimination of poisons from the body?

> The following methods are used to increase elimination of poisons from the body:
>
> **1.** Urinary alkalization
> **2.** Multiple-dose activated charcoal
> **3.** Extracorporeal techniques
> **4.** Diaphoresis

Q. How do you classify antidotes?

> Antidotes can be classified according to the mode of action of chemicals/drugs.

Q. Give some examples of some toxins and their antidotes.

Q. Important examples of some toxins and their antidotes are summarized in Tables 16.6 and 16.7.

Table 16.6 Common Antidotes and Toxins Based on the Mode/Mechanism of Action

Toxin	Antidote
Acetaminophen	N-acetylcysteine
Benzodiazepines	Flumazenil[a]
Lockers	Glucagon
Ca channel blockers	Ca, IV insulin in high doses with IV glucose
Organophosphates and (cholinesterase inhibitors)	Pralidoxime, physostigmine[a]
Carbamates	Atropine and protopam
Heparin	Protamine
Ethylene glycol	Ethanol fomepizole
Tricyclic antidepressants	NaHCO$_3$
Isoniazid	Pyridoxine (vitamin B$_6$)
Digitalis glycosides(digoxin, digitoxin, oleander, fox glove)	Steroid binding resins; Potassium salts; beta adrenergic blocking agents; procaine amide
Formaldehyde	Ammonia (by mouth)
Cyanide	Methehemoglobin (formed by nitrite administration), thiocyanide
Botulinum	Botulinus antitoxin; Guanidine
Methyl alcohol	Ethanol
Selenocysthionine	Cystine
Fluoroacetate	Acetate; monoacetin
Bromide	Chloride
Strontium, radium	Calcium salts
Neuromuscular blocking agents, e.g., curare	Neostigmine; edrophonium
Morphine and other related narcotics (opioids)	Naloxone and other related

(*Continued*)

Table 16.6 *(Continued)*

Toxin	Antidote
Coumarin anticoagulants	Vitamin K
Thallium	Potassium salts
Amino acid analogs	Amino acids
Carbon monoxide	Oxygen
Cyclopropane	Alpha adrenergic blocking agents, i.e., haloalkylamine; antihistamines
Histamine	Antihistamines
Agents that produce methemoglobinemia (e.g., aniline dyes, some local anesthetics, nitrites, nitrates, phenacetin, and sulfonamides	Methylene blue
Antitumor agents such as methotrexate and other folic acid antagonists	Glycine
5-Fluorouracil	Thymidine
6-Mercaptopurine	Purines

[a]*Use is controversial.*

Table 16.7 Metals that Make Complexes (Inert Complex Formation) with Poison: Guidelines for their Therapy

Metal	Chelating Drug[a]	Dosage[b]
Antimony, Arsenic, Bismuth, Chromates,[c] Chromic acid,[c] Chromium trioxide,[c] Copper salts, Gold, Nickel, Tungsten, Zinc salts	Dimercaprol 10% in oil	3−4 mg/kg via deep IM injection q. 4 hours on day 1, 2 mg/kg q. 4 hours on day 2, 3 mg/kg IM q. 6 hours on day 3, then 3 mg/kg q. 12 hours for 7−10 days until recovery
Cadmium, Lead, Zinc, Zinc salts	Edentate Ca disodium edathamil), diluted to 5 %	25−35 mg/kg IV slowly (1 hour) q. 12 hours for 5−7 days, followed 7 days without the drug; then repeated
Arsenic, Copper salts, Gold, Lead, Mercury,[c] Nickel, Zinc salts	Penicillamine	20−30 mg/kg/day in 3−4 divided doses (usual starting dose is 250 mg q.i.d.) to a maximum adult dose of 2 g/day
Arsenic, occupational exposure in Bismuth, lead if children have blood levels >45 µg/dL (>2.15 µmol/L); Lead occupational exposure in adults; Mercury, occupational exposure in adults	Succimer	10 mg/kg p.o. q 8 hours for 5 days, then 10 mg/kg p.o. q. 12 hours for 14 days

q. stands for every.
[a]*Iron and Thallium salts are not chelated effectively.*
[b]*Dosages depend on type and severity of poisoning.*
[c]*Chelating drug of choice.*

16.6 QUESTION AND ANSWER EXERCISES
16.6.1 SHORT QUESTIONS AND ANSWERS
Exercise 1

Q.1 What are the three aims of emergency care when someone is bitten or stung by a poisonous animal?

  The aims of the emergency care are:
  1. to minimize systemic absorption of the venom,
  2. to maintain life support, and
  3. to facilitate the neutralization of the toxins by the immune system.

Q.2 List groups of chemicals that are nonnaturally produced toxicants.
  1. Pesticides
  2. Pharmaceuticals
  3. Food additives
  4. Solvents
  5. Environment contaminants

Q.3 Give four examples of naturally produced toxicants.
  1. Plants (plant toxins)
  2. Fungus (mycotoxins)
  3. Bacteria (exotoxins)
  4. Animal/insects (venoms)

Q.4 What are the top four causes of poisonings for animal or human control centers?

  Pesticides > Plants > Household products > Medicines

Q.5 In which season toxicant exposures have the highest incidence?

  In summer: May−August

  In December: young and adult dogs

Q.6 Name top three toxicant exposure agents causing death.
  1. Organophosphate insecticides
  2. Ethylene glycol (antifreeze)
  3. Anticoagulant rodenticides

Q.7 In animal exposure by toxicants, what percent develop major signs or deaths?

  1−3%.

Q.8 Indicate the circumstances under which activated charcoal should *not* be administered.

  It is ineffective in cases of heavy metal or corrosive chemical poisoning.

Q.9 Indicate the circumstances under which iso-osmotic laxative should *not* be administered.

  Suspected or proven obstruction or perforation of the bowel.

Q.10 Indicate the circumstances under which penicillamine should *not* be administered.

  A person with a hypersensitivity to penicillamine.

Exercise 2

Q.1 What is a chelating agent?

A substance that binds strongly to metal ions, facilitating its elimination.

Q.2 What is the antidote of copper poisoning?

Stomach wash with potassium ferrocyanide 1% solution in water acts as an antidote by forming cupric ferrocyanide. Calcium EDTA or BAL is the recommended antidote. Electrolyte and fluid balance to be maintained.

Q.3 Name the agent(s) used in the treatment of poisoning by cyanide.

Amyl nitrite, sodium nitrite, and sodium thiosulfate.

Q.4 Name the agent(s) used in the treatment of poisoning by lead.

Penicillamine

Q.5 Name the agent(s) used in the treatment of poisoning by mercury.

Penicillamine

Q.6 Name the agent(s) used in the treatment of poisoning by pesticides.

The organophosphate pesticides can be treated using atropine and pralidoxime iodide.

Q.7 Your neighbor visits you in an extremely distressed state. A young child of 3 years old has swallowed an unknown quantity of paracetamol tablets. What would you advise his/her parents to do? Why?

Contact the ambulance straight away. The child must be taken to hospital immediately. Paracetamol must be removed immediately to prevent liver damage.

If Ipecac syrup is available, this may be administered to induce vomiting although it appears that this drug is not routinely used to remove drugs from the body because of problems such as aspiration.

Q.8 Farmer A, 60 years old, is brought into the emergency department with organophosphate poisoning. How would this form of poisoning be treated?

1. Respiratory support of the farmer by mechanical ventilation,

2. blockade of the cholinergic receptors by the administration of atropine, and

3. the reactivation of the enzyme cholinesterase by the administration of pralidoxime iodide.

Q.9 Describe briefly the four principles underlying the management of acute clinical overdose.

There are four principles underlying the management of clinical over dosage:

1. life support,

2. client assessment,

3. drug decontamination/detoxification, and

4. drug neutralization/elimination.

Life Support—minimizing the onset of life-threatening emergencies that can be induced by drugs include seizures, cardiac arrhythmias, circulatory shock, and often as a consequence of coma, airway obstruction, and respiratory arrest. Massive damage to vital organs such as the liver, lungs, or kidneys caused by drug toxicity can also lead to death within a relatively short period of time.

Client Assessment—This involves drug identification and dosage taken, assessing the set of clinical manifestations, and laboratory testing.

Drug Decontamination/Detoxification—This involves reducing the rate of drug absorption.

Drug Neutralization and Elimination—Once the drug is identified there may be specific antidotes to counteract the effects of the drug overdose and/or ways to facilitate drug excretion.

Q.10 Explain the supportive care and management of adverse effects for a client who has taken ketamine for recreational purposes.

Treatment for its adverse effects may include the use of oral antihypertensive agents such as angiotensin-converting enzyme inhibitors and calcium antagonists, or intravenous vasodilators such as glyceryl trinitrate and sodium nitroprusside. Supportive care for clients who wish to reduce their dependence on ketamine include the use of cognitive behavioral therapy and benzodiazepine agents such as diazepam. Benzodiazepines may also help clients who are under the influence of hallucinations associated with ketamine misuse.

Exercise 3

Q.1 What are the main tools used in client assessment to identify the specific agent in a suspected drug overdose?
1. Taking a client history
2. Noting the set of clinical manifestations
3. Laboratory testing of blood samples

Q.2 Name the specific antidote(s) for overdose of warfarin poisoning.
Vitamin K

Q.3 Name the specific antidote(s) for overdose of digoxin poisoning.
Digoxin antibody fragments

Q.4 Name the specific antidote(s) for overdose of pethidine poisoning.
Narcotic antagonist, naloxone.

Q.5 Name the specific antidote(s) for overdose of heparin toxicity.
Protamine sulfate

Q.6 Describe in brief different mechanism of specific antidotal therapy.
1. Agents that specifically interact with the toxicant, e.g., iron (deasferrioxamine) and silver nitrate (sodium chloride).
2. Complex formation, e.g., methanol, fluoroacetate, and heparin.
3. Metabolic activation, e.g., enhance metabolic conversion.
4. Pharmacological antidotes, e.g., morphine, warfarin, and curare.
5. Enhancement of excretion of the toxicants, e.g., bromide, copper, lead, and arsenic.

Q.7 Under what circumstances might you use gastric lavage or hemodialysis to facilitate the elimination of a drug in overdose?

It can be used where most of the drug dose is present in the bloodstream rather than in tissues or in interstitial fluid. The apparent volume of distribution (V_d), can be a useful indicator of this.

Q.8 Describe the management of a young woman admitted to the emergency department following ingestion of ecstasy at a street party. She is extremely agitated and anxious but her fluid status and electrolyte levels are normal.

In treating individuals suffering from the effects of stimulants, deescalation techniques are used through verbal communication, group negotiation with affected individuals, and physical restraint. Sedation may also need to be administered to reduce the risk of the individuals harming themselves and others. In giving sedating medication, benzodiazepines are usually preferred compared with antipsychotic drugs because benzodiazepines are more sedating and have fewer side effects.

Q.9 What is the problem associated with the detection of some banned substances through urine testing of sports people?

Some banned substances are naturally present in the body.

Q.10 What is an antidote?

An antidote a medicine taken or given to counteract a particular poison that may be chemical, pharmacological, or physiological in nature.

Exercise 4

Q.1 What are the symptoms of ciguatera poisoning?

Ciguatera poisoning results in a variety of symptoms, such as diaphoresis, bradycardia, hypotension, abdominal pain, nausea, vomiting, diarrhea, metallic taste, myalgias, arthralgias, weakness, headache, ataxia, vertigo, sensation of loose and painful teeth, reversal of temperature sensation, peripheral and perioral paresthesias, and visual disturbances.

Q.2 What is the mode of action of ciguatoxin toxicity?

Ciguatoxin (found on warm water, bottom-dwelling fish, including barracudas, sea bass, red snappers, grouper, and sturgeons, among others) binds to sodium channels and increases sodium channel permeability.

Q.3 What are the symptoms of scombroid poisoning?

Flushing is a classic symptom of scombroid toxicity. Scombroid poisoning is caused by histamine-producing bacteria on the surface of improperly stored dark, tropical fish (e.g., tuna, mackerel, and mahi-mahi). Symptoms include headache, abdominal pain, nausea, vomiting, diarrhea, perioral and peripheral paresthesias, dizziness, palpitations, and diffuse flushing of the skin.

Q.4 Why ethylene toxicity causes renal toxicity?

Ethylene glycol toxicity is caused by its conversion to oxalic acid, which causes renal toxicity.

Q.5 Why methanol toxicity causes renal and ocular toxicity?
Methanol toxicity is caused by its conversion to formic acid, which causes both renal and ocular toxicity.

Q.6 Why fomepizole is a good option for alcohol poisoning?
Fomepizole is an alcohol dehydrogenase inhibitor, which blocks the initial conversion of ethylene glycol to glycoaldehyde and methanol to formaldehyde, thus decreasing the precursors to oxalic and formic acid, which are responsible for toxicity.

Q.7 How does herbicide paraquat act to cause lung toxicity?
Paraquat acts on NADH to create superoxides.

Q.8 Which organ is most affected by diquat herbicide?
Kidney

Q.9 Which chelating agent is preferred for copper poisoning?
Penicillamine

Q.10 How do methemoglobinemia causes cyanosis?
Methemoglobinemia causes cyanosis due to the oxidation of the iron molecule in hemoglobin, thereby reducing its oxygen carrying capacity.

16.6.2 MULTIPLE CHOICE QUESTIONS (CHOOSE THE BEST STATEMENT, IT CAN BE ONE, TWO OR ALL OR NONE)

Exercise 5

Q.1 Administration by oral gavage of a test compound that is highly metabolized by the liver versus subcutaneous injection will most likely result in
   a. less parent compound present in the systemic circulation
   b. more local irritation at the site of administration caused by the compound
   c. lower levels of metabolites in the systemic circulation
   d. more systemic toxicity
   e. less systemic toxicity

Q.2 Intoxication from consumption of wild cherry or apricot pits would best be treated by
   a. hyperbaric oxygen
   b. artificial respiration
   c. inhalation of amyl nitrite
   d. intravenous sodium nitrite and sodium thiosulfate
   e. oral sodium nitrate

Q.3 The most useful bedside test to suggest snakebite is
   a. envenomation
   b. Prothrombin time
   c. 20 min whole blood clotting time

d. International normalized ratio

e. platelet count

Q.4 A 12-year-old boy had an alleged history of snakebite and presented to the hospital with inability to open eyes well and difficulty in breathing. He is very anxious and is having tachycardia and tachypnea. On examination, bite mark cannot be visualized and there is no swelling of the limb. He has bilateral ptosis. His 20-minute whole blood clotting test is good quality. What is the next course of action?

a. Do not give anti-snake venom (ASV), but observe the patient.

b. Give ASV and keep the patient in observation.

c. Give ASV, and give neostigmine and observe the patient.

d. Reassure the patient and send him home with anxiolytic.

Q.5 Magnan's symptoms are characteristic symptoms with which poisoning?

a. Alcohol

b. Charas

c. Cocaine

d. Ecstasy

Q.6 Which of the following is the correct xenobiotic: toxicity pair?

a. Adriamycin: tubular proteinuria

b. Polyvinyl alcohol: disseminated intravascular coagulation

c. Hydralazine: renal papillary necrosis

d. Maleic acid: mesangial fibrosis

e. Gold: glomerulonephritis

Q.7 The primary site of kidney damage resulting from acute exposure to inorganic mercury salts is the

a. glomerulus

b. proximal tubule

c. loop of Henle

d. renal papilla

e. entire nephron

Q.8 Which substance has been identified as a respiratory tract carcinogen in humans?

a. Kaolin

b. Hydrogen fluoride

c. Arsenic

d. Cotton dust

e. Vanadium

Q.9 Chloracne is associated with

a. prominent hyperkeratosis of the follicular canal

b. production of excessive sebum

c. exposure to halogenated aliphatic hydrocarbons

d. exposure to chlorine gas

e. increases in serum androgen levels

Q.10 Toxic injury to the cell body, axon, and surrounding Schwann cells of peripheral nerves are referred to, respectively, as
   a. neuropathy, axonopathy, and myelopathy
   b. neuronopathy, axonopathy, and myelinopathy
   c. neuropathy, axonopathy, and gliosis
   d. neuronopathy, dying-back neuropathy, and myelopathy
   e. chromatolysis, axonopathy, and glia cells

Answers

1. a; 2. d; 3. b; 4. c; 5. C; 6. e; 7. b; 8. c; 9. a; 10. b.

Exercise 6

Q.1 A person was brought by police from the railway platform. He is talking irrelevant. He is having dry mouth with hot skin, dilated pupils, staggering gait, and slurred speech. The most probable diagnosis is
   a. alcohol intoxication
   b. carbamates poisoning
   c. organophosphorus poisoning
   d. datura poisoning

Q.2 Regarding methanol poisoning:
   Assertion: Administration of ethanol is one of the treatment modalities.
   Reason: Ethanol inhibits alcohol dehydrogenase.
   Please select the most correct option from the following:
   a. Both assertion and reason are true, and the reason is the correct explanation for the assertion.
   b. Both assertion and reason are true, and the reason is not the correct explanation for the assertion.
   c. Assertion is true, but the reason is false.
   d. Assertion is false, but the reason is true.

Q.3 In methyl alcohol poisoning, there is CNS depression, cardiac depression, and optic nerve atrophy. These effects are produced due to:
   a. formaldehyde and formic acid
   b. acetaldehyde
   c. pyridine
   d. acetic acid

Q.4 A 39-year-old carpenter has taken two bottles of liquor from the local shop. After about an hour, he develops confusion, vomiting, and blurring of vision. He has been brought to the emergency department. He should be given
   a. naloxone
   b. diazepam
   c. flumazenil
   d. ethyl alcohol

Q.5 Phosphine liberated in the stomach in Aluminum phosphide poisoning is toxic to all except
  a. lungs
  b. kidneys
  c. liver
  d. heart

Q.6 Paraquat poisoning causes
  a. renal failure
  b. cardiac failure
  c. respiratory failure
  d. multiple organ failure

Q.7 Ecstasy toxicity causes
  a. hyperreflexia
  b. trismus
  c. dilated pupils
  d. visual hallucinations
  e. All of the above

Q.8 A housewife ingests a rodenticide white powder accidentally. She is brought to hospital where the examination shows generalized, flaccid paralysis and an irregular pulse. Electrocardiogram shows multiple ventricular ectopics, generalized changes with ST-T. Serum potassium is 2.5 mEq/L. The most likely ingested poison is:
  a. barium carbonate
  b. super warfarins
  c. zinc phosphide
  d. aluminum phosphide

Q.9 All of the following are treatment options for toxic alcohol poisoning except
  a. fomepizole
  b. hydroxycobalamin
  c. thiamine
  d. folic acid
  e. pyridoxine

Q.10 Hyperthermia in a patient of poisoning is a pointer to all except
  a. ecstasy
  b. selective serotonin reuptake inhibitor
  c. salicylates
  d. chlorpromazine

Answer

1.d; 2. a; 3. a; 4. d; 5. b; 6. d; 7. e; 8. a; 9. b; 10. d.

Exercise 7

Q.1 Digoxin immune Fab therapy is NOT indicated in which of the following natural teas/broths
  a. Oleander
  b. Lily of the valley
  c. Cane toad
  d. Sea Horse

Q.2 With respect to theophylline toxicity, which is FALSE
  a. Anxiety, vomiting, and tremor are early manifestations.
  b. It can precipitate supraventricular tachycardia.
  c. Hypoglycemia, hypophosphatemia, and hypomagnesaemia are complications.
  d. Beta blockers are contraindicated.

Q.3 Which of the following paired agents or syndrome/interventions is FALSE
  a. Anticholinergic agents: Physostigmine
  b. Neuroleptic Malignant syndrome: Bromocryptine
  c. Serotonin syndrome: Cyproheptadine
  d. Organophosphates: Atropine, pyridoxine

Q.4 Regarding clozapine overdose, which is TRUE:
  a. Ingestion of a single tablet in a child needs assessment in hospital.
  b. Acute poisoning is associated with agranulocytosis.
  c. Patients typically become comatose and require endotracheal intubation with significant overdose.
  d. Overdose is not associated with anticholinergic effects.

Q.5 All of the following is true regarding iron overdose, EXCEPT:
  a. a serum iron level should be done 12 hours following ingestion.
  b. an anion-gap metabolic acidosis is typical.
  c. activated charcoal is not indicated as it does not adsorb iron.
  d. abdominal x-ray may be useful.

Q.6 With regard to iron overdose which statement is FALSE?
  a. Accidental childhood ingestion is usually not serious.
  b. Desferrioxamine is indicated if there are signs of systemic toxicity or a 4- to 6-hour level of >90 μmol/L
  c. Whole Bowel Irrigation is recommended for ingestions of >60 mg/kg confirmed on x-ray.
  d. Significant toxicity causes a normal anion-gap acidosis.

Q.7 Which of the following significant toxic ingestions would NOT require early activated charcoal to ensure a good outcome?
  a. Paraquat $>$ 50 mg/kg
  b. Sodium Valproate $>$ 1 g/kg
  c. Colchicine $>$ 0.8 mg/kg
  d. Bupropion $>$ 9 g

Q.8 Common causes of toxic seizures in Australia include all EXCEPT
  a. alcohol
  b. tramadol
  c. venlafaxine
  d. bupropion
Q.9 A drug that can mimic brain death when taken in overdose is?
  a. thiopentone
  b. propranolol
  c. quetiapine
  d. baclofen
Q.10 Which of the following statements regarding clozapine overdose is TRUE:
  a. A child that ingested a single tablet needs to be assessed and observed in hospital.
  b. Acute poisoning is associated with agranulocytosis.
  c. Patients typically become comatose and require endotracheal intubation with significant overdose.
  d. Patients need to be observed in hospital for at least 24 hours.

Answers

1. d; 2. d; 3. d; 4. a; 5. a; 6. d; 7. b; 8. a; 9. d; 10. a.

Exercise 8

Q.1 All of the following is true regarding iron overdose, EXCEPT:
  a. A serum iron level should be done 12 hours following ingestion.
  b. An anion-gap metabolic acidosis is typical.
  c. Activated charcoal is not indicated as it does not adsorb iron.
  d. Hypoglycemia is a rare feature of severe iron poisoning.
Q.2 Which of the following is NOT a benign presentation?
  a. A child with a normal GIT who bites a mercury thermometer and swallows some mercury
  b. A child who ingests 30 mg/kg of elemental iron
  c. A child who ingests one of her brother's risperidone tablets
  d. A child who ingests 1 g metformin
Q.3 Which pairing is INCORRECT?
  a. Lead encephalopathy—sodium calcium edetate
  b. Isoniazid overdose—pyridoxine
  c. Methemoglobinemia—methylene blue
  d. Methotrexate overdose—cyproheptadine
Q.4 Amisulpride overdose commonly results in:
  a. abrupt cardiovascular collapse up to 12 hours postingestion with large
  b. overdoses
  c. torsades at doses of 2–4 g
  d. serotonin syndrome if coingested with a serotonergic compound
  e. seizures with massive overdose

Q.5 Which of the following statements regarding sympathomimetic toxicity is INCORRECT?
  a. MDMA may cause SIADH.
  b. Cocaine is a sodium channel blocker.
  c. Lignocaine is used as a second-line agent to control ventricular dysrhythmias in cocaine overdose.
  d. Beta blockers are used as a first-line agent to control hypertension and tachycardia in methamphetamine overdose.

Q.6 Which of the following is TRUE regarding β-blocker toxicity?
  a. Propranolol facilitates sodium entry into cells resulting in QT prolongation on ECG.
  b. Significant toxicity is usually apparent within 6 hours.
  c. Sotalol is the only β-blocker, which causes QT prolongation.
  d. β-Blocker overdose causes decreased intracellular cAMP concentrations.

Q.7 Regarding calcium channel blockers (CCB):
  a. Nifedipine produces more cardiotoxic effects than verapamil.
  b. Activated charcoal therapy is not indicated in CCB overdose.
  c. Calcium and glucagon form the mainstay of treatment in CCB overdose.
  d. Standard CCB preparations are rapidly absorbed from the GI tract with onset of action within 30 minutes.

Q.8 Regarding warfarin, which is FALSE?
  a. Activated charcoal may be useful for decontamination.
  b. A normal INR at 48 hours excludes acute warfarin ingestion.
  c. Prothrombinex contains Factors II, IX, and X.
  d. Superwarfarin ingestion is rarely fatal.

Q.9 Regarding β-blocker toxicity, which is FALSE?
  a. Activated charcoal may be useful for decontamination.
  b. Sotalol is associated with prolonged QRS.
  c. Seizures are seen in propranolol poisoning.
  d. PR prolongation is an early sign of toxicity.

Q.10 Which medication is NOT implicated in serotonin syndrome?
  a. Fentanyl
  b. Ondansetron
  c. Valproic acid
  d. Mirtazapine

Answer

1. a; 2. c; 3. d; 4. a; 5. b; 6. d; 7. b; 8. c; 9. b; 10. d.

Exercise 9

Q.1 Which one of the following is true concerning salicylate intoxication?
  a. High blood levels cannot be removed by dialysis.
  b. If a respiratory alkalosis is present, do not administer intravenous bicarbonate.

    c. Salicylate intoxication causes both a metabolic acidosis and a metabolic alkalosis.

    d. The recommended treatment is intravenous fluids without dextrose.

    e. Oil of wintergreen can cause salicylate poisoning.

Q.2 A 35-year-old woman presents with an acute lithium overdose. Which one of the following statements concerning lithium is true?

    a. Aggressive diuresis is needed to augment lithium excretion.

    b. Hypocalcemia can be seen as a side effect of lithium.

    c. Lithium cannot be removed by dialysis.

    d. It is recommended that you avoid the use of saline in lithium intoxication.

    e. You should evaluate thyroid function in anyone taking lithium.

Q.3 Which one of the following is the treatment for a heparin overdose?

    a. Vitamin K

    b. Fresh frozen plasma

    c. Protamine sulfate

    d. Desmopressin acetate (DDAVP)

    e. Cryoprecipitate

Q.4 Which one of the following antidotes matches the underlying toxicity?

    a. Benzodiazepines—naloxone (Narcan)

    b. Narcotics—flumazenil (Romazicon)

    c. Ethylene glycol—ethanol (booze)

    d. Acetaminophen—fomepizole (4-methylpyrazole)

    e. High carboxyhemoglobin—methylene blue

Q.5 Which one of the following statements concerning digoxin is true?

    a. Digoxin is used in treating diastolic heart failure.

    b. Digoxin toxicity is treated with dialysis.

    c. Digoxin dosing must be increased when kidney disease is present.

    d. Amiodarone and quinidine can decrease digoxin levels.

    e. Hypokalemia can exacerbate digoxin toxicity.

Q.6 A patient had a fever and altered mental status. He was recently started on fluphenazine (Prolixin). He is agitated and his temperature is 39.4°C (103°F). His blood pressure is 160/100 mmHg. A CPK level is 50,000. What is the most appropriate treatment at this time?

    a. Urgent hemodialysis

    b. Intravenous saline alone for the rhabdomyolysis

    c. Lorazepam (Ativan) for agitation

    d. Dantrolene

    e. Cyproheptadine

Q.7 Humans have died from an immune reaction, referred to as _____ caused by fly bites.

    a. diphtheria toxic shock

    b. heart inflammation

    c. typhoid fever

    d. anaphylactic shock

Q.8 All of the following symptoms are commonly found in sympathomimetic intoxications except _____.

a. agitation

b. tachycardia and hypertension

c. hyperthermia

d. dry, flushed skin

e. mydriasis

Q.9 All of the following are effectively bound to activated charcoal except

_____.

a. acetaminophen

b. tricyclic antidepressant

c. iron

d. theophylline

e. salicylates

Q.10 What is the most important therapy in the management of a serious benzodiazepine ingestion?

a. Multidose activated charcoal

b. Alkaline diuresis

c. Aggressive airway management

d. Cardiac monitoring

e. Hemodialysis

Answers

1. e; 2. e; 3. c; 4.c; 5. e; 6.d; 7.d; 8. d; 9. c; 10. c.

Exercise 10

Q.1 Which of the following is not a side effect of digoxin toxicity?

a. Bradycardia

b. Yellow vision changes

c. Scooping of the T-segment on ECG

d. Hypokalemia

e. Gynecomastia

Q.2 Which of the following chelating agents is recommended for acute lead poisoning with signs of encephalopathy?

a. Succimer

b. Penicillamine

c. Dimercaprol

d. Calcium EDTA

e. Dimercaprol + Calcium EDTA

Q.3 Which of the following dermatologic findings and potential causes is incorrect?

a. Cyanosis—Methemoglobinemia

b. Erythroderma—Boric Acid

    c. Pallor—Carbon Monoxide

    d. Jaundice—Hypercarotenemia (excess carrot intake)

    e. Brightly flushed skin—Niacin

Q.4 All of the following symptoms can occur with ciguatera poisoning except

_____.

    a. myalgias

    b. flushing

    c. metallic taste

    d. reversal of temperature sensation

    e. sensation of loose, painful teeth

Q.5 Which of the following is true with regard to acetaminophen toxicity?

    a. The Rumack-Matthew nomogram may be used for both acute and chronic ingestions.

    b. The APAP level should ideally be checked within 1–4 hours of ingestion.

    c. The Rumack-Matthew nomogram applies for ingestions up to 48 hours postingestion.

    d. N-acetylcysteine should be started within 8 hours of ingestion if an APAP level cannot be obtained.

    e. Activated charcoal should be used for all sustained release ingestions.

Q.6 All of the following statements concerning acetaminophen toxicity are except:

    a. Hepatotoxicity occurs because of a depletion of glutathione.

    b. Drugs that enhance the cytochrome P450 system diminish the toxic potential.

    c. Signs of hepatotoxicity do not occur until at least 8 hours postingestion.

    d. Hepatic necrosis is centrilobular in distribution.

    e. Cimetidine may be protective because of its ability to diminish hepatic metabolism.

Q.7 Ophotoxemia refers to:

    a. organophosphorus poisoning

    b. heavy metal poisoning

    c. scorpion venom poisoning

    d. snake venom poisoning

Q.8 Elapidaes are:

    a. vasculotoxic

    b. neurotoxic

    c. musculotoxic

    d. nontoxic

Q.9 All of the following are treatment options for toxic alcohol poisoning, except:

    a. fomepizole

    b. hydroxocobalamin

    c. thiamine

   d. folic Acid

   e. pyridoxine

Answer

1. d; 2. e; 3.c; 4. b; 5. d; 6. b; 7. d; 8. b; 9. b.

Exercise 11

Q.1 Which is FALSE regarding paraquat poisoning?
  a. Supplemental oxygen should be avoided.
  b. It is associated with "paraquat tongue."
  c. A raised creatinine carries a poor prognosis.
  d. Paraquat has an effect on the neuromuscular junction.

Q.2 Which of the following drug:antidote pairs is least appropriate in the ED
  a. Hydrofluoric acid burn:calcium chloride
  b. Cyanide poisoning:thiosulfate
  c. Clonidine overdose:naloxone
  d. Benzodiazepine overdose: flumazenil

Q.3 Which statement is FALSE?
  a. In anticholinergic syndrome death may result from hyperthermia and dysrhythmias.
  b. Oil of wintergreen ingestion is associated with altered mental state, respiratory alkalosis, metabolic acidosis, and tinnitus.
  c. Serotonin syndrome is associated with ocular myoclonus and hyperreflexia.
  d. Cyproheptadine may be of benefit in neuroleptic malignant syndrome.

Q.4 Which statement is FALSE in regard to lithium poisoning?
  a. Peak serum levels occur within 2−4 hours of oral ingestion.
  b. Significant ECG changes only occur at very high serum levels.
  c. Clinical features of lithium toxicity can be observed even when serum levels are in the normal range.
  d. Neurological features dominate the clinical presentation.

Q.5 Which statement is FALSE in regard to theophylline poisoning?
  a. The precise mechanism of toxicity is unknown.
  b. Serum levels will confirm poisoning and are invaluable in ongoing management.
  c. Seizures refractory to benzodiazepines should be treated with second-line agents including phenytoin and phenobarbitone.
  d. Poisoning associated with chronic use is more common than acute ingestions.

Q.6 Which of the following is NOT a feature of pure fast sodium channel blockade
  a. QRS widening
  b. Tachycardia
  c. VT
  d. VF

Q.7 In regards to β-blockers, which is FALSE?
  a. Poisoning with most β-blockers is usually benign.
  b. Insulin:dextrose therapy may have a role.
  c. NaHCO3 has an occasional role.
  d. Most symptomatic overdoses exhibit bradycardia.

Q.8 Regarding activated charcoal, which is INCORRECT:
  a. The enormous surface area provided by these particles of charcoal irreversibly absorbs most ingested toxins preventing further absorption from the GI tract.
  b. The major risk is charcoal pulmonary aspiration due to loss of airway reflexes associated with impaired consciousness or seizures.
  c. Ileus is not a contraindication to single dose activated charcoal.
  d. Multiple dose activated charcoal has the potential to enhance drug elimination by interruption to enterohepatic circulation and gastrointestinal dialysis.
  e. There are no data to support the use of activated charcoal in sorbitol or other cathartic agent over activated charcoal in water.

Q.9 Regarding urinary alkalinization, which is INCORRECT:
  a. Production of alkaline urine prevents reabsorption across the renal tubular epithelium thus promoting excretion in the urine.
  b. In salicylate overdose metabolism is saturated and the elimination half-life greatly prolonged.
  c. Severe established salicylate toxicity warrants a trial of urinary alkalinization rather than immediate hemodialysis.
  d. In phenobarbitone coma, multidose activated charcoal is superior to urinary alkalinization as first line.

Q.10 Which of the following statements is FALSE with regards the toxicokinetics of phenytoin?
  a. HONK is a recognized complication.
  b. Is a Na Channel blocker.
  c. Causes QRS widening.
  d. Shares the same order of elimination kinetics as salicylate.

Answer

1. d; 2. d; 3. d; 4. b; 5. c; 6. b; 7. d; 8. a; 9. c; 10. c.

16.6.3 FILL IN THE BLANKS

Exercise 12

Q.1 The type of evidence seen at the time of poisoning is referred as _____.

Q.2 The most common feed contaminant that can be expected during improper storage is _____.

Q.3 Pink coloration in urine is suggestive of poisoning due to _____.
Q.4 Phenols and cresols produce _____ coloration of urine.
Q.5 The symptoms or lesions that are characteristic to a particular toxicant are known as _____.
Q.6 The evidence that is obtained during postmortem examination is known as _____ evidence.
Q.7 Bitter almond smell of ruminal contents is suggestive of _____.
Q.8 Poisoning with phosphorus results in _____ odor during postmortem examination.
Q.9 The detection of toxic material in body using laboratory methods constitutes _____ evidence.
Q.10 The evidence that is obtained by feeding suspected material (feed) to healthy animals to ascertain the presence of toxicant is _____.

Answers
1. CIRCUMSTANCIAL EVIDENCE; 2. MYCOTOXINS (Aflatoxin); 3. PHENOTHIAZINES; 4. GREEN; 5. PATHOGNOMONIC (symptom or lesion); 6. PATHOLOGICAL; 7. CYANIDE POISONING; 8. GARLIC-LIKE; 9. ANALYTICAL; 10. EXPERIMENTAL EVIDENCE.

Exercise 13
Q.1 The aim of treatment during poisoning is to _____ the threshold of the toxicant.
Q.2 The time versus concentration curve of toxicant in the body is shaped _____.
Q.3 The AP of the time—concentration of toxicant curve represents _____.
Q.4 The DP of the time—concentration of toxicant curve represents _____.
Q.5 When emesis is contraindicated, the safest alternative is _____.
Q.6 The most commonly used adsorbing agent to bind toxicants in GIT is _____.
Q.7 The type of diuretics or purgatives that are preferred in cases of poisoning is _____.
Q.8 When a large amount of toxicant is absorbed into the body or when renal failure occurs ensues, the method of choice employed for elimination of the toxicant is _____.
Q.9 The mechanism involved in the enhanced elimination of acidic agents in alkalized urine and basic agents in acidified urine is _____.
Q.10 The substance that counteracts or neutralizes a toxicant is known as _____.

Answers

1. INCREASE (Measures are directed to create a situation where more toxicant is required to produce the toxicity); 2. BELL OR INVERTED "U"; 3. ABSORPTION; 4. EXCRETION; 5. GASTRIC LAVAGE (In case of ruminants, rumen lavage or rumenotomy can be performed); 6. ACTIVATED CHARCOAL (Charcoal should be activated through burning (oxidation) which increases the number of pores and thus the surface area); 7. OSMOTIC/SALINE TYPE (Osmotic or saline type of agents are the only category, which actually drag water from the organs or body. However, for prompt action, furosemide, which is a loop diuretic is also used); 8. DYLASIS; 9. ION TRAPPING (The process of ion trapping also occurs for basic drugs in the acidic pH of rumen, due to the production of volatile fatty acid); 10. ANTIDOTE.

Exercise 14

Q.1 Ethanol acts as an antidote for methanol poisoning by _____.

Q.2 The antidote for alkaloids is _____.

Q.3 The antidote for paracetamol (acetaminophen) toxicity is _____.

Q.4 The agents, which are used in case of CNS depression and respiratory arrest, are called as _____.

Q.5 Secondary photosensitization in Lantana camara is mainly due to _____.

Q.6 The phytoconstituents of *Lantana camara*, which cause bile duct occlusion and liver damage, are _____.

Q.7 Hepatic lesions such as _____ and _____ are diagnostic in differentiation primary and secondary photosensitization.

Q.8 Plasma from blood can be prepared by adding _____ in the blood.

Q.9 Serum can be prepared by letting the collected patient's blood clot. The resulting supernatant is called _____.

Q.10 Elapidaes (snakes) are _____.

Answers

1. COMPETITIVE INHIBITION (Mechanism); 2. POTASSIUM PERMANGANATE (KMNO4 acts by oxidizing the alkaloids); 3. N-ACETYL CYSTEINE (Paracetamol toxicity is common worldwide and is leading cause for acute liver failure in the United Kingdom and the United States. Continuous use for a week is likely to cause hepatotoxicity. The toxicity is due to depletion of liver stores of glutathione, which is required for conjugation of metabolite of paracetamol); 4. ANALEPTICS. (e.g., doxapram); 5. BILE DUCT OCCLUSION; 6. LANTADENE A and B; 7. FIBROSIS and BILIARY HYPERPLASIA; 8. ANTICOAGULANT; 9. SERUM; 10. NUEROTOXIC.

16.6.4 MATCH THE STATEMENTS

Exercise 15

Q. Match the column A with column B.

Q	Column A (Poison)		Column B (Antidote/Antagonist)
1	Arsenic	A	Atropine/pralidoxime
2	Cyanide	B	Fuller's earth
3	Methanol	C	Dimercaprol
4	Paraquat	D	Ethanol
5	Parathion	E	Sodium nitrite/sodium thiosulfate
6	Lead	F	N-acetyl cysteine
7	Paracetamol	G	EDTA
8	LSD	H	Gun metal kidney
9	Thalidomide	I	Abuse
10	Copper	J	Teratogenicity

Answer

	Column A (Poison)		Column B (Antidote/Antagonist)
1	Arsenic	A	Dimercaprol
2	Cyanide	B	Sodium nitrite/sodium thiosulfate
3	Methanol	C	Ethanol
4	Paraquat	D	Fuller's earth
5	Parathion	E	Atropine/pralidoxime
6	Lead	F	EDTA
7	Paracetamol	G	N-acetyl cysteine
8	LSD	H	Abuse
9	Thalidomide	I	Teratogenicity
10	Copper	J	Gun metal kidney

FURTHER READING

Branch, S., 2010. Forensic and clinical toxicology. In: Hodgson, E.A. (Ed.), A Text book of Modern Toxicology, 4th edition John Wiley, New Jersey, pp. 399–409.

Cantilena Jr., L.R., 2013. Clinical toxicology. In: Klaassen, C.D. (Ed.), Casarett and Doull's Toxicology: The Basic Science of Poisons, 8th ed McGraw-Hill, New York, pp. 1375–1390.

Gupta, P.K., 1988. Veterinary Toxicology. Cosmo Publications, New Delhi, India, Chapter 15.

Gupta, P.K., 1988. Veterinary Toxicology. Cosmo Publications, New Delhi, India (Chapter 11).

Gupta, P.K., 2010. Mechanism of antidotal therapy. In: 2nd reprint Gupta, P.K. (Ed.), Modern Toxicology: The Adverse Effects of Xenobiotics, Vol. 3. PharmaMed Press, Hyderabad, India, pp. 244–264.

Gupta, P.K., 2010. Principles of non-specific therapy. In: 2nd reprint Gupta, P.K. (Ed.), Modern Toxicology: The Adverse Effects of Xenobiotics, Vol. 3. PharmaMed Press, Hyderabad, India, pp. 210–243.

Gupta, P.K., 2016. Fundamental in Toxicology: Essential Concepts and Applications in Toxicology. Elsevier/BSP, San Diego, USA.

Leidy, R.B., 2010. Toxicant Analysis and Quality Assurance Principles. In: Hodgson, E.A. (Ed.), A Text book of Modern Toxicology, 4th edition John Wiley, New Jersey, pp. 23–28.

Leidy, R.B., 2010. Analytical Methods in Toxicology. In: Hodgson, E.A. (Ed.), A Text book of Modern Toxicology, 4th edition John Wiley, New Jersey, pp. 441–461.

Manual, M., 2006. Poisoning. Merck Research Laboratories, Merck & Co. Inc., pp. 2651–2695.

Pillay, V.V., 2008. Comprehensive Medical Toxicology, 2nd edition Paras Medical Publisher, Hyderabad, India, Chapter 3.

Poklis, A., 2013. Analytical and Forensic Toxicology. In: Klaassen, C.D. (Ed.), Casarett and Doull's Toxicology: The Basic Science of Poisons, 8th ed McGraw-Hill, New York, pp. 1357–1374.

Rao, G.N., 2010. Textbook of Forensic Medicine & Toxicology. Jaypee Brothers Medical Publishers, New Delhi, India (Chapter 31).

Brainstorming: Toxicology question bank

Illustrated Toxicology. DOI: http://dx.doi.org/10.1016/B978-0-12-813213-5.00017-1

17.1 SHORT QUESTIONS

Exercise 1

Q.1 Write short notes on classification of poisons.
Q.2 Write short notes on chronicity factor.
Q.3 Write short notes on clinical evidences for diagnosis of poisoning.
Q.4 Write short notes on distribution of toxicants.
Q.5 Write short notes on universal antidote.
Q.6 Define toxicoepidemiology.
Q.7 Define mutagenicity.
Q.8 Define RfD.
Q.9 Differentiate between toxin and venom.
Q.10 Differentiate between subacute and chronic poisoning.

Exercise 2

Q.1 Differentiate between toxicokinetics and toxicodynamics.
Q.2 Differentiate between exposure-related factors and animal-related factors that modify toxicant action.
Q.3 Define enterotoxin.
Q.4 Define radiation.
Q.5 Define cyanogenetic glycosides.
Q.6 Define resinoids.

Q.7 Write short notes on gastric lavage.
Q.8 Write short notes on copper poisoning.
Q.9 Write short notes on molybdenum poisoning.
Q.10 Write short notes on treatment of cyanide poisoning.

Exercise 3

Q.1 Write short notes on treatment of nitrite poisoning.
Q.2 Define pyrethroids.
Q.3 Define peat scour.
Q.4 Define blind staggers.
Q.5 Define alkali disease.
Q.6 Define sui or sutari poisoning.
Q.7 Differentiate between blind staggers and alkali disease.
Q.8 Differentiate between ionizing and nonionizing radiation.
Q.9 Differentiate between risk and hazard.
Q.10 Differentiate between bracken fern toxicity in ruminants and nonruminants.

Exercise 4

Q.1 Write short notes on the treatment of organophophorus (OP) compound poisoning.
Q.2 Write short notes on residue analysis.
Q.3 Write short notes on abrus poisoning.
Q.4 Differentiate between treatment of OP compound and carbamate poisoning.
Q.5 Differentiate between natural hazards and man-made hazards.
Q.6 Differentiate between phase I and phase II metabolism with relation to toxicokinetics.
Q.7 Differentiate between elapid venom and crotalid venom.
Q.8 Differentiate between clinical signs of lead poisoning in cattle and horses.
Q.9 Write short notes on treatment of OP compound poisoning.
Q.10 Write short notes on residue analysis.

Exercise 5

Q.1 Why are potently toxic chemicals sometimes used as antidotes? Give two examples.
Q.2 Barbiturate (sodium barbituric acid, pKa = 7.3) overdose is often treated with i.v. sodium bicarbonate. Explain the basis for this therapy.
Q.3 Why sometimes the very young or the health-conscious person gets cancer, while the 95-year-old lifelong smoker does not?
Q.4 Give two main reasons why amphibole is regarded as the more potent and higher risk form of asbestos compared to serpentine type 17.
Q.5 Why thallium is a popular poison for murders?
Q.6 Why unbleached (brown) paper is increasingly used for consumer items like coffee filters.
Q.7 Why warfarin poisoning in people is rare?

Q.8 Why "Bay region" Polycyclic aromatic hydrocarbons (PAHs) are more carcinogenic than those without a bay region?

Q.9 Why Pralidoxime (2-PAM) not used in treatment of malathion poisoning?

Q.10 Why terracing gardens with used railroad ties is a bad idea?

Exercise 6

Q.1 Why PAHs naturally occur in the environment?

Q.2 Why would omission of trace histidine cause a false-negative response in the Ames assay?

Q.3 Plasma clearance (Pc) and volume of distribution (Vd) values of drugs are often correlated. Why?

Q.4 Vinyl chloride is carcinogenic; polyvinyl chloride is not. Why?

Q.5 Methanol is only mildly potent but can be very hazardous. Why?

Q.6 The new designer aerosol rodent spray "A," has an oral LD50 in rats of 20 mg/kg, an LD2 of 1 mg/kg, and an LD99 of 38 mg/kg. Draw the dose—response curves for spray "A" when (1) the x-axis is plotted with an arithmetic and logarithmic scales (i.e., show two curves) and (2) a curve when the response is plotted using a probit scale. Label all curves and show how the LD values are obtained.

Q.7 It is found that a toxin is more toxic when it is given in one large dose than when it is administered in small doses given at 6- to 8-hour intervals. It takes a larger total dose to produce the same effect when it is given in small increments than when the toxin is given as one large dose. Give at least three reasons to explain this phenomenon.

Q.8 Repair is an important process that may ultimately determine whether a chemical will manifest toxicity. Describe briefly the three levels of repair and give an example of each.

Q.9 Discuss four major anatomic and physiological properties that are responsible for the "blood—brain barrier" in the central nervous system (CNS).

Q.10 Explain what is an LD50 or ED50. Why are these values used to compare toxic responses of organisms to chemicals instead of lower or higher values?

Exercise 7

Q.1 Describe four potential storage depots for toxicants. Provide an example of a storage mechanism or a type of toxicant that is stored in each depot.

Q.2 A contaminant in the local drinking water is at a concentration of 0.2 mg/mL. What will be the average daily dose (mg/kg) of the contaminant for a mouse? Mouse water consumption per day is 5 mL and the mouse weight is 30 g.

Q.3 Explain the various aspects of nitrite poisoning.

Q.4 Give an account of urea toxicity.

Q.5 What are the various sources of cyanide poisoning?

Q.6 Mention the various groups of alkaloids that are toxic and give an account of any three alkaloidal toxicity.

Q.7 Write a brief account of aflatoxins.

Q.8 Describe briefly mechanism of cyanide poisoning.

Q.9 Explain how cyanide toxicity could be treated.

Q.10 Explain the mode of action of selenium poisoning.

Exercise 8

Q.1 What are some general considerations for dermal decontamination?

Q.2 What are the sources of thiaminase affecting horses?

Q.3 What are the most common clinical signs of Bufo toad poisoning?

Q.4 What are the proper samples to be sent to a laboratory to rule out cholinesterase inhibitors?

Q.5 Describe in brief absorption and fate of arsenic poisoning.

Q.6 Describe in brief clinical symptoms of arsenic poisoning.

Q.7 What is the treatment of arsenic poisoning in human beings?

Q.8 Give a detailed account of lead poisoning.

Q.9 How does selenium poisoning occur?

Q.10 Explain in brief how iron causes toxicity.

Exercise 9

Q.1 Write short notes on abrus poisoning.

Q.2 Write short notes on treatment of OP compound poisoning.

Q.3 What is the mechanism of action of carbamate insecticides?

Q.4 What is the most common cause of death due to Bufo toad poisoning?

Q.5 Why is zinc phosphide less toxic on an empty stomach?

Q.6 Explain in brief the common causes of poisoning in animals.

Q.7 What are general approaches for the diagnosis of poisoning?

Q.8 Explain the various mechanisms by which toxicants act.

Q.9 Explain how various factors modify the action of toxicants.

Q.10 Give an account of the general line of treatment of poisoning.

Exercise 10

Q.1 Describe lethal synthesis with an example.

Q.2 Discuss when will you use gastric lavage and when will you use emetics.

Q.3 Write short notes on use of chelators in veterinary practice.

Q.4 Write short notes on enzootic hematuria.

Q.5 Write short notes on residue analysis.

Q.6 Write short notes on abrus poisoning.

Q.7 Write short notes on treatment of OP compound poisoning.

Q.8 Write short note on nitrate poisoning in cattle.

Q.9 What is the best method of treatment for nitrate poisoning.

Q.10 Write short notes on castor bean poisoning.

Exercise 11

Q.1 Explain how the specific antidotes produce their action and give a detailed account of the various specific antidotes available for veterinary practice.

Q.2 Give an account of the sources of arsenic poisoning.

Q.3 Describe in mechanism of toxicity of arsenic poisoning.

Q.4 Write short notes on nerium poisoning

Q.5 Write short notes on acceptable daily intake.

Q.6 Write short notes on preservatives in animal feed.

Q.7 Write short notes on Minamata disease.

Q.8 Describe clinical signs associated with botulinum poisoning.

Q.9 What causes a pH of more than 8.5 in ruminant and how will you treat this case?

Q.10 Write short notes on when an animal comes after being drenched in insecticide.

17.2 MULTIPLE CHOICE QUESTIONS

None, one, or more of the selections may be correct (Choose one, two, or all correct answers).

Exercise 12

Q.1 What is toxicology?
   a. The field that studies the adverse effects on humans and animals.
   b. The field that studies the adverse effects of chemicals on living organisms.
   c. The field that studies the adverse effects of chemicals and microorganisms.
   d. The field that studies the risk−benefit balance of chemicals for living organisms.

Q.2 Indicate which persons played an important role in the history of toxicology.
   a. Hippocrates
   b. *Atropa belladonna*
   c. Paracelsus
   d. Van 't Hoff
   e. Rachel Carson
   f. St. Anthony
   g. Orfila

Q.3 Indicate which chemicals played an important role in the history of modern toxicology (indicate all that apply).
   a. Mercury
   b. Dioxins

    c. DDT

    d. Alcohol

    e. Softanon

Q.4 Which of the following areas of study is not part of preclinical trials?

    a. Toxicology

    b. Drug metabolism

    c. Pharmacology

    d. Structure–activity relationships

Q.5 Which of the following terms is used to describe the dose of a drug required to produce a measurable effect in 50% of the animals tested?

    a. LD50

    b. LD1

    c. ED50

    d. ED99

Q.6 Which of the following terms is used to describe the dose of a drug required to kill 50% of a group of animals?

    a. LD50

    b. LD1

    c. ED50

    d. ED99

Q.7 What is meant by the therapeutic ratio or index?

    a. The ratio of LD50 to ED99

    b. The ratio of LD50 to ED50

    c. The ratio of LD1 to LD50

    d. The ratio of ED99 to ED50

Q.8 What is true about the acceptable daily intake (ADI) or total daily intake (TDI)?

    a. The ADI is for nongenotoxic compounds, the TDI for genotoxic compounds.

    b. The ADI is used for additives and therefore larger safety factors are used to derive it from the no observed adverse effect level (NOAEL).

    c. The ADI may vary depending on the study from which the NOAEL is taken.

    d. The ADI and TDI are health-based safety limits and independent from the experimental design of the animal study from which it is derived.

    e. The TDI for a compound is generally higher than its ADI.

Q.9 What is true about in vitro testing?

    a. In vitro test alternatives for all in vivo end parameters will be available in the near future.

    b. Present in vitro tests can predict the carcinogenic potential of a compound.

    c. The hypoxanthine guanine phosphoribosyl transferase (HGPRT) test predicts genotoxicity for mammalian cells.

    d. The Mouse Lymphoma TK assay can predict both gene mutations as well as several chromosomal adverse effects.

    e. In vitro toxicity testing is most useful for genotoxicity and toxicokinetics.

Q.10 What are in vitro tests for detecting gene mutations?
  a. Comet assay
  b. Mouse Lymphoma TK assay
  c. S9 incubations
  d. Micronucleus test
  e. SCE test
  f. HGPRT test
  g. Microarray test
  h. Breast cell proliferation

Exercise 13

Q.1 What is (are) true about environmental risk assessment?
  a. In the quotient method the Predicted Estimated Concentration (PEC) is compared to the Predicted No Effect Concentration (PNEC).
  b. The PNEC is the equivalent of the NOAEL in food safety assessment.
  c. The PNEC is the equivalent of the ADI in food safety assessment.
  d. The PNEC is equivalent to the lowest observed adverse effect level in food safety assessment.

Q.2 What is true about human risk assessment?
  a. Well-conducted epidemiological studies can provide convincing evidence for human risk.
  b. Ames tests provide insight in human cancer risks.
  c. Interspecies and intraspecies differences are not taken into account when calculating cancer risks.
  d. For quantitative risk assessment, the benchmark dose provides an estimate that is less dependent on the experimental setup than the NOAEL approach.
  e. Exposure assessment is often a key area of uncertainty in human risk assessment.

Q.3 What is the best description for the benchmark dose?
  a. A dose that can be interpreted as a NOAEL but is defined in a better way.
  b. The dose that results in a defined, for example, 10% response.
  c. The dose that defines the sensitivity of a part of the population.
  d. A dose that defines the margin of safety, taking the statistical uncertainty into account.

Q.4 The role of safety factors is to take into account: (Indicate **all** that apply)
  a. Differences in life style factors
  b. Differences between species
  c. Differences in methods for exposure assessment
  d. Suboptimal study designs
  e. Differences in intake levels

Q.5 Which of the following techniques is the most suitable for detecting a metabolite labeled with 13C?
  a. Infrared spectroscopy
  b. Nuclear magnetic resonance spectroscopy
  c. Scintillation counting (detection of radioactivity)
  d. Mass spectrometry

Q.6 Which of the following techniques would be used to detect a metabolite labeled with 3H?
  a. Infrared spectroscopy
  b. Nuclear magnetic resonance spectroscopy
  c. Scintillation counting (detection of radioactivity)

Q.7 Which of the following techniques would be used to detect a metabolite labeled with 14C?
  a. Infrared spectroscopy
  b. Nuclear magnetic resonance spectroscopy
  c. Scintillation counting (detection of radioactivity)
  d. Mass spectrometry

Q.8 Which of the following techniques would be used to detect a metabolite labeled with 2H?
  a. Infrared spectroscopy
  b. Nuclear magnetic resonance spectroscopy
  c. Scintillation counting (detection of radioactivity)
  d. Mass spectrometry

Q.9 What sort of factors might affect the stability of a compound in a pharmaceutical preparation?
  a. Temperature and humidity
  b. UV and visible light
  c. Container and labels
  d. All of the above

Q.10 What term is applied to a drug which is effective against a relatively rare medical problem?
  a. New chemical entity
  b. Orphan drug
  c. Lead compound
  d. Parent drug

Exercise 14

Q.1 All of the following statements are true of the P-gp, Mrp2, Mrp4, and Bcrp transport systems that contribute to the blood−brain barrier except:
  a. They are located on the luminal side of the capillary endothelial cell.
  b. They can efflux uncharged molecules.
  c. They do not require energy from ATP.
  d. Some can efflux anionic or cationic molecules.

Q.2 All of the following statements are true of the blood—brain barrier except:
   a. It is not fully developed at birth.
   b. It is remarkably constant throughout all areas of the brain.
   c. Lipid-soluble chemicals will penetrate faster.
   d. Ionized chemicals will penetrate slower.

Q.3 Elemental mercury is poorly absorbed orally because of
   a. large particle size
   b. efflux transporters
   c. formation of insoluble complexes with phosphate
   d. All of the above

Q.4 Aqueous pores are primarily involved in the transport of _____
   a. small hydrophobic molecules
   b. large hydrophobic molecules
   c. small hydrophilic molecules
   d. large hydrophilic molecules

Q.5 The agent with the largest octane/water partition coefficient is

   _____
   a. paraquat
   b. ethylene
   c. acetic acid
   d. 2,3,7,8-TETRACHLORODIBENZO-P-DIOXIN (TCDD)

Q.6 In renal glomeruli, pores allow molecules to pass through that are smaller than _____
   a. 60 kDa
   b. 30 kDa
   c. 15 kDa
   d. 5 kDa

Q.7 Most of the vital nutrients essential for fetal development are delivered by

   _____
   a. simple diffusion
   b. facilitated diffusion
   c. active transport
   d. ion trapping

Q.8 Most toxicants cross the placenta by _____
   a. simple diffusion
   b. facilitated diffusion
   c. active transport
   d. ion trapping

Q.9 All of the following protect the fetus from toxicant exposure except ____.
   a. tight endothelial cell junctions similar to the blood—brain barrier
   b. multiple tissue layers in the placenta
   c. biotransformation ability of the placenta
   d. the presence of transporter systems in the placenta

Q.10 The higher pH of the infant gastrointestinal (GI) tract causes infants to be more susceptible to ____.
a. reflux disease
b. toxic megacolon
c. methemoglobinemia
d. GI erosions

Exercise 15

Q.1 A transport process that removes particles from alveoli is _____
a. phagocytosis
b. phospholipidosis
c. mediated through BCRP
d. mediated through MDRI/P-gp

Q.2 P-gp, MDRI, and BCRP on enterocyte brush border membranes function as _____
a. influx transporters
b. bile acid binders
c. metal transporters
d. efflux transporters

Q.3 Substrates for P-gp include all of the following except _____
a. cyclosporin
b. paclitaxel
c. ethanol
d. colchicines

Q.4 The transfer of toxicants by simple diffusion from areas of high concentration to areas of lower concentration is called _____
a. Dalton's law
b. Priestley's law
c. Fick's law
d. Henderson's law

Q.5 The fluid character of cell membranes is somewhat dependent on the amount of _____
a. saturated fatty acids
b. transmembrane proteins
c. ion channels
d. unsaturated fatty acids

Q.6 Grapefruit juices affects _____
a. activity of CYP3A4
b. function of P-gp
c. absorption of lovastatin
d. All of the above

Q.7 Species differences in GI absorption are due to _____
a. anatomical factors
b. GI pH differences

   c. differences in GI microflora
   d. All of the above

Q.8 All of the following are true of absorption of gases in the lung except
   _____.
   a. lipid solubility is more important than in GI absorption
   b. degree of ionization is less important than in GI absorption
   c. diffusion through cell membranes is usually not rate limiting
   d. very water-soluble molecules can be removed in the nose before
      reaching the lungs

Q.9 the most characterized transplacental carcinogen is _____
   a. warfarin
   b. phenytoin
   c. diethylstilbestrol
   d. vitamin A

Q.10 Enzymes in the intestinal microflora may hydrolyze conjugates of organic
   compounds with _____
   a. UDP-glucuronic acid
   b. sulfate
   c. Both
   d. Neither

Exercise 16

Q.1 The process of hydrolysis of an organic conjugate in the gut and
   reabsorption of the liberated parent compound is called _____.
   a. gastric bypass
   b. enterohepatic cycling
   c. first-pass effect
   d. well-stirred effect

Q.2 The substance with the highest bile-to-plasma concentration ratio is _____.
   a. arsenic
   b. albumin
   c. iron
   d. gold

Q.3 All of the following are transporters involved in biliary excretion except
   _____.
   a. P-gp
   b. Mrp2
   c. Bcrp
   d. Ras

Q.4 The organ that receives the smallest of cardiac output is _____.
   a. liver
   b. lung
   c. kidney
   d. skin

Q.5 A major route for the excretion of TCDD is _____.
   a. urinary excretion
   b. exhalation
   c. diffusion into fecal fat
   d. saliva

Q.6 Xenobiotics can enter the gut by all of the following mechanisms except _____.
   a. excretion across the gut wall
   b. patent ductus arteriosis
   c. elimination in the saliva
   d. elimination in pancreatic juice

Q.7 The major plasma proteins that bind xenobiotics are _____.
   a. ferritin and transferrin
   b. ceruloplasmin and retinal-binding protein
   c. albumin and acid glycoprotein
   d. gamma globulin and fibrin

Q.8 All of the following are true of the lung except:
   a. It is a major barrier to the absorption of chemicals into the blood.
   b. It has large surface area and a thin membrane.
   c. It is a major site of inactivation of certain peptides and prostaglandins.
   d. It has less capacity to metabolize foreign compounds than the liver does.

Q.9 All of the following contribute to the blood—brain barrier except _____.
   a. low protein concentration of brain interstitial fluid
   b. tight junctions between endothelial capillary cell
   c. significant endocytosis
   d. the presence of afflux transporters

Q.10 A person was brought by police from the railway platform. He is talking irrelevant. He is having dry mouth with hot skin, dilated pupils, staggering gait, and slurred speech. The most probable diagnosis is _____.
   a. alcohol intoxication
   b. carbamates poisoning
   c. organophosphorus poisoning
   d. datura poisoning

Exercise 17

Q.1 Regarding methanol poisoning:
   Assertion: Administration of ethanol is one of the treatment modalities.
   Reason: Ethanol inhibits alcohol dehydrogenase Please select the most correct option from the following:
   a. Both assertion and reason are true, and the reason is the correct explanation for the assertion.
   b. Both assertion and reason are true, and the reason is not the correct explanation for the assertion.

    c. Assertion is true, but the reason is false.

    d. Assertion is false, but the reason is true.

Q.2 In methyl alcohol poisoning, there is CNS depression, cardiac depression, and optic nerve atrophy. These effects are produced due to:

    a. formaldehyde and formic acid

    b. acetaldehyde

    c. pyridine

    d. acetic acid

Q.3 A 39-year-old carpenter has taken two bottles of liquor from the local shop. After about an hour, he develops confusion, vomiting, and blurring of vision. He has been brought to the emergency department. He should be given

    a. naloxone

    b. diazepam

    c. flumazenil

    d. ethyl alcohol

Q.4 Phosphine liberated in the stomach in aluminum phosphide poisoning is toxic to all except _____

    a. lungs

    b. kidneys

    c. liver

    d. heart

Q.5 Paraquat poisoning causes:

    a. renal failure

    b. cardiac failure

    c. respiratory failure

    d. multiple organ failure

Q.6 Ecstasy toxicity causes:

    a. hyperreflexia

    b. trismus

    c. dilated pupils

    d. visual hallucinations

    e. All of the above

Q.7 A housewife ingests a rodenticide white powder accidentally. She is brought to hospital where the examination shows generalized, flaccid paralysis, and an irregular pulse. Electrocardiogram shows multiple ventricular ectopics, generalized changes with ST-T. Serum potassium is 2.5 mEq/L. The most likely ingested poison is:

    a. barium carbonate

    b. super warfarins

    c. zinc phosphide

    d. aluminum phosphide

Q.8 All of the following are treatment options for toxic alcohol poisoning except:

    a. fomepizole

    b. hydroxocobalamin

    c. thiamine
    d. folic acid
    e. pyridoxine

Q.9 Hyperthermia in a patient of poisoning is a pointer to all except:
    a. ecstasy
    b. selective serotonin reuptake inhibitor
    c. salicylates
    d. chlorpromazine

Q.10 Excessive secretions refers to:
    a. organophosphorus poisoning
    b. heavy metal poisoning
    c. scorpion venom poisoning
    d. snake venom poisoning

Exercise 18

Q.1 Elapidaes are:
    a. vasculotoxic
    b. neurotoxic
    c. musculotoxic
    d. nontoxic

Q.2 The most useful bedside test to suggest snakebite envenomation is:
    a. prothrombin time
    b. 20-minute whole blood clotting time
    c. International normalized ratio
    d. platelet count

Q.3 A 12-year-old boy had an alleged history of snakebite and presented to the hospital with inability to open eyes well and difficulty in breathing. He is very anxious and is having tachycardia and tachypnea. On examination, bite mark cannot be visualized and there is no swelling of the limb. He has bilateral ptosis. His 20-minute whole blood clotting test is good quality. What is the next course of action?
    a. Do not give anti-snake venom (ASV), but observe the patient.
    b. Give ASV and keep the patient in observation.
    c. Give ASV, and give neostigmine and observe the patient.
    d. Reassure the patient and send him home with anxiolytic.

Q.4 Magnan's symptoms are characteristic symptoms with which poisoning?
    a. Alcohol
    b. Charas
    c. Cocaine
    d. Ecstasy

Q.5 The primary site of kidney damage resulting from acute exposure to inorganic mercury salts is the _____.
    a. glomerulus
    b. proximal tubule

    c. loop of Henle

    d. renal papilla

    e. entire nephron

Q.6 Which substance has been identified as a respiratory tract carcinogen in humans?

    a. Kaolin

    b. Hydrogen fluoride

    c. Arsenic

    d. Cotton dust

    e. Vanadium

Q.7 The following are true for dioxin:

    a. Contaminants from paper bleaching

    b. Major source is municipal waste incineration

    c. People less susceptible than rodents

    d. Caused disaster at Three Mile Beach

    e. Affinity for cytosolic receptor about same in rats and people

Q.8 The following are true for xenoestrogens:

    a. Bisphenol A is an estrogenic food additive.

    b. TCDD is potent estrogen.

    c. Cell growth in estrogen-sensitive tissues protects against cancer.

    d. They are foreign chemicals that bind with estrogen receptor.

    e. Males do not have estrogen receptors, so are not at risk to these chemicals.

Q.9 The following are correct toxin: mechanism pairs:

    a. CN: blocks TCA cycle

    b. Benzene: DNA binding

    c. Warfarin: inhibits $Ca+2$ uptake

    d. DNOC: uncouples oxidative phosphorylation

Q.10 The following are characteristics of aromatic amines:

    a. Amino group endocyclic

    b. In dyes, cigarette smoke

    c. Nitrene is a reactive intermediate

    d. Some are known bladder carcinogens

    e. α-amino less carcinogenic than β

Exercise 19

Q.1 If Trichloroethylene (TCE) has a zero-order intake of 0.02 μg/day and eliminated at 0.001 Day 1, then:

    a. $t\frac{1}{2} = 693$ days

    b. $t\frac{1}{2} = 346$ days

    c. Xmax = 20 mg

    d. Xmax = 0.02 mg

    e. time-to-Xmax = 4851 days

Q.2 Which of these groups is usually designated as one of the most sensitive subpopulations for exposures to toxic substances?
   a. Adult women
   b. Infants
   c. Adult men
   d. Adolescents

Q.3 You have worked at a chemical facility for 10 years. The facility does not require protective equipment, and you have developed a number of serious health affects in the last 7 years. You are possibly experiencing what type of exposure?
   a. Chronic
   b. Acute

Q.4 You are worried about contamination of vegetables grown in contaminated soils. What type of toxicologist would you contact?
   a. Descriptive
   b. Environmental
   c. Regulatory
   d. Food

Q.5 You are concerned about risks associated with growing vegetables in soil with high lead and arsenic concentrations. You are speaking of what type of substance?
   a. Toxin
   b. Toxicant

Q.6 The larger the amount of exposure and the greater the dose, the greater the observed response or effect.
   a. True
   b. False

Q.7 What type of toxicologist takes samples of your blood, urine, and hair for testing?
   a. Descriptive
   b. Analytical
   c. Mechanistic
   d. Forensic

Q.8 Toxic agents can be classified in terms of their physical state, their effects, and their source.
   a. True
   b. False

Q.9 Which agency deals with the health effects that may occur from environmental exposure to toxic chemicals?
   a. The Environmental Protection Agency
   b. The Centers for Disease Control and Prevention
   c. The Agency for Toxic Substances and Disease Registry
   d. The Nuclear Regulatory Commission

Q.10 Which database has information on emergency handling procedures, environmental data, regulatory status, and human exposure?
a. TOXNET
b. HazDat
c. IRIS
d. CHEMTREC

Exercise 20

Q.1 HazDat contains information on hazardous substances found at NPL and non-NPL waste sites, and on emergency events.
a. True
b. False

Q.2 The NOAEL is the same as the no observed effect level (NOEL).
a. True
b. False

Q.3 The term "toxicant" is used when talking about toxic substances that are produced by or are as byproduct of human-made activities.
a. True
b. False

Q.4 The following are correct toxin: antidote (or treatment) combinations:
a. strychnine: KMnO4
b. carbaryl: 2-PAM
c. DNOC: atropine
d. malathion: atropine
e. Rotenone: 2-PAM

Q.5 The following are true for organophosphates:
a. inactivated with tap water
b. require metabolism to the phosphorthioate for toxicity
c. phosphoryl group binds to anionic site in acetylcholinesterase
d. invented by Iraqi scientists
e. tri-ortho-tolyl phosphate (TOTP) causative agent of "Ginger Jake Shuffle"

Q.6 The following are true for organophosphates:
a. p-Nitrophenol is a biomarker for parathion exposure.
b. The two antidotes can be given in any order—just as long as both are given.
c. Short environmental half-life
d. Symptoms begin almost immediately
e. Less groundwater residues than DDT

Q.7 The following statements are true for methylisocyanate (MIC):
a. Few persistent effects in exposed people.
b. Longer $t\frac{1}{2}$ in the body if food is in the stomach.
c. Starting material to produce the rodenticide Sevin.
d. Indiscriminate toxin due to extreme chemical reactivity.
e. Increased PCO2 in exposed people.

Q.8 The following are from natural sources:
  a. Strychnine
  b. Sarin
  c. Rotenone
  d. Atropine
  e. Warfarin
Q.9 The following form epoxide intermediates:
  a. Aromatic amines
  b. Organophosphates
  c. PAHs
  d. MIC
  e. Benzene

Exercise 21

Q.1 The following must be metabolically activated for toxicity:
  a. Aromatic amines
  b. PAHs
  c. Carbaryl
  d. MIC
  e. Vinyl chloride
Q.2 The "first pass effect" refers to:
  a. rejection on a first date
  b. a toxicant passing through the circulation for one cycle
  c. elimination of a toxicant before it is distributed by the blood stream
  d. successfully completing this course the first time
  e. None of the above
Q.3 For a gas with a high solubility in plasma, absorption in the lungs depends more on respiration rate than on pulmonary blood flow.
  a. True
  b. False
Q.4 Chemicals are more readily absorbed through the skin or GI tract if they are:
  a. polar compounds
  b. ionic compounds
  c. lipid soluble
  d. nonionic, neutral compounds
  e. Both (c) and (d)
Q.5 Metallothionein is a special protein that binds metals in the ____.
  a. liver
  b. GI tract
  c. type I pneumocytes
  d. nasal passages

Q.6 With respect to excretion of toxic substances, which of the following is the correct order of importance of the three major routes?
   a. fecal > lung > kidney
   b. lung > fecal > kidney
   c. fecal > kidney > lung
   d. kidney > fecal > lung

Q.7 Which of the following processes or interactions would interfere with the delivery of the ultimate toxicant to its target site (intracellular molecule) where it produces the toxic effect?
   a. Increased porosity of capillaries
   b. Reabsorption
   c. Specialized membrane transporters
   d. Activation of the toxicant (toxication)
   e. Excretion

Q.8 Excretion of weak organic bases by the kidney is favored by _____ and reabsorption of weak organic acids by the kidney tubule epithelium is favored by _____ in the forming urine.
   a. high pH, high pH
   b. low pH, low pH
   c. high pH, low pH
   d. low pH, high pH

Q.9 Which of the following would be considered a detoxication biotransformation process?
   a. Formation of electrophiles
   b. Formation of free radicals
   c. Conjugation with glucuronic acid
   d. Formation of redox-active reactants
   e. Both (a) and (b)

Q.10 Dysregulation of gene expression can result from _____ by the toxicant.
   a. disruption of DNA transcription B
   b. interference with promoter regions of genes
   c. interference with phosphorylation networks involved in signal transduction
   d. interference with signal production
   e. All of the above.

Exercise 22

Q.1 Class B substances that are excreted by the liver have a bile-to-plasma concentration ratio that is greater than 1. These substances are probably
   a. excreted by passive processes if they are lipophilic.
   b. actively transported by the hepatocytes.
   c. reabsorbed in the bile ducts.
   d. not excreted rapidly.

Q.2 Which of the following would enhance the absorption of a toxicant through the various skin layers.
  a. Hydrophilicity
  b. Lipophilicity
  c. Active transport mechanisms
  d. Hydration of the skin
  e. Both (b) and (d)

Q.3 Toxins get across the placenta to the developing fetus
  a. by active transport processes
  b. by simple diffusion
  c. by paracellular transport
  d. through fenestrated capillaries
  e. with difficulty because the placenta acts as a barrier much like the blood−brain barrier.

Q.4 The most important contributing source for excretion of toxicants via the fecal route is:
  a. intestinal secretion
  b. exfoliation of intestinal cells
  c. biliary excretion
  d. pancreatic excretion
  e. None of the above

Q.5 Disposition refers to the _____ of toxic substances.
  a. absorption
  b. distribution
  c. biotransformation
  d. excretion
  e. All of these processes

Q.6 What are important types of lung toxicity?
  a. Cancer, mesothelioma, and cirrhosis.
  b. Silicosis, inflammation, and hypersensitivity.
  c. Inflammation, methemoglobinemia, and asbestosis.
  d. Emphysema, fibrosis, and edema.

Q.7 Indicate which compounds may cause lung toxicity.
  a. NO_2
  b. CO_2
  c. Asbestos
  d. Dioxins
  e. Radon
  f. CO
  g. Mustard gas

Q.8 What is true about hypersensitivity?
  a. Type III hypersensitivity is also called antibody-mediated cytotoxic hypersensitivity.
  b. Histamine release plays a role in type IV hypersensitivity.

    c. Immunosuppressive drugs can be used for the treatment of type IV hypersensitivity.

    d. Anaphylactic shock is a Type I hypersensitivity.

Q.9 Which compounds may cause immunosuppression?

    a. Tributyltin oxide (TBTO)

    b. Drugs for cancer patients

    c. Drugs for transplant patients

    d. Penicillin

    e. PCBs and dioxins

    f. Poison ivy

    g. Bee venom

Q.10 What are chemicals that cause liver toxicity?

    a. Dioxins, PCBs, and furans

    b. Acetaminophen and bromobenzene

    c. Fatty acids and mycotoxins

    d. Alcohol and bile acids

Exercise 23

Q.1 Which types of effect on the liver are chemically induced?

    a. Porphyria

    b. Steatosis

    c. Cholestasis

    d. Glomerular injury

    e. Emphysema

    f. Lymphatic necrosis

    g. Mucous excretion

    h. Cirrhosis

Q.2 What is true about toxic effects of chemicals on the liver?

    a. The toxic effect is often increased because activated macrophages excrete reactive oxygen species (ROS).

    b. Kupffer cells, the fixed macrophages in the liver, are most sensitive to chemical compounds because they have the most active metabolism of xenobiotics.

    c. Most compounds that cause toxic effects on the liver interact with bile formation.

    d. Zone 3 hepatocytes are especially sensitive to chemicals that require bioactivation by cytochromes P450.

    e. Porphyria results from chemicals that interfere with heme biosynthesis.

Q.3 Indicate what is true about the mechanism of liver damage caused by aflatoxin.

    a. The ultimate toxic effect is liver necrosis.

    b. Aflatoxin requires bioactivation before it can exert its adverse effect on the liver.

    c. Mutation of the gene for the p53 tumor suppressor gene plays a role in the mechanism of toxic action.

    d. Mutation of the Ras oncogene plays a role in the mechanism of toxic action.

    e. The ultimate toxic effect is mesothelioma.

Q.4 Give the right sequential order of the following steps (Number the steps from 1 to 4 on the dots).

    a. Risk assessment. . . . . .

    b. Hazard identification. . . . . .

    c. Risk management. . . . . .

    d. Hazard characterization. . . . . .

Q.5 indicate what is true about the process of risk evaluation as defined by the FAO and WHO.

    a. Risk assessment consists of risk characterization, exposure assessment, risk management, and risk communication.

    b. Risk assessment integrates hazard characterization and exposure assessment.

    c. Risk management is part of risk assessment.

    d. Exposure assessment follows hazard characterization.

    e. Risk management follows risk assessment.

Q.6 What is true about the process of risk assessment?

    a. Acute exposure and chronic exposure from a chemical result in effects on a similar target organ, but only at a single high or a repeated low dose of exposure, respectively.

    b. DNA can be a toxicological receptor.

    c. A dose−response curve is important to establish the LD50 that is an important parameter in modern toxicological risk assessment.

    d. The LD50 is a constant parameter reflecting the acute toxicity of a chemical for different species.

Q.7 What is true about mechanisms of toxicity?

    a. Methemoglobinemia is caused by chemicals that cause electron transfer that oxidizes the Fe in hemoglobin from $Fe2+$ to $Fe3+$.

    b. Lipid peroxidation is initiated by hydrogen abstraction.

    c. ROS damage only unsaturated membrane lipids.

    d. Sarin and soman act by binding to the acetylcholine receptor.

    e. An antagonist does not require structural similarity to the natural ligand to block the receptor.

    f. Inhibition of oxygen binding to hemoglobin by CO is an example of noncovalent binding causing toxicity.

Q.8 What is true for absorption, distribution, metabolism and excretion (ADME) characteristics?

    a. ADME characteristics describe what happens to a compound when it has entered the body.

    b. ADME characteristics describe the toxicodynamic phase.

    c. ADME characteristics determine the bioavailability of a compound upon oral intake.

    d. ADME characteristics describe how a compound becomes toxic including the mechanism of action.

Q.9 What is true about the biotransformation of xenobiotics?

    a. Phase I modification can follow phase II conjugation.

    b. Phase I modification makes a compound water-soluble.

    c. Phase I modification results in bioactivation of a xenobiotic.

    d. Hydrophilic metabolites do not require phase I or phase II metabolism to be excreted in the urine.

    e. Biotransformation can be part of the mechanism of toxicity of a chemical.

Q.10 What type of biotransformation reactions are phase I reactions?

    a. N-acetylation, glucuronidation, epoxidation

    b. Hydroxylation, sulfation, glutathione conjugation

    c. Methylation, N-oxidation, nitroreduction

    d. Heteroatom dealkylation, epoxidation, hydroxylation

Exercise 24

Q.1 What is true about toxicokinetics?

    a. Toxicokinetics describes dose−response curves.

    b. Toxicokinetics describes plasma concentrations as a function of time.

    c. Toxicokinetics describes models for bioavailability.

    d. Toxicokinetics is part of the toxicodynamic phase.

    e. Toxicokinetics includes Physiologically based pharmacokinetic (PBPK) modeling.

Q.2 What are the advantages of PBPK modeling over classical toxicokinetic modeling?

    a. PBPK models can predict the concentration of a chemical in all relevant organs.

    b. PBPK models can calculate the apparent volume of distribution.

    c. PBPK models can be used to predict interspecies differences.

    d. PBPK models can be used to predict chronic toxicity.

    e. PBPK models can be used to model plasma levels.

Q.3 What is true about mutagenesis?

    a. Mutagenesis consistently predicts carcinogenesis.

    b. Mutagenesis includes initiation, promotion, and progression.

    c. Mutagenesis occurs more often in germ cells than in somatic cells.

    d. Mutagenesis can result from oxidative stress.

Q.4 What is true about developmental toxicology?

    a. Mutation can be a mechanism underlying teratogenesis.

    b. Decreased nutrient supply can be a mechanism underlying teratogenesis.

    c. Teratogenicity of a chemical is usually reflected by growth retardation at low dose and lethality at high dose.

   d. The majority of the birth defects are caused by exposure to radiation, drugs, chemicals, or maternal metabolic imbalances.

   e. Teratogenic agents can have an effect on the placenta only.

Q.5 Indicate what is true about neurotoxicity.

   a. Neurons are especially sensitive towards the consequences of CO or cyanide poisoning.

   b. For neurotoxicity, chronic effects are of larger concern than acute effects.

   c. Methylmercury causes neurotoxicity and thereby loss of coordination (ataxia).

   d. Neuronopathy may cause a stocking and glove-like distribution of effects.

   e. Neuronopathy of dopaminergic neurons may cause Parkinson-like effects.

Q.6 Indicate which effects represent neurotransmission toxicity.

   a. Effects on neurotransmitter biosynthesis

   b. Effects on neurotransmitter release

   c. Effects on the postsynaptic receptor

   d. Effects on acetylcholine esterase

   e. Effects on sodium (Na^+) channels

   f. Effects on neuronal mitochondria

   g. Receptor antagonists

Q.7 Indicate what are the targets for direct effects on the heart function.

   a. Effects on neurotransmitters

   b. Effects on calcium channels

   c. Effects on Na/K pumps

   d. Effects on fatty acid biosynthesis

   e. Effects on oxidative phosphorylation

   f. Effects on the electron transport system in the mitochondria

   g. Artherosclerosis

Q.8 Which are chemicals known for their heart toxicity?

   a. Digitalis glycosides

   b. Adriamycin

   c. Polycyclic hydrocarbons

   d. Unsaturated fatty acids

   e. Chlorinated dioxins

Q.9 Indicate what is true about cardiovascular toxicity.

   a. The mechanism by which arteriosclerosis develops is generally agreed upon.

   b. The somatic mutation theory predicts that atherosclerotic plaques represent malignant tumor sites.

   c. In the response to injury theory endothelial cells develop into atherosclerotic plaques.

d. Atherosclerotic plaque formation may represent an effect resulting from immune stimulation.

e. Vasoconstriction and vasodilatation are early stages in the development of arthrosclerosis.

Q.10 What is true about absorption of toxicant by the lungs?

  a. The mucociliary escalator plays a role.
  b. The first pass effect plays a role.
  c. Particle water solubility plays a role.
  d. Ionization plays an important role.
  e. Diffusion through cell membranes is rate limiting.

Exercise 25

Q.1 What parameters are used as input in PBPK models?

  a. Apparent volume of distribution, plasma concentrations, dose administered
  b. Plasma concentrations, urinary levels, metabolite levels
  c. Blood flow rates, tissue volumes, kinetic parameters for biotransformation
  d. Tissue concentrations, species dependent parameters, first-order elimination constants

Q.2 What are characteristic toxic effects of chemicals on the skin?

  a. Contact dermatitis, skin necrosis, skin colorization
  b. Atopic contact dermatitis, urticaria, phototoxicity
  c. Acne, steatosis, skin cancer
  d. Hydratation, edema, melanoma

Q.3 What is NOT true about toxic effects of chemicals on the skin?

  a. The skin is highly sensitive because it has a large surface where exposure can occur.
  b. The skin is highly sensitive because it is easily penetrated by water-soluble compounds.
  c. The skin is especially sensitive to corrosive agents.
  d. UV light can play a role in the skin toxicity of chemical compounds.
  e. Toxic effects on the skin may occur due to systemic exposure.

Q.4 Which compounds are known for their skin toxicity?

  a. TCDD
  b. PCBs
  c. Sarin
  d. Soman
  e. Arsenic
  f. Methyl mercury
  g. PAHs

Q.5 What is true about endocrine disruption?

  a. Compounds causing endocrine disruption originate from a very narrow class of chemical compounds.
  b. Compounds causing endocrine disruption are present in our food and environment.

    c. Compounds causing endocrine disruption are toxic to one of the hormone-producing organs.

    d. Compounds causing endocrine disruption can be a risk factor for cancer incidences.

Q.6 What are effects that can be caused by endocrine disruptors?

    a. Skin rashes

    b. Increased changes on liver cancer

    c. Increased changes on breast cancer

    d. Imposex

    e. Reduced changes on pregnancy

Q.7 Give the right sequential order of the following steps (Number the steps from 1 to 5 on the dots).

    a. Tumor development......

    b. Activation of gene expression......

    c. Exposure to an endocrine disruptor......

    d. Activation of cell proliferation......

    e. Activation of the estrogen receptor......

Q.8 What are important cancer-inducing factors?

    a. Environmental contaminants

    b. RNA viruses

    c. Ionizing radiation

    d. Pesticides

    e. Food additives

    f. Food colors

    g. Genetic factors

Q.9 What is true about induction of cancer by asbestos?

    a. It requires metabolic biotransformation (bioactivation) by macrophages.

    b. It occurs in lungs and liver and results in mesotheliomas.

    c. It is initiated by the fact that asbestos fibers become surrounded by glycoprotein and cannot be adequately removed by macrophages.

    d. It only occurs in combination with heavy smoking.

Q.10 What are important classes of cancer-inducing chemicals?

    a. Nitrosamines

    b. Films and fibers

    c. Polycyclic hydrocarbons

    d. Bacterial toxins

    e. Mycotoxins

    f. Carotenes

Exercise 26

Q.1 What is true about mutagenesis?

    a. Mutagenesis consistently predicts carcinogenesis.

    b. Mutagenesis includes initiation, promotion, and progression.

    c. Mutagenesis occurs more often in germ cells than in somatic cells.

    d. Mutagenesis can result from oxidative stress.

    e. Mutagenesis is a reversible process.

Q.2 What are chromosome aberrations, i.e., changes at the individual chromosome level?

    a. Aneuploidy

    b. Frameshift mutations

    c. Base-pair substitutions

    d. Translocations

    e. Sister chromatid exchanges

Q.3 What is true about gene mutations?

    a. Genetic abnormalities resulting from mutations can be placed in two categories: frameshift mutations and chromosome aberrations.

    b. Changes in the number of chromosomes, aneuploidy or polyploidy are not considered genetic abnormalities resulting from mutations.

    c. Transitions and transversions are frameshift mutations.

    d. Most chemical carcinogens with cancer initiating activity are also mutagenic.

Q.4 Indicate which principles are part of Wilson's general principles of teratology.

    a. Susceptibility toward teratogenic agents depends on the genotype of the conceptus.

    b. Susceptibility varies with the developmental stage at time of exposure.

    c. There is no threshold and no NOAEL for teratogenic effects.

    d. With increasing concentration of the teratogen, observed effects change from growth retardation to malformations to death.

    e. Mechanisms that initiate the teratogenic effect are compound specific.

    f. There is homology in development and thus in developmental stages for different organisms.

Q.5 What is the most important principle underlying the investigation of the teratogenicity of chemical compounds for men by doing animal experiments?

    a. Susceptibility varies only marginally with the species investigated.

    b. There is homology in development for different mammalian species.

    c. Dose–response curves show the same characteristics in different mammalian species.

    d. Mechanisms of teratogenicity are similar in different mammalian species.

Q.6 What is true about toxicogenomics?

    a. Toxicogenomics studies use DNA microarray techniques.

    b. Toxicogenomics studies describe the effects of chemical compounds on DNA.

    c. Toxicogenomics studies are an in vitro approach that can replace in vivo animal studies for toxicity.

    d. Toxicogenomics studies use real-time RT-PCR to validate mRNA expression patterns.

    e. Toxicogenomics studies use real-time PCR to quantify protein expression.

Q.7 What is the best description of a reporter gene assay?
   a. An assay that detects DNA damage and thus genotoxicity.
   b. An assay that quantifies the activation of a receptor protein.
   c. An assay that quantifies expression levels of the cellular proteins.
   d. An assay that is based on real-time RT-PCR.

Q.8 Give the right sequential order of the following steps (Number the steps from 1 to 5 on the dots).
   a. Binding to the dioxin responsive elements . . . . . .
   b. Binding to the aryl hydrocarbon (Ah) receptor. . . . . .
   c. Expression of a reporter gene. . . . . .
   d. Translocation to the nucleus. . . . . .
   e. Luciferase activity. . . . . .

Q.9 What is true about RT-PCR?
   a. RT stands for Reverse Transcription.
   b. RT stands for Real Time.
   c. When measured real-time the original amount of cDNA can be calculated from the number of amplification cycles it takes to reach a threshold level for detectable DNA-associated fluorescence.
   d. It quantifies the amount of mRNA.
   e. It quantifies the amount of DNA.

Q.10 Although poisoning is popular in murder mysteries and detective stories, it is:
   a. not a common form of murder
   b. a common form of suicide
   c. a common form of murder
   d. a common form of manslaughter

Exercise 27

Q.1 Hallucinogens are:
   a. always derived from plants
   b. often derived from plants
   c. never derived from plants
   d. rarely derived from plants

Q.2 Lysergic Acid Diathylamide (LSD) was originally found in a fungus that grows on rye and other grains in 1938 and is one of the most potent mood-changing chemicals. It is:
   a. colorless
   b. odorless, colorless, and tasteless
   c. odorless
   d. None of these choices

Q.3 Narcotics act to:
   a. reduce pain by suppressing the brain's ability to relay pain messages to the CNS
   b. reduce pain by suppressing the CNS's ability to relay pain messages to the brain
   c. increase pain by increasing the CNS's ability to relay pain messages to the brain
   d. None of these choices

Q.4 Controlled substances are defined as:
   a. illegal drugs whose sale, possession, and use are prohibited because of the mind-altering effect of the drugs and the potential
   b. legal drugs whose sale, possession, and use are restricted because of the mind-altering effect of the drugs and the potential
   c. legal drugs whose sale, possession, and use are permitted
   d. None of these

Q.5 Stimulants:
   a. increase feelings of energy and alertness, while increasing appetite
   b. increase feelings of energy and alertness, while suppressing appetite
   c. increase feelings of lethargy and alertness, while increasing appetite
   d. decrease feelings of energy and alertness, while suppressing appetite

Q.6 Botulism is the:
   a. least poisonous biological substance known to man
   b. most poisonous artificial substance known to man
   c. most poisonous biological substance known to man
   d. None of these

Q.7 Marijuana is considered to be a:
   a. stimulant
   b. narcotic
   c. depressant
   d. hallucinogen

Q.8 Ethyl alcohol is considered to be a _____
   a. hallucinogen
   b. narcotic
   c. depressant
   d. stimulant

Q.9 Over the counter drugs such as ibuprofen, acetaminophen, acetylsalicylic acid, and naproxen are considered:
   a. highly addictive
   b. analgesics
   c. harmless
   d. narcotics

Q.10 A patient is admitted to the emergency room with the following symptoms: dry mouth and skin; weak, rapid pulse (130 beats/minute); elevated body temperature (103°F); and mydriasis. He is excited and disoriented. In his

pocket is a bottle of pills labeled: "take one as necessary for stomach pain." This patient is most likely to be suffering from an overdose of
a. a narcotic analgesic
b. a nonnarcotic analgesic
c. an antacid
d. an antimuscarinic agent
e. a benzodiazepine tranquilizer

Exercise 28

Q.1 Toxicology is the study of:
a. prevalence of disease and death in a population
b. adverse effects of chemicals on living organisms
c. the appearance of symptoms produced by infectious agents
d. word origins
e. None of the above

Q.2 In the human body, toxicological processes ultimately take place at which level?
a. Cell
b. Tissue
c. Organ
d. Organ system
e. The whole organism

Q.3 Which type of toxicologist is concerned with the use of toxicants by the public and in the workplace?
a. Descriptive toxicologist
b. Mechanistic toxicologist
c. Regulatory toxicologist

Q.4 Which is the best definition of the term toxicant?
a. A chemical that causes no adverse effects
b. A substance produced as a result of human activities
c. A branch of toxicology
d. An agent that neutralizes the effects of a poison
e. A substance that is naturally produced

Q.5 The statement, "All substances are poisons; there is none which is not a poison." Only the dose determines that a thing is not a poison, is attributed to which of the following?
a. Hippocrates
b. Theophrastus
c. Mithridates
d. Paracelsus
e. Catherine De Medici

Q.6 Toxicity is recognized when on the administration of a chemical an observable and quantifiable is identified.
a. Mutagen
b. Waste product

  c. Dose

  d. End-effect or response

  e. Safety factor

Q.7 A substance that is being tested for toxicity is injected intramuscularly mixed with peanut oil. The term vehicle in this case refers to:

  a. the syringe used

  b. the needle type used

  c. the manner in which the substance was transported to the laboratory

  d. the peanut oil

  e. None of the above

Q.8 Which of the following are true statements about toxicity testing?

  a. Acute lethal tests do not predict carcinogenicity.

  b. People are generally 10 times less susceptible than animals to most toxins.

  c. The Draize test predicts chemical irritation.

  d. Chronic toxicity tests generally use two rodent species for their lifetime.

  e. Dose levels are often corrected between species by surface area calculations.

  f. All of the above

Q.9 The following are true statements about cytochrome P450.

  a. The "P" in cytochrome P-450 stands for "protein."

  b. Catalyzes the replacement of sulfur for potassium in parathion.

  c. The heme requires reduction to the $+2$ state before substrate binding can occur.

  d. It is highest in liver.

  e. Catalyzes reactions resulting in increased toxicity.

Q.10 The following are true statements about phase I reactions:

  a. Cytochrome P-450 often generates epoxides that are often unstable, but are generally nontoxic.

  b. Para hydroxylation is the main result of cytochrome P-450—mediated metabolism of toluene.

  c. Cytochrome P-450 may hydroxylate aliphatic C and N atoms.

  d. Removal of chlorine from DDT produces DDE that is nearly as toxic as DDT.

  e. Phase I metabolite, phenol, is more water soluble and therefore more easily excreted than benzene.

Exercise 29

Q.1 In the Ames assay:

  a. S9 refers to the sediment from the $9000 \times g$ centrifuge spin of liver homogenate.

  b. Mutagens that do not require metabolic activation are not detected.

  c. "rfa" is a feature that increases error-prone repair.

  d. Radioactive thymidine is added to top agar.

  e. A positive response means that the test chemical is a carcinogen.

Q.2 What is the most important factor that determines chemical toxicity?
  a. Dose
  b. Route of exposure
  c. The metabolic profile of the chemical
  d. Potency
  e. Possible synergistic effects with other chemicals

Q.3 The following are true for absorption of lipid-soluble chemicals:
  a. Is significantly affected by the partition coefficient of the chemical; the higher the value, the more hydrophilic the chemical.
  b. Dermal absorption can be accelerated by physical exertion.
  c. Ocular absorption is generally more rapid than oral.
  d. GI absorption will probably be greater in an obese person with an empty stomach than in a lean person who just had a meal.
  e. Is generally better with compounds of smaller molecular size.
  f. All of the above

Q.4 The sigmoid(s) dose−response curve for a toxicant indicates a threshold dose below where no effects are observed. A threshold occurs because of

_____.
  a. saturation of biotransformation pathways
  b. saturation of protein binding sites
  c. saturation of receptor sites
  d. depletion of cofactors
  e. All the above

Q.5 In the figure below, drug A is _____ than drug B, and drug C is _____ than drug D.
  a. less potent, less efficacious
  b. more potent, more efficacious
  c. less potent, more efficacious
  d. more potent, less efficacious

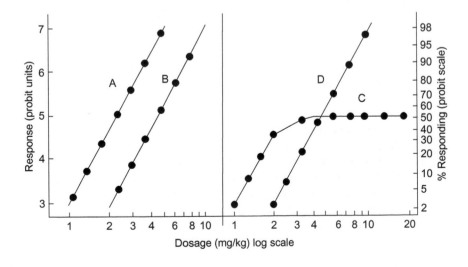

Q.6 The sigmoid(s) dose–response curve is usually converted into a probit–probability presentation. Each probit unit of the transformed data represents
  a. 50% of the population
  b. 99.7% of the population
  c. one standard deviation
  d. two standard deviations
  e. the LD50 value obtained from the plot

Q.7 A weak organic acid with a pKa of 5.5 would be expected to be:
  a. more ionized at low pH
  b. more ionized at high pH
  c. nonionized at low pH
  d. nonionized at high pH
  e. Both (b) and (c) are true

Q.8 A toxic substance produced by biological systems is specifically referred to as a _____.
  a. toxicant
  b. toxin
  c. xenobiotic
  d. poison

Q.9 A newly formed hapten protein complex usually stimulates the formation of a significant amount of antibodies in:
  a. 1–2 minutes
  b. 1–2 hours
  c. 1–2 days
  d. 1–2 weeks

Q.10 Prolonged muscle relaxation after succinylcholine is an example of a/an:
  a. IGE-mediated allergic reaction
  b. idiosyncratic reaction
  c. immune complex reaction
  d. reaction related to a genetic increase in the activity

Exercise 30

Q.1 Which of the following is not a side effect of digoxin toxicity?
  a. Bradycardia
  b. Yellow vision changes
  c. Scooping of the T segment on ECG
  d. Hypokalemia
  e. Gynecomastia

Q.2 Which of the following chelating agents is recommended for acute lead poisoning with signs of encephalopathy?
  a. Succimer
  b. Penicillamine
  c. Dimercaprol

    d. Calcium EDTA

    e. Dimercaprol + Calcium EDTA

Q.3 Which of the following dermatologic findings and potential causes is incorrect?

    a. Cyanosis—Methemoglobinemia

    b. Erythroderma—Boric Acid

    c. Pallor—Carbon Monoxide

    d. Jaundice—Hypercarotinemia (excess carrot intake)

    e. Brightly flushed skin—Niacin

Q.4 All of the following symptoms can occur with Ciguatera poisoning except:

    a. myalgias

    b. flushing

    c. metallic taste

    d. reversal of temperature sensation

    e. sensation of loose, painful teeth

Q.5 Which of the following is true with regard to acetaminophen toxicity?

    a. The Rumack-Matthew Nomogram may be used for both acute and chronic ingestions.

    b. The APAP level should ideally be checked within 1–4 hours of ingestion.

    c. The Rumack-Matthew Nomogram applies for ingestions up to 48 hours postingestion.

    d. N-Acetylcysteine should be started within 8 hours of ingestion if an APAP level cannot be obtained.

    e. Activated charcoal should be used for all sustained release ingestions.

Q.6 Cholinesterase inhibitor toxicity is due to:

    a. excessive levels of the enzyme acetylcholinesterase

    b. depressed activity of the enzyme acetylcholinesterase

    c. excessive levels of the neurotransmitter acetylcholine

    d. depressed levels of the neurotransmitter acetylcholine

    e. None of the above

Q.7 Which of the following are true about organophosphates?

    a. They include pesticides.

    b. They include nerve agents.

    c. They are less toxic than carbamates.

    d. They have a longer duration of action than carbamates.

    e. None of the above

Q.8 Cholinesterase inhibitors block the ability of acetylcholinesterase to break down acetylcholine by:

    a. occupying the binding site on cholinesterase to which the acetylcholine would attach

    b. preventing the release of acetylcholine from its attachment on cholinesterase

    c. attaching to acetylcholine that prevents its attachment to cholinesterase

    d. None of the above

Q.9 Nicotinic and muscarinic receptors:
  a. are both acetylcholine receptors
  b. have the same structure
  c. have different physiology
  d. have different functions
  e. None of the above

Q.10 What causes the cholinergic toxidrome?
  a. Elevated levels of acetylcholinesterase
  b. Elevated levels of acetylcholine
  c. Acetylcholine deficiency
  d. None of the above

Exercise 31

Q.1 Cholinergic receptors are found in which of the following locations?
  a. The CNS
  b. The sympathetic nervous system
  c. The parasympathetic nervous system
  d. The skeletal neuromuscular junctions
  e. None of the above

Q.2 Why do excessive levels of acetylcholine ("The cholinergic toxidrome") cause different signs and symptoms, depending on whether the nicotinic or muscarinic receptors are involved?
  a. Because some nicotinic and muscarinic receptors are located in and affect different anatomic structures
  b. Because nicotinic and muscarinic receptors are triggered by different neurotransmitters
  c. Because nicotinic and muscarinic receptors have different mechanisms of action
  d. None of the above

Q.3 Nicotinic receptors:
  a. trigger rapid neural transmission
  b. trigger rapid neuromuscular transmission
  c. become stimulated then paralyzed by toxic levels of acetylcholine
  d. are found only in the autonomic nervous system
  e. None of the above

Q.4 Overstimulation of nicotinic receptors can cause:
  a. tachycardia
  b. fasciculations
  c. mydriasis (pupillary dilation)
  d. leucopenia
  e. None of the above

Q.5 Nicotinic receptors are found in which of the following locations:
  a. Sympathetic nervous system
  b. Parasympathetic nervous system

    c. CNS

    d. All of the above

    e. None of the above

Q.6 When compared with the action of nicotinic receptors, muscarinic receptors:

    a. are faster

    b. initiate rather than modulate smooth muscle activity

    c. have primarily parasympathetic effects on the peripheral nervous system

    d. stimulate sweating via the sympathetic nervous system

    e. None of the above

Q.7 Cholinesterase inhibitor toxicity leads to the following clinical findings mediated by muscarinic receptors:

    a. Miosis (pupillary constriction)

    b. Bronchorrhea

    c. Nausea

    d. Bronchospasm

    e. None of the above

Q.8 Muscarinic receptors are found in:

    a. Skeletal muscle

    b. Smooth muscle

    c. Exocrine glands

    d. Sweat glands

    e. None of the above

Q.9 Signs and symptoms of cholinesterase inhibitor poisoning:

    a. may vary depending on the specific chemical involved

    b. are dominated by nicotinic findings in pediatric cases

    c. involving the CNS are primarily due to the presence of muscarinic receptors

    d. may mimic mental illness

    e. None of the above

Q.10 Death from cholinesterase inhibitor poisoning is usually due to:

    a. cardiac failure

    b. respiratory failure

    c. renal failure

    d. hepatic failure

    e. None of the above

Exercise 32

Q.1 Which of the following are true about the CNS effects of cholinesterase inhibitors?

    a. The pathology can be explained on the basis of increased muscarinic, as opposed to nicotinic, receptor activity.

    b. The pathology can be explained on the basis of increased nicotinic, as opposed to muscarinic, receptor activity.

    c. The pathology is poorly understood but involves both nicotinic and muscarinic receptors.

    d. None of the above.

Q.2 Which of the following CNS signs and symptoms have been reported in cases of cholinesterase inhibitor poisoning?

    a. Anxiety

    b. Emotional liability

    c. Convulsions

    d. Excess dreaming

    e. None of the above

Q.3 Potential sources of exposure to cholinesterase inhibitors include which of the following:

    a. Pesticides

    b. Pyridostigmine

    c. Castor beans

    d. Potato sprouts

    e. None of the above

Q.4 What is true about toxic effects of chemicals on the kidney?

    a. The kidney is extra susceptible to toxic injury because nontoxic concentrations in plasma may reach toxic concentrations in the kidney.

    b. The glomerulus is the part of the kidney most sensitive to toxic damage.

    c. Chemicals that require bioactivation are toxic to the kidney upon metabolism in the liver.

    d. Beta-lyase is an enzyme involved in bioactivation of several kidney toxins.

    e. The distal tubule is the most common site for renal injury by chemicals.

Q.5 Give the right sequential order of the following steps (Number the steps from 1 to 5 on the dots).

    a. Transport to the kidney......

    b. Conversion by glutathione S-transferases......

    c. Conversion by beta-lyase......

    d. Transport to the liver......

    e. Conversion in the mercapturic acid pathway......

Q.6 What are the most important enzymes for bioactivation of halogenated hydrocarbons causing kidney toxicity?

    a. Cytochromes P450, dehalogenases, epoxide hydroxylases.

    b. Beta-lyase, cytochrome P450s, glutathione S-transferases.

    c. Mercapturic acid pathway enzymes.

    d. The correct answer is not given.

Q.7 What are the important types of lung toxicity? (Indicate the one best answer).

    a. Cancer, mesothelioma, and cirrhosis

    b. Silicosis, inflammation, and hypersensitivity

    c. Inflammation, methemoglobinemia, and asbestosis

    d. Emphysema, fibrosis, and edema

17.3 FILL THE BLANKS
(WRITE YOUR ANSWER ON THE BLANK SPACE)

Exercise 33

Q.1 The concept of dose in toxicology was introduced in by _____.

Q.2 The target organ concept was introduced in toxicology by _____.

Q.3 The affair with _____ introduced emphasis on teratology and reproduction toxicology in safety testing of drugs and chemicals.

Q.4 Modern toxicology especially developed because of the many new drugs, pesticides, munitions, and industrial chemicals developed during the periods of the _____ and _____.

Q.5 The process in which compounds pass cell membranes against a concentration gradient is called _____.

Q.6 The phase in which the toxic effect of a chemical or its metabolite is generated is called _____ phase.

Q.7 Absorption of gasses is dependent on their _____.

Q.8 Absorption of particles is especially dependent on their _____.

Q.9 The process in which compounds are modified into metabolites that are more toxic than the parent compound is called _____.

Q.10 The most important enzyme system for the phase I biotransformation reaction is _____.

Exercise 34

Q.1 The most important enzymes for phase II metabolism of xenobiotics with hydroxyl groups are _____ and _____.

Q.2 The mechanism for phase I hydroxylation of aliphatics by P450 proceeding by H-radical abstraction followed by OH-radical coupling to the aliphatic radical is called the _____ mechanism.

Q.3 The process in which compounds are modified into metabolites that are more toxic than the parent compound is called _____.

Q.4 The most important enzyme system for the phase I biotransformation reaction is _____.

Q.5 The most important enzymes for phase II metabolism of xenobiotics with hydroxyl groups are _____ and _____.

Q.6 The mechanism for phase I hydroxylation of aliphatics by P450 proceeding by H-radical abstraction followed by OH-radical coupling to the aliphatic radical is called the _____ mechanism.

Q.7 Minamata disease is caused by the chemical compound _____.

Q.8 Q.8 A stocking-and-glove—like distribution of neurotoxic effect can be due to a type of neurotoxicity that is also called _____.

Q.9 Q.8 Neurotoxicity caused by effects of chemicals on the myelin layer produced by the myelinating cells is called _____

Q.10 Neurotoxicity caused by an adverse effect directly on the central cell body of the neuron is also called _____.

Q.11 Q.10 The process in which compounds pass cell membranes against a concentration gradient is called _____.

Exercise 35

Q.1 The phase in which the toxic effect of a chemical or its metabolite is generated is called _____ phase.

Q.2 Absorption of gasses is dependent on their _____.

Q.3 Absorption of particles is especially dependent on their _____.

Q.4 The two types of contact dermatitis that can be caused by chemical compounds are called _____ and _____ contact dermatitis.

Q.5 Necrosis without secondary inflammation caused by extremely corrosive agents is also called _____.

Q.6 The type of skin toxicity caused by psoralenes in combination with UV-A is called _____.

Q.7 The very characteristic skin toxicity caused by dioxins is called

_____.

Q.8 The process of carcinogenesis requires often more than one mutation and is therefore considered a _____ process.

Q.9 The process of carcinogenesis requires activation of _____ genes and inactivation of _____ genes.

Q.10 The three stages in the process of carcinogenesis are called

_____, _____, and _____.

Exercise 36

Q.1 Interaction of a chemical with the immune system resulting in an impaired immune function is called _____.

Q.2 Hypersensitivity mediated by mast cells and IgEs is called type _____ (choose: I, II, III, or IV) hypersensitivity or _____ hypersensitivity.

Q.3 Type IV hypersensitivity is also called _____ hypersensitivity.

Q.4 A sudden very severe allergic reaction that involves the whole body is also called _____.

Q.5 The cells in the alveoli most sensitive to chemical damage are the _____ pneumocytes, and when damaged they can be replaced by _____ pneumocytes.

Q.6 The Clara cells in the lung are of importance for toxicity because they contain the highest level of _____.

Q.7 A factor determining how deep gasses can penetrate into the lungs is their

_____.

Q.8 A factor determining how deep particles can penetrate into the lungs is

_____.

17.4 MATCH THE STATEMENTS

Exercise 37

Select the most appropriate answer from column B for each description of the toxic effect in Column A. The terms may be used once, more than once, or not at all.

Description of the Toxic Effect: Column A	Column B
Q. 1 Acute toxicity	A. Symptoms restricted to the site of initial exposure
Q. 2 Systemic toxicity	B. Toxicity occurring within less than 24 hours
Q. 3 Local toxicity	C. Toxic effects occur within the body
Q. 4 Delayed toxicity	D. Dead and lost cells replaced by cell division
Q. 5 Reversible toxic effect	E. The appearance of cancerous tumors 25–30 years after exposure to a toxin.
Q. 6 Additive effects	F. Equal to the sum of effects of each agent given alone
Q. 7 Potentiation effects	G. Combined effect of two chemicals is greater than the sum of effects of each
Q. 8 Antagonistic effects	H. One substance is not toxic but when added to another toxic chemical it makes that chemical more toxic
Q. 9 Synergistic effects	I. When two chemicals interfere with each other's actions

Exercise 38

Description of the Toxic Effect: Column A	Column B
Q. 1 Integrating hazard characteristics with exposure data	A. Risk assessment
Q. 2 The probability that an adverse effect will occur	B. Hazard
Q. 3 Integrating risk assessment with social, economic, and political aspects	C. Receptor
Q. 4 The molecular structure affected by a toxic agent	D. Risk
Q. 5 A potential danger of a compound or a process	E. Risk management
Q. 6 Compound causing lipid peroxidation	F. Electron abstraction
Q. 7 Electrophile causing a DNA mutation	G. Hydrogen abstraction
Q. 8 Compound causing methemoglobinemia	H. Covalent bonding
Q. 9 Compound inhibiting acetylcholinesterase	I. Agonist action
Q. 10 Compound binding and activating an acetylcholine receptor in the same way as done by acetylcholine	J. Modulating action

Exercise 39

Description of the Toxic Effect: Column A		Column B
Q. 1	Process requiring energy	A. Facilitated diffusion
Q. 2	ADME characteristics	B. Toxicokinetics
Q. 3	Transport by a carrier	C. First pass effect
Q. 4	Process preventing systemic effects	D. Toxicodynamics
Q. 5	Reaction with the toxicological receptor	E. Active transport

Exercise 40

Description of the Toxic Effect: Column A		Column B
Q. 1	A. Kinetic model in which plasma levels and tissue levels of a chemical are modeled to be similar	1. PBPK model
Q. 2	B. Kinetic model in which all relevant tissues are described as separate compartments	2. One compartment model
Q. 3	C. Kinetic model in which the amount of compound eliminated is constant with time	3. Zero-order kinetics
Q. 4	D. Kinetic model in which the rate of elimination of a compound is proportional to the amount of the compound in the body	4. Apparent volume of distribution
Q. 5	E. The amount of drug in the body divided by the plasma drug concentration	5. First-order kinetics

Exercise 41

Description of the Toxic Effect: Column A		Column B
Q. 1	Enzymatic undo of damage	A. Mismatch repair
Q. 2	Removal of damaged base followed by DNA polymerase and DNA ligase activity	B. Error-prone repair
Q. 3	Incorporation of random nucleotides to fill up a lesion	C. Excision repair
Q. 4	Repair of action of DNA polymerase III resulting in one wrong base pair incorporated per 108 bases synthesized	D. Reversal of damage

Exercise 42

Description of the Toxic Effect: Column A	Column B
Q. 1 Synthetic estrogen	A. Zearalenone
Q. 2 Mycoestrogen	B. Genistein
Q. 3 Metabolite with estrogen activity	C. Hydroxyl-PCB
Q. 4 Phytoestrogen	D. Diethylstilbestrol (DES)
Q. 5 Industrial chemical with estrogen activity	E. Bisphenol A

Exercise 43

Description of the Toxic Effect: Column A	Column B
Q. 1 Teratogenic chemotherapeutic agent that causes DNA crosslinks	A. Cyclophosphamide
Q. 2 Vitamin A analog with teratogenic potential	B. Thalidomide
Q. 3 Teratogenic because of placental toxicity	C. Cadmium
Q. 4 Chemical that introduced the concept of teratology in the field of safety testing	D. DES
Q. 5 Teratogenic chemical causing vaginal cancer in female offspring and also effects in male second generation	E. Isotretinoin

Exercise 44

Description of the Toxic Effect: Column A	Column B
Q. 1 Effect on bone marrow	A. Benzene
Q. 2 Type IV hypersensitivity	B. Penicillin
Q. 3 Effect on thymus (thymus atrophy)	C. Tributyltin oxide (TBTO)
Q. 4 Type I hypersensitivity	D. Urushiol from poison ivy

Exercise 45

Description of the Toxic Effect: Column A		Column B
Q. 1	Therapeutic agents for which use levels are limited by nephrotoxicity	A. Chloroform
Q. 2	Chemical that requires cytochrome P450 bioactivation to become toxic	B. Ochratoxin A
Q. 3	Chemical requiring beta-lyase activity to become nephrotoxic	C. Cadmium
Q. 4	Chemical causing nephrotoxicity produced by a fungus	D. Halogenated hydrocarbon
Q. 5	Chemical that becomes nephrotoxic because it accumulates in the kidney	E. Aminoglycoside antibiotics

Exercise 46

Description of the Toxic Effect: Column A		Column B
Q. 1	Accumulation of macrophages	A. Emphysema
Q. 2	Accumulation of water	B. Edema
Q. 3	Accumulation of collagen	C. Mesothelioma
Q. 4	Accumulation of damage to alveolar walls	D. Inflammation
Q. 5	Accumulation of malignant tissue	E. Fibrosis

Exercise 47

Description of the Toxic Effect: Column A		Column B
Q. 1	Effects on contraction frequency of the heart	A. Inotropy
Q. 2	Effects on heart rhythm	B. Chronotropy
Q. 3	Effects on contraction intensity of the heart	C. Bathmotropy
Q. 4	Effects on excitability of the heart	D. Dromotropy
Q. 5	Effects on impulse conductivity of the heart	E. Arrhythmia

Exercise 48

Description		Number of Term
Q. 1	Single dose test	A. Semichronic test
Q. 2	90 days test	B. Chronic test
Q. 3	28 days test	C. Acute test
Q. 4	Carcinogenicity test	D. Short-term test
Q. 5	Skin irritation test	E. Specific test

FURTHER READING

Bert Hakkinen, P.J., Kennedy, G., Stoss, F.W., 2000. Information Resources in Toxicology, 3rd ed. Academic Press, San Diego, CA.

Boelsterli, U.A., 2007. Mechanistic Toxicology: The Molecular Basis of How Chemicals Disrupt Biological Targets, 2nd ed. CRC Press, Boca Raton, FL.

Fruncillo, R.J., 2011. 2,000 Toxicology Board Review Questions. Xlibris Corporation LLC, USA, p. 498.

Gupta, P.K. (Ed.), 2010. Modern Toxicology: Basis of Organ and Reproduction Toxicity, Vol. 1. PharmaMed Press, Hyderabad, India. (2nd reprint).

Gupta, P.K., 2014. Essential Concepts in Toxicology. BSP Pvt Ltd, Hyderabad, India.

Gupta, P.K., 2016. Fundamental in Toxicology: Essential Concepts and Applications in Toxicology. Elsevier/BSP, San Diego, USA.

Gupta, R.C. (Ed.), 2018. Veterinary Toxicology: Basic and Clinical Principles. 3rd ed. Academic Press/Elsevier, San Diego, USA.

Hodgson, E.A. (Ed.), 2010. A Textbook of Modern Toxicology. 4th ed. John Wiley, New Jersey.

Klaassen, C.D. (Ed.), 2013. Casarett and Doull's Toxicology: The Basic Science of Poisons. 8th ed McGraw-Hill, New York.

Merck Veterinary Manual, 2016. Poisonous and Venomous Animals. Merck Research Laboratories, Merck & Co. Inc., pp. 3157–3165.

Nelson, L.S. (Ed.), 2011. Goldfrank's Toxicologic Emergencies. 9th ed McGraw-Hill, New York.

Püssa, T., 2013. Principles of Food Toxicology, 2nd ed. CRC Press, Boca Raton. FL, USA, p. 414.

Rao, G.N., 2010. Textbook of Forensic Medicine & Toxicology. Jaypee Brothers Medical Publishers, New Delhi, India.

Timbrell, J., 1997. Study Toxicology Through Questions. CRC Press, 144 pages.

Timbrell, J.A. (Ed.), 2009. Principles of Biochemical Toxicology. 4th ed. Informa, New York.

Index

Note: Page numbers followed by "*f*" and "*t*" refer to figures and tables, respectively.

593